When your child is sick

CANADIAN EDITION

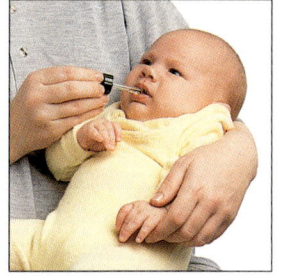

When your child is sick

DR. PAUL MUNK
SENIOR STAFF PHYSICIAN, HOSPITAL FOR SICK CHILDREN, TORONTO
ASSISTANT PROFESSOR OF PAEDIATRICS, UNIVERSITY OF TORONTO

•

DR. BERNARD VALMAN

DK

DK

Editor, Canada Julia Roles
Project Editor, Canada Ian Whitelaw

Editors Jill Hamilton, Mary Lindsay
Design Schermuly Design Co.
Illustrator Joanna Cameron
Senior Managing Editor Martyn Page
Managing Art Editor Louise Dick
DTP Designer Julian Dams
Production Wendy Penn

DK INDIA
DTP Co-ordinator Pankaj Sharma
DTP Designer Balwant Singh, Sunil Sharma

Canadian Edition 2005
Copyright © 1997, 2002, 2005 Dorling Kindersley Limited
Text copyright © 1997, 2002, 2005 Bernard Valman

Dorling Kindersley is represented in Canada by
Tourmaline Editions Inc.
662 King Street West, Suite 304
Toronto, Ontario M5V 1M7

Dr. Bernard Valman has asserted his moral right to
be identified as the author of this work.

Adapted for Canada by Dr. Paul Munk

Library and Archives Canada Cataloguing in Publication

When your child is sick / Canadian editor, Paul Munk. -- Canadian ed.

Includes index.
ISBN 1-55363-047-5

1. Pediatrics--Popular works. I. Munk, Paul

RJ61.W44 2005   618.92   C2004-906450-9

Reproduced by GRB Editrice, Italy
Printed and bound by Star Standard, Singapore

05 06 07 08 6 5 4 3 2 1

Discover more at
www.dk.com

FOREWORD

Childhood is a time of continuing growth and development with, inevitably, some illnesses and injuries. There are few greater challenges to parenting than the sick, non-verbal infant, although the non-communicating adolescent is perhaps a match.

This Canadian edition of *When Your Child Is Sick* is intended to help you interpret any signs of illness and provide you with the facts you need to make decisions about your child's health. The Symptom Charts will enable you to distinguish between minor problems and emergencies, and to know when to seek medical help. They also offer suggestions for safe home management where appropriate. The Diseases and Disorders section will answer most of your questions about the causes, treatment, and prognosis of many childhood illnesses.

Dealing specifically with Canadian guidelines and current approaches, *When Your Child Is Sick* presents precise information to enable you to provide compassionate parenting during sickness and as your child develops. Please remember that this book is not a substitute for medical diagnosis and should be used as a guideline only. I would ask you to consult your child's own physician on personal health matters.

Paul Munk

Paul Munk, MD, FRCP(C)
Senior Staff Physician, Hospital for Sick Children, Toronto
Assistant Professor of Paediatrics, University of Toronto

CONTENTS

HOW TO USE THIS BOOK

The book is divided into four sections that provide information on the child's body and how it works, and what can go wrong. The first section, Your Child's Body, concentrates on the basics of anatomy, growth, and development. The second section, which is the core of the book, comprises Symptom Charts. When your child is ill, the question-and-answer charts will help you to determine the possible cause and decide whether medical attention is required. The third section, Diseases and Disorders, provides details of more than 140 conditions. The final section covers essential first-aid techniques and emergency procedures.

Your Child's Body
The first section of the book describes the anatomy, growth, and development of children. Following on from this general introduction are guidelines for safe and healthy living for children of all ages. Problems in babies, being different from those that affect older children, are covered in the final part of this opening section.

Fully annotated artworks show details of a child's body

Clear text explains the basics of anatomy, growth, and development

"Danger signs" box alerts you to potentially life-threatening symptoms

Pathways lead you from one question to the next, to a possible cause, or to an endpoint

Charts are color-coded according to age group

Each "button" contains a possible answer to the question above

"Go to" box refers you to another chart

List of articles in section

Symptom Charts
The core of the book consists of 41 charts, which are arranged in three groups: those for children under 1 year; those for children over 1 year; and those for children of all ages. Starting with your child's symptoms you can use these charts to identify the possible cause of the problem and follow the medical and/or self-help action suggested.

Diseases and Disorders
Arranged by body system, each of the articles in this section describes a disease or disorder. The articles include information about the symptoms and causes of the problem, whether and when you should seek medical help, what the doctor might do, self-help measures you can follow at home, and the outlook.

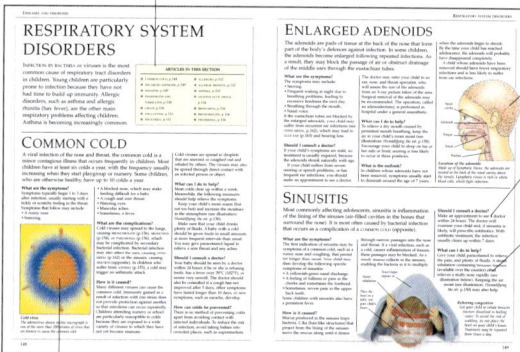

Annotated artwork explains what the problem is or where it occurs

This section explains if and when you should consult a doctor

Self-help measures give simple remedies you can use at home

Photograph illustrates the cause or appearance of the disease

Clear, step-by-step photographs show first-aid techniques

Boxes highlight special information or alternative methods or situations

First Aid and Nursing a sick child
The final part of the book demonstrates first-aid methods for life-threatening emergencies. Also included is first-aid treatment for broken bones and some other injuries before going to hospital. Nursing a Sick Child gives the basic instructions for looking after a child who is not well.

HOW TO USE THE CHARTS

Find the chart that matches your child's main symptom. Beginning at the box labeled "Start here," follow the pathway to the first question. Choose the appropriate answer, and take the pathway leading from that answer. It may go to another question; a possible cause, which directs you to information elsewhere in the book and also tells you what action to take –

whether to obtain medical help and what self-help measures might be helpful, a reference to another symptom chart, or an endpoint.

CAUTION Remember that the charts provide only likely diagnoses. If you have any doubts about either the diagnosis or the treatment of any symptoms, always consult your doctor.

"Go to" box
You may look up your child's symptoms on one chart but find that the pathway leads to one of these boxes, referring you to another chart that is more appropriate for your child's illness

"Danger signs" box
Symptoms that may indicate a serious condition are listed in these boxes. If you notice any of these symptoms, you should follow the instructions to phone your doctor at once

Question box
Each question is followed by two or more possible answers. Choose the one that most closely matches your child's symptoms, and follow the pathway leading from it to another location on the chart

Possible causes
The possible causes of your child's symptoms are given here. They are usually accompanied by cross-references to further information given in other sections of the book

Action needed
The necessary medical and self-help measures are described under the heading "Action needed." You may be instructed to obtain medical help (see below) and/or use self-help procedures

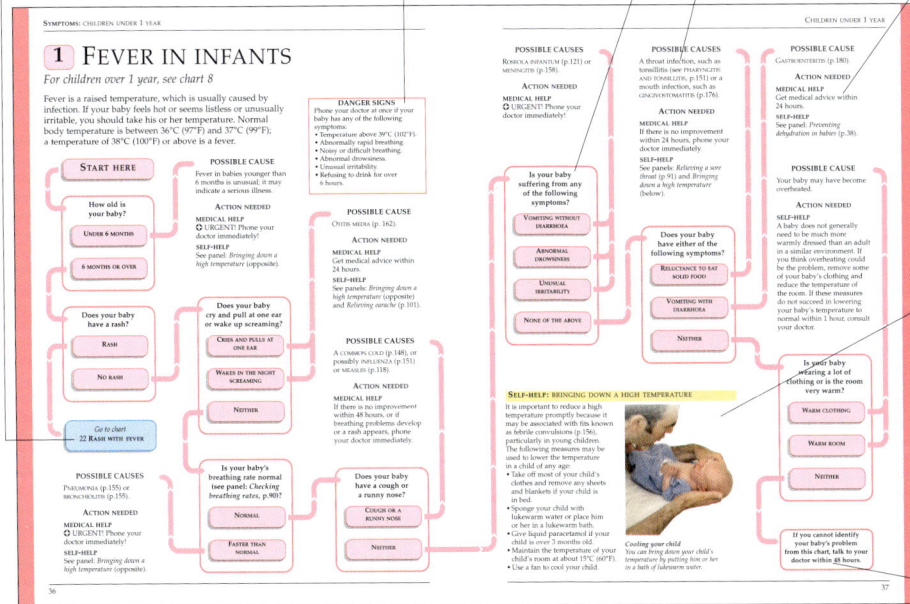

Self-help panel
These panels describe in detail various self-help measures that you can use to help relieve your child's symptoms. Some charts have assessment panels, which show you how to evaluate your child's breathing rate, growth, vision, and hearing ability

Endpoint box
Some pathways may lead to an endpoint, rather than a possible cause. This endpoint tells you when you should seek medical assistance if it is not possible to identify your child's problem from the symptom chart

Medical Help

There are five levels of medical help, depending on the severity of your child's condition. If a problem can be remedied by self-help measures alone, the medical help category is omitted.

⊕ EMERGENCY! Call an ambulance!
Your child's condition may be life-threatening or lead to permanent disability. Get medical help immediately, by calling an ambulance. Sometimes, you may prefer to call your doctor or take your child to the hospital yourself.

⊕ URGENT! Phone your doctor immediately!
Your child may have a serious illness that requires prompt medical treatment. You should phone your doctor or an emergency room without delay.

Get medical advice within 24 hours.
Your child may be suffering from a condition that requires urgent medical assessment and should be seen by a doctor within 24 hours. If you cannot see the doctor, you should speak to him or her on the phone.

Make an appointment to see your doctor.
Your child's condition requires medical treatment, but your child will not be adversely affected if the next available appointment is not for 3 or 4 days.

Consult your doctor.
There is no need for you to make a special appointment or to contact the doctor with any haste; discuss your child's symptoms at the next appointment, or phone your doctor sooner if you become concerned.

YOUR CHILD'S BODY

EARLY STIMULATION MAY PROMOTE
MENTAL DEVELOPMENT

A BASIC KNOWLEDGE of a child's anatomy and normal physical, emotional, and mental development gives parents a clearer understanding of the many common problems or illnesses that tend to affect children. This section begins with a brief look at the development of children from birth to adolescence. The section continues with advice on infant feeding and weaning, and provides nutritional guidelines for growing children. To maximize a child's chance of a safe, healthy life, information about immunization, prevention of accidents, and care in the sun is also included. Babies tend to have a different set of problems from toddlers and older children and some of these, such as feeding and sleeping problems, are covered at the end of the section.

SECTION THROUGH THE EYE

ANATOMY AND DEVELOPMENT

TO DECIDE WHEN SOMETHING IS WRONG with your child, it may help if you know what constitutes normal anatomy and healthy development. The following section provides an overview of body systems and how they work, skeletal development, the senses and how they work, growth, and milestones of infant, child, and adolescent development.

BODY SYSTEMS

The systems of the body work in harmony to perform the many different functions necessary for life. These functions include respiration, digestion, movement, circulation of oxygen and nutrients, and removal of waste products. Each system consists of a particular set of organs, tissues, and cells that work together to perform vital life-giving functions. Some components, such as the pulmonary vessels, have a role in more than one system.

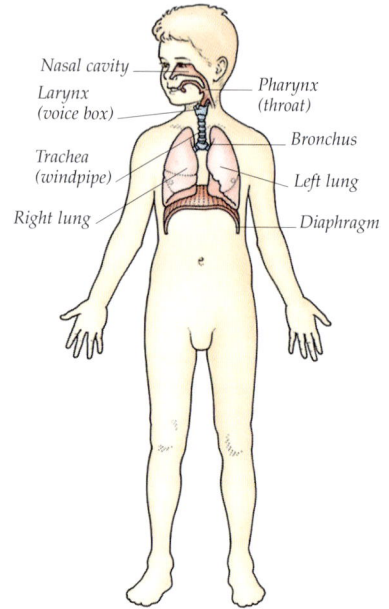

Respiratory system
The lungs, air passages such as the nose and trachea, and breathing muscles, including the diaphragm, comprise the respiratory system. Associated blood vessels supply oxygen to the body tissues and remove waste carbon dioxide and take it to the lungs for exhalation.

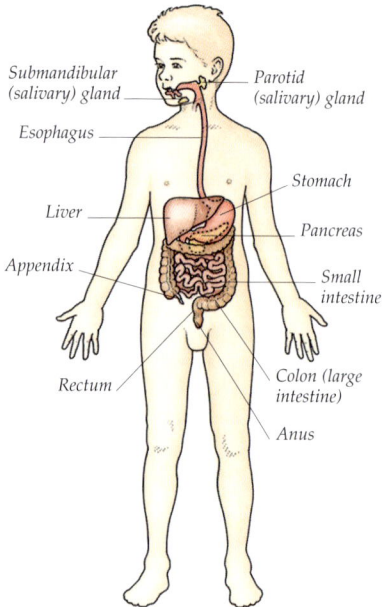

Nasal cavity
Larynx (voice box)
Pharynx (throat)
Trachea (windpipe)
Bronchus
Left lung
Right lung
Diaphragm

Digestive system
The digestive tract consists of a long tube that extends from the mouth to the anus. As food passes along this tube, it is broken down into minute molecules that can be absorbed into the bloodstream. Associated organs secrete chemicals to assist in the digestive process.

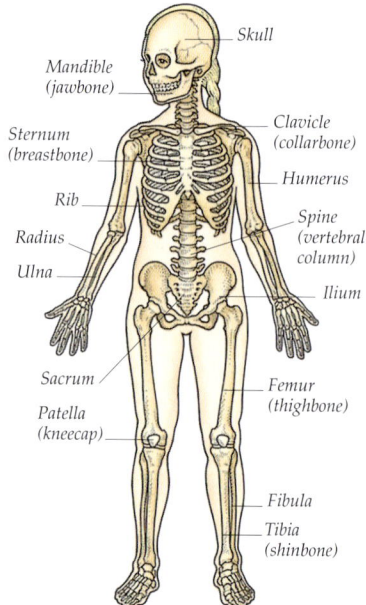

Submandibular (salivary) gland
Parotid (salivary) gland
Esophagus
Stomach
Liver
Pancreas
Appendix
Small intestine
Rectum
Colon (large intestine)
Anus

Skeletal system
The skeleton is the strong internal framework that provides support for the body. As well as supporting the soft tissues, the skeleton also protects the organs and provides anchorage for muscles. During childhood, the skeleton is continually growing and changing shape.

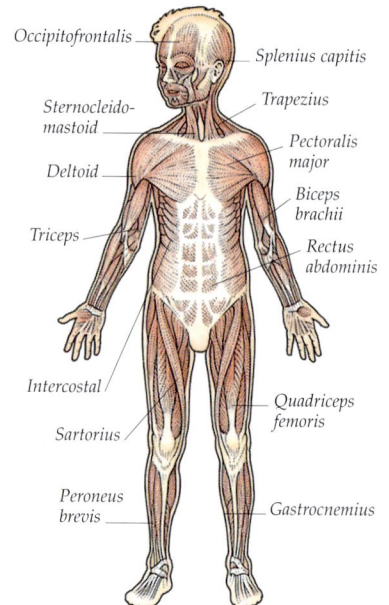

Skull
Mandible (jawbone)
Clavicle (collarbone)
Sternum (breastbone)
Humerus
Rib
Spine (vertebral column)
Radius
Ulna
Ilium
Sacrum
Femur (thighbone)
Patella (kneecap)
Fibula
Tibia (shinbone)

Muscular system
There are three types of muscle: voluntary, involuntary, and cardiac. Voluntary muscles (above) work with the skeleton to enable the body to move. Involuntary muscles surround hollow organs, such as the intestines and stomach. The heart is made of cardiac muscle.

Occipitofrontalis
Splenius capitis
Sternocleido-mastoid
Trapezius
Deltoid
Pectoralis major
Biceps brachii
Triceps
Rectus abdominis
Intercostal
Quadriceps femoris
Sartorius
Peroneus brevis
Gastrocnemius

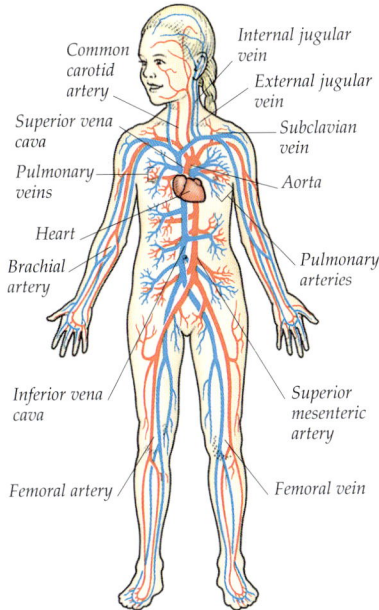

Cardiovascular system

Common carotid artery
Internal jugular vein
External jugular vein
Superior vena cava
Subclavian vein
Pulmonary veins
Aorta
Heart
Brachial artery
Pulmonary arteries
Inferior vena cava
Superior mesenteric artery
Femoral artery
Femoral vein

The heart pumps blood through the arteries, veins, and capillaries. Oxygen and nutrients are delivered by the blood to all parts of the body and waste products are removed. Blood is returned to the lungs for reoxygenation and elimination of carbon dioxide.

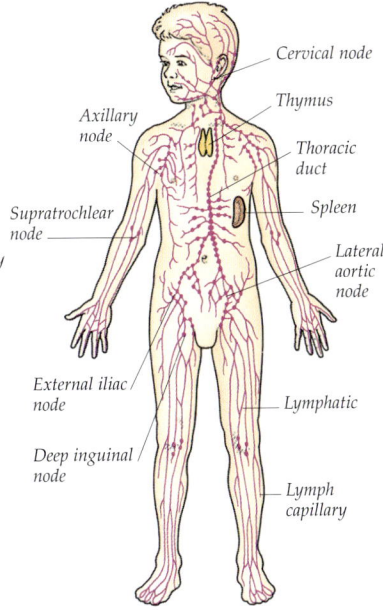

Lymphatic system

Cervical node
Thymus
Axillary node
Thoracic duct
Spleen
Supratrochlear node
Lateral aortic node
External iliac node
Lymphatic
Deep inguinal node
Lymph capillary

The lymphatic system, a major part of the body's immune system, is made up of a network of vessels (lymphatics) and filters (lymph nodes). Lymph, a fluid of white blood cells that flows through the vessels, destroys microorganisms trapped in the nodes.

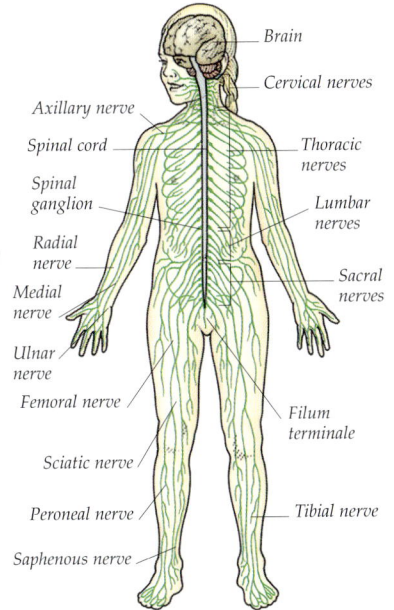

Nervous system

Brain
Cervical nerves
Axillary nerve
Spinal cord
Thoracic nerves
Spinal ganglion
Radial nerve
Lumbar nerves
Medial nerve
Sacral nerves
Ulnar nerve
Femoral nerve
Filum terminale
Sciatic nerve
Peroneal nerve
Tibial nerve
Saphenous nerve

Comprising the brain, spinal cord, and many millions of nerve cells, the nervous system is the control center for all voluntary activities and involuntary bodily functions. Nerves are responsible for perception of sensations, such as touch, taste, smell, vision, and hearing.

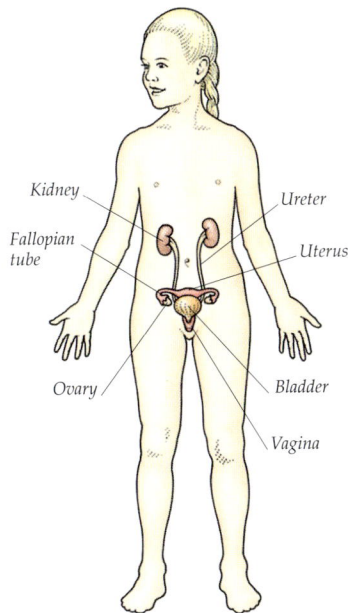

Girl's genitourinary system

Kidney
Ureter
Fallopian tube
Uterus
Ovary
Bladder
Vagina

The urinary system – kidneys, ureters, and bladder – filters waste products, surplus water, and excess salts from the blood. The genital system, composed of two ovaries, the uterus, and various ducts, produces hormones and, from puberty, one or more eggs every month.

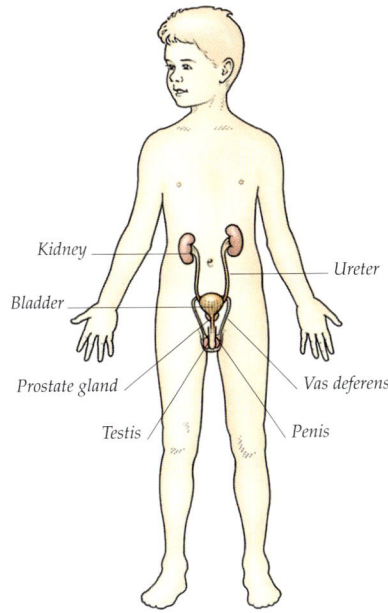

Boy's genitourinary system

Kidney
Ureter
Bladder
Prostate gland
Vas deferens
Testis
Penis

As in a girl, a boy's urinary system comprises kidneys, ureters, and bladder. Urine and, after puberty, semen pass out of the body through the urethra and penis. The testes produce hormones that are responsible for the male characteristics that appear at puberty.

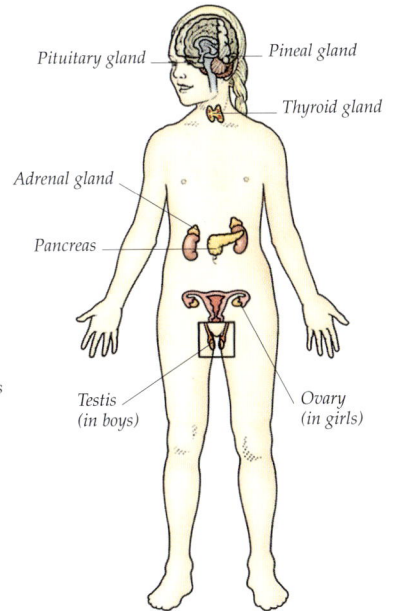

Endocrine system

Pituitary gland
Pineal gland
Thyroid gland
Adrenal gland
Pancreas
Testis (in boys)
Ovary (in girls)

The endocrine glands manufacture hormones, the body's chemical messengers. Hormones are distributed to all parts of the body by the blood and help to regulate internal processes, such as growth. Some glands, such as the testis and ovary, are inactive until puberty.

SKELETAL DEVELOPMENT

At birth most of a baby's skeleton is composed of bone, but some parts, notably the ends of the arm, leg, hand, and foot bones, are made of cartilage and do not ossify (turn into bone) until late adolescence. The cartilage continues to grow before ossifying, which allows the rapid growth of childhood to take place; this process continues through childhood until adult size is reached. The number of individual bones in the body decreases as adulthood approaches: a newborn baby may have over 300 distinct bones, but many of these fuse together as the child grows, resulting in an adult skeleton of 206 bones.

GROWTH OF THE SKULL

At birth, a baby's skull is not fully ossified – the individual bones making up the cranium (brain case) are joined by flexible bands of fibrous tissue. These areas allow the skull to change shape during childbirth and enable rapid growth of the brain during the first year or two of life. The anterior fontanelle towards the front of the skull is the largest band of fibrous tissue and it is clearly visible through the skin.

The bones of the face enlarge at the same rate as the rest of the skull so that when growth is complete, the head is in proportion to the rest of the body.

DEVELOPMENT OF THE TEETH

At birth, the primary teeth are already developing in the jaws. The first of these erupt by about 6 months, and by the age of approximately 3 years the entire set of 20 primary teeth has come through. Meanwhile, the secondary set of 32 teeth is developing in the jaws and will appear between the ages of 6 and 16 years. As these teeth erupt, the primary teeth are displaced and fall out. The third molars (wisdom teeth) usually break through at 16 or older, although sometimes they never appear.

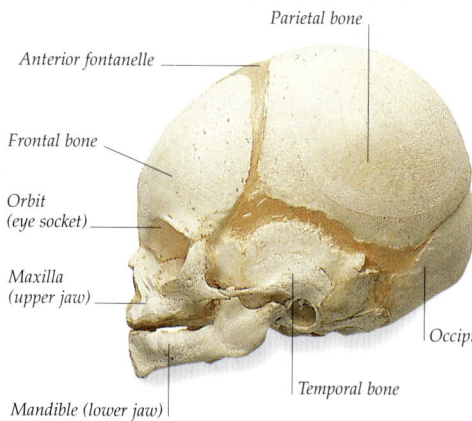

Skull of a newborn baby
Ossification of the skull begins long before birth, but the fontanelles, formed of fibrous tissue, persist between the bones, allowing the skull to accommodate the growing brain. The facial bones of a newborn baby are small, and the teeth have not started to erupt.

Skull of a 6-year-old
By the age of 6 years, the fontanelles have ossified, and they are no longer visible. All the primary teeth have erupted and the secondary teeth are just beginning to emerge. The maxilla is lower and further forward than in the newborn baby's skull, and the eye sockets and the nasal region have expanded. The mandible has grown downward and forward.

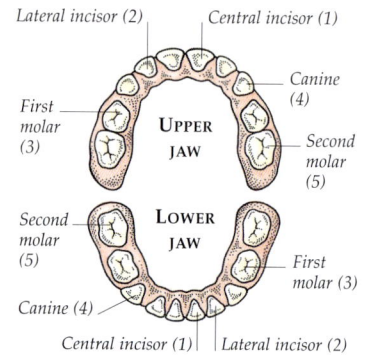

Primary teeth
Deciduous, or primary, teeth erupt between the ages of 6 months and 3 years in a specific order (as shown in brackets, above). The pattern is the same in upper and lower jaws.

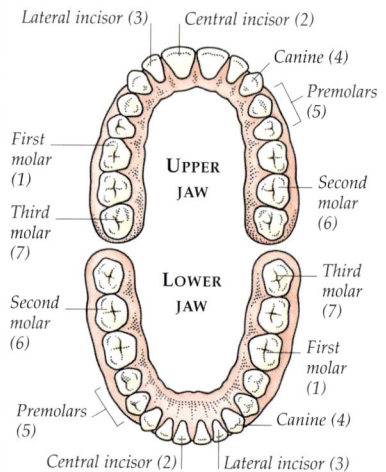

Secondary teeth
Permanent, or secondary, teeth erupt between the ages of 6 and 16 years in the order shown in brackets (above). The premolars, canines, and incisors directly replace primary teeth.

MAIN AREAS OF BONE GROWTH

In childhood, most of the long bones contain cartilage, which allows the bones to grow. The cartilage in these areas grows and absorbs calcium to develop into bone. Limb, hand, and foot bones, the areas in which most growth occurs, are made up of a diaphysis (shaft), which is the main part of the bone, and an epiphysis (growing region) at either one or both ends. During the course of a child's growing years, the epiphyses gradually ossify, leaving a cartilage plate where growth continues until adult height and size is reached in late adolescence.

Bony and ossifying areas are clearly visible on an X ray, whereas cartilage does not show up very clearly. X rays, therefore, can be used by a doctor to tell the age of a child and also to decide whether his or her growth is normal. This type of assessment is possible because the areas of ossification appear in a particular sequence in every child. For example, at the age of 1 year, a child will develop areas of ossification in the shoulder, hand, hip, and foot. From the age of 2 years, additional areas of ossification are formed in the shoulder, elbow, hand, hip, knee, and foot bones. Additional ossification centers are established each year, and growth continues in the old areas as well as in the new ones.

Shoulder
Elbow
Hand and wrist
Foot and ankle

Epiphysis at end of finger bone
Epiphysis at end of hand bone
Early ossification of hand bone
Early ossification of wrist bones

NEW OSSIFICATION AREAS IN A CHILD OF 2½ YEARS

X RAY OF HAND AT 2½ YEARS

Bone growth in a 2½-year-old
New areas of ossification include bones in the shoulder, elbow, wrist, hand, foot, and ankle; areas of ossification established earlier continue to grow. The X ray of the hand shows the shafts of the bones (opaque areas) have ossified but the ends (transparent areas) are still growing.

Elbow
Hand and wrist
Knee

Epiphysis at end of finger bone
Epiphysis at end of hand bone
Advanced ossification of hand bones
Advanced ossification of wrist bones

NEW OSSIFICATION AREAS IN A CHILD OF 6 YEARS

X RAY OF HAND AT 6 YEARS

Bone growth in a 6-year-old
By the age of 6 years, ossification sites in other elbow, hand, and wrist bones have formed; a new site appears in the knee. The hand X ray shows many ossified wrist bones (opaque areas) but there are still growing centers at the top ends of the hand bones (transparent areas).

BONE REPAIR

Children are naturally curious and adventurous, with the result that they are particularly prone to falls and dislocated and broken bones. When a bone is fractured, the natural healing process begins immediately and, in children, the whole sequence may take a few weeks. To prevent a broken bone from reforming in a misaligned position – thus leaving a crooked, unstable bone that is liable to further injury – the displaced edges of bone must be lined up and fixed promptly. A fracture that occurs at the growing end of a bone may disrupt its growth, causing the bone to be short.

Repair and regeneration of a bone after it has been broken is a type of ossification. It differs from the formation of completely new bone from cartilage in that the damaged area has to be cleared of wound debris before new bone can grow. This process is done by specialized blood cells and connective tissue cells, which invade the site and absorb the debris. New bone is laid down between the bone ends, and after a few weeks the bone is completely repaired.

Fractured humerus
The humerus in the upper part of the picture has broken close to the elbow joint. This is one type of fracture that very commonly affects children of all ages.

Healed fracture
A few weeks later the bone has reformed and is correctly positioned for optimum mobility of the elbow. The repaired site is as strong as the original bone prior to the injury.

THE SENSES

The five senses – sight, hearing, touch, smell, and taste – are responsible for giving your child vital information about his or her surroundings. The eyes and ears are the most important of the sensory organs. Touch relies on receptors in the skin that detect temperature, pressure, and pain. The related senses of smell and taste, as detected by the nose and tongue, differentiate the main tastes and warn against potentially noxious substances in food and air. Smell also activates secretion of saliva for digesting food.

All senses are normally present at birth, but they need adequate stimulation to develop fully. Taste and smell are often more acute in children than in adults because they have not been subjected to pollutants, such as smoke.

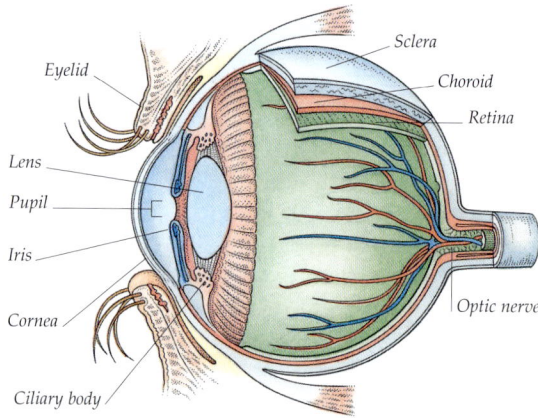

SECTION THROUGH THE EYE

Eye structure and vision
Sight is the most complex of the senses. Light rays enter through the pupil at the front of the eye and register on the retina at the back. The light rays are converted to nerve impulses that are passed, via the optic nerve, to the brain, where they are interpreted as images.

SECTION THROUGH THE EAR

Ear structure and hearing
The ears are the organs of hearing. Sound waves pass from the outer to the middle ear, where a system of membranes and tiny bones conveys vibrations to the inner ear. Vibrations are converted to nerve impulses in the cochlea and passed, via the auditory nerve, to the brain.

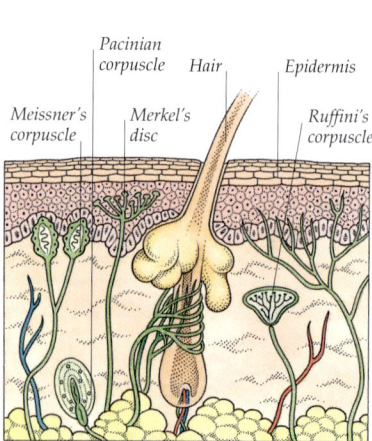

SECTION THROUGH THE SKIN

Skin structure and touch
Specialized skin cells, which detect pressure, pain, and temperature, are free nerve endings or bulblike structures. These receptors are not related exclusively to one touch sensation.

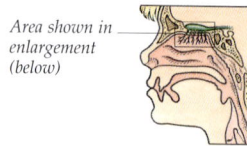

SECTION THROUGH THE NASAL REGION

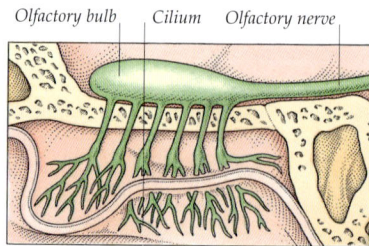

ENLARGED NASAL REGION

Nose structure and smell
Smells dissolve in mucus in the nasal cavity and stimulate the hairlike cilia of specialized nerve cells. The nerve impulses generated travel along the olfactory nerve to the brain.

UPPER SURFACE OF THE TONGUE

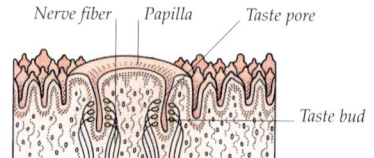

SECTION THROUGH A PAPILLA

Tongue structure and taste
Taste buds are located mainly within papillae on the surface of the tongue. Different types of papillae arranged over the tongue can detect bitter, sour, salty, or sweet tastes.

GROWTH CHARTS

The growth charts on the following pages allow you to record and plot your child's growth. By plotting head circumference, weight, and height against age, you can compare your child's growth with the normal range for that age. Growth in babies should be monitored by regular attendance at a doctor's office so that any growth problems are picked up early. If any of your child's measurements fall outside the shaded area, or if the growth curve is erratic, make an appointment to see your doctor.

HOW TO USE THE CHARTS

First, measure your child using the illustrations in the box below as a guide. Use the weight measurements recorded at the clinic if your child is too young or too small to be weighed on your bathroom scale.

The charts on the following pages cover all the measurements and ages required to track your child's growth: head circumference and weight for boys and girls from birth to 2 years, and height and weight for boys and girls between 2 and 18 years. Find your child's age along the bottom of the chart and draw an imaginary vertical line until it meets head circumference, height, or weight, found on the side of the chart. Note the measurement; plot the point first with a pencil dot and then overwrite with a pen once you are sure the point is in the correct place.

Take measurements regularly and draw a line connecting the dots to form a "growth curve." The charts will show you how your child compares to the average for all children of the same age, which is represented by the 50th percentile line. If the curve does not run parallel to the 50th percentile line, or fails to keep within the shaded area, have a doctor see your child.

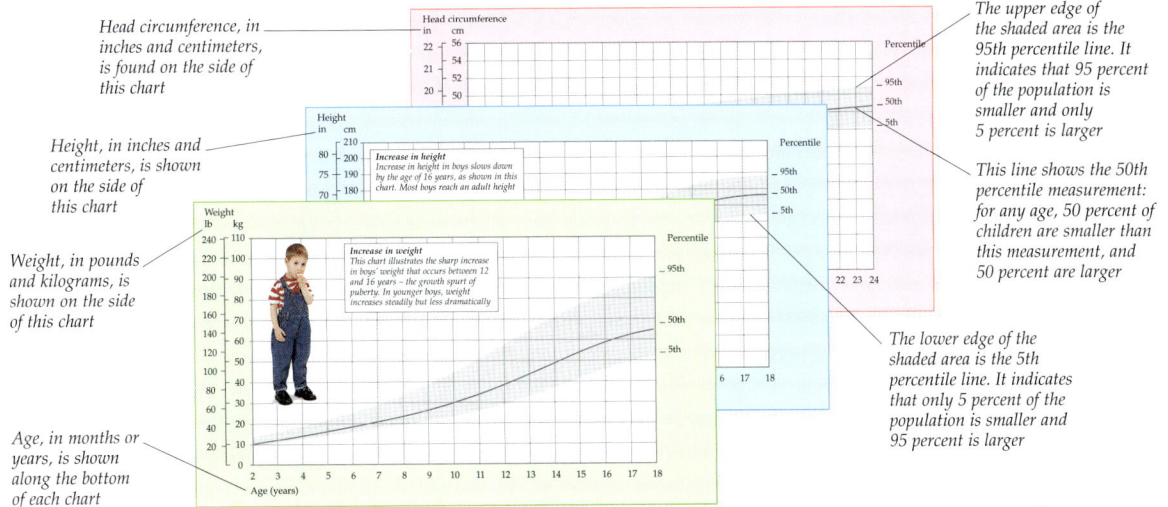

Head circumference, in inches and centimeters, is found on the side of this chart

Height, in inches and centimeters, is shown on the side of this chart

Weight, in pounds and kilograms, is shown on the side of this chart

Age, in months or years, is shown along the bottom of each chart

The upper edge of the shaded area is the 95th percentile line. It indicates that 95 percent of the population is smaller and only 5 percent is larger

This line shows the 50th percentile measurement: for any age, 50 percent of children are smaller than this measurement, and 50 percent are larger

The lower edge of the shaded area is the 5th percentile line. It indicates that only 5 percent of the population is smaller and 95 percent is larger

Increase in height
Increase in height in boys slows down by the age of 16 years, as shown in this chart. Most boys reach an adult height.

Increase in weight
This chart illustrates the sharp increase in boys' weight that occurs between 12 and 16 years – the growth spurt of puberty. In younger boys, weight increases steadily but less dramatically.

MEASURING YOUR CHILD

These illustrations show you how to measure your child's height and head circumference. If your child is too small to be weighed accurately on a bathroom scale, measure him or her on the special infants' scale at the doctor's office. If you want to weigh an older child using a domestic bathroom scale, make sure that it is accurate or has been recently calibrated. Keep a written record of the actual measurements and the dates on which they were taken. They may be an invaluable record of your child's physical development.

Measuring a child's head circumference
Wrap a paper or plastic tape measure around the largest part of the head, from a point midway between the hairline and eyebrows at the front to the bony protuberance at the back.

Measuring a child's height
Stand your child, in bare feet, against a wall or door. Lower a book, with the spine against the wall, or a cereal or similar package, narrow side to the wall, onto his or her head. Mark with a pencil the position where the base of the book's spine or lower edge of the package meets the wall. Measure the distance from the floor with a metal tape measure that can be locked to ensure that an accurate reading is taken.

BOYS' GROWTH CHARTS

BOYS' HEAD CIRCUMFERENCE FROM BIRTH TO 2 YEARS

Head circumference
in   cm

Percentile

— 95th

— 50th

— 5th

Increase in head circumference
This chart shows the normal range of growth in the head circumference of boys. This measurement is an effective substitute for height in assessing rate of growth up to 2 years of age.

Age (months)

BOYS' WEIGHT FROM BIRTH TO 2 YEARS

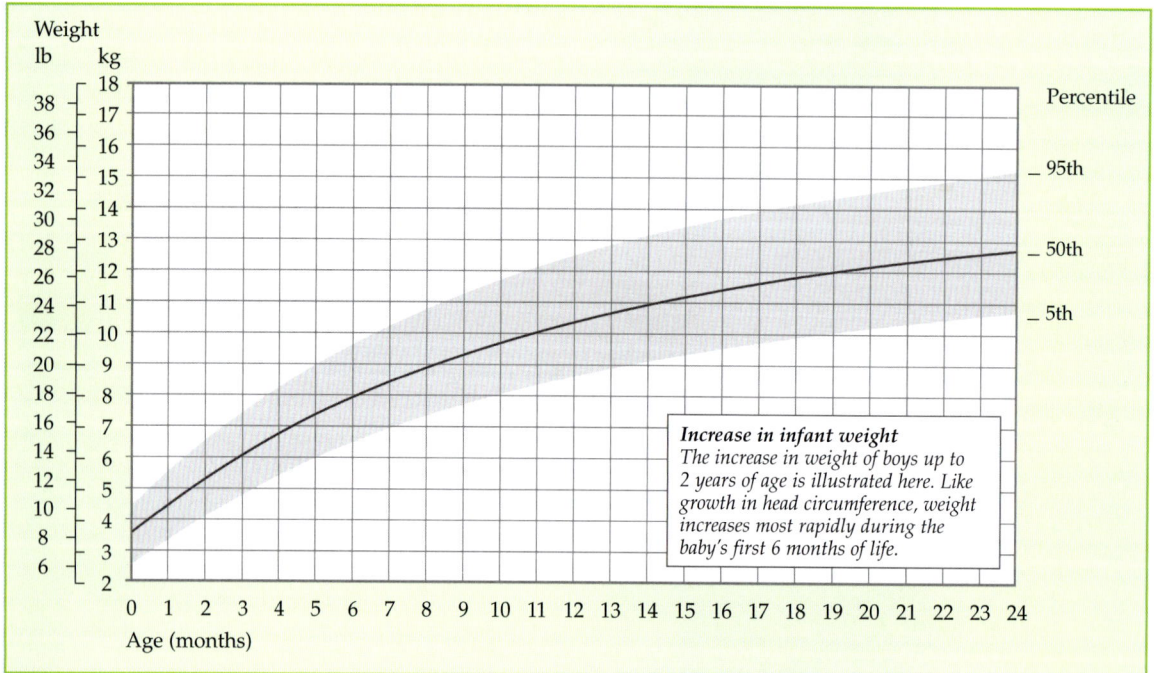

Weight
lb   kg

Percentile

— 95th

— 50th

— 5th

Increase in infant weight
The increase in weight of boys up to 2 years of age is illustrated here. Like growth in head circumference, weight increases most rapidly during the baby's first 6 months of life.

Age (months)

BOYS' HEIGHT FROM 2 TO 18 YEARS

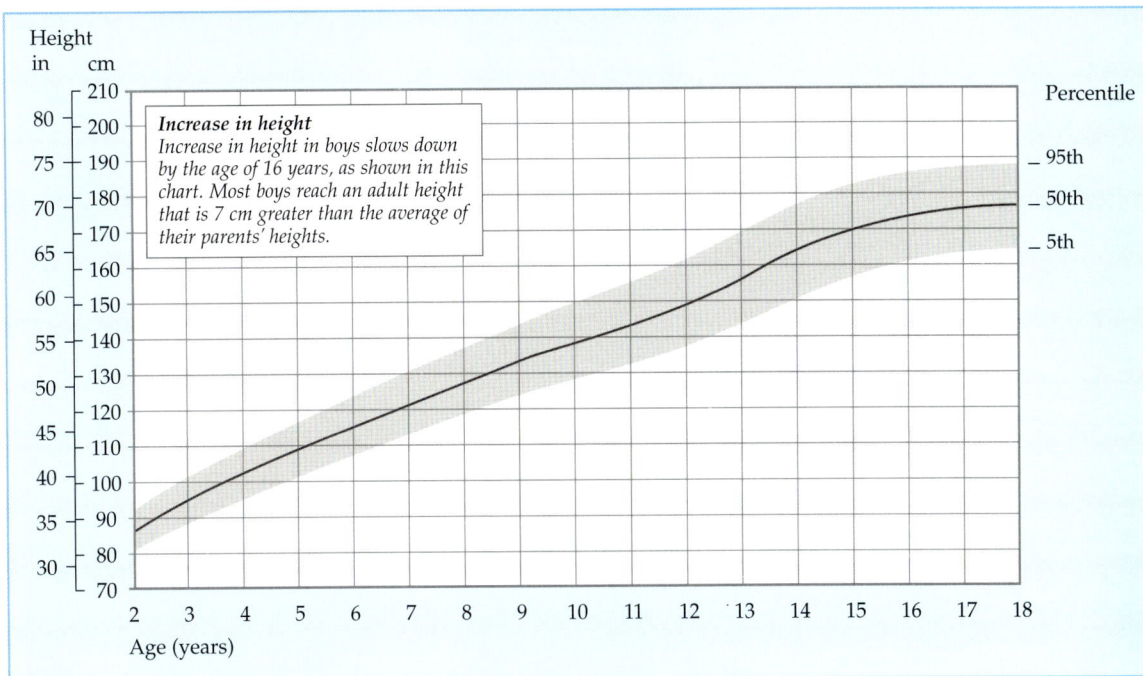

Height
in   cm

Increase in height
*Increase in height in boys slows down
by the age of 16 years, as shown in this
chart. Most boys reach an adult height
that is 7 cm greater than the average of
their parents' heights.*

Percentile

— 95th

— 50th

— 5th

Age (years)

BOYS' WEIGHT FROM 2 TO 18 YEARS

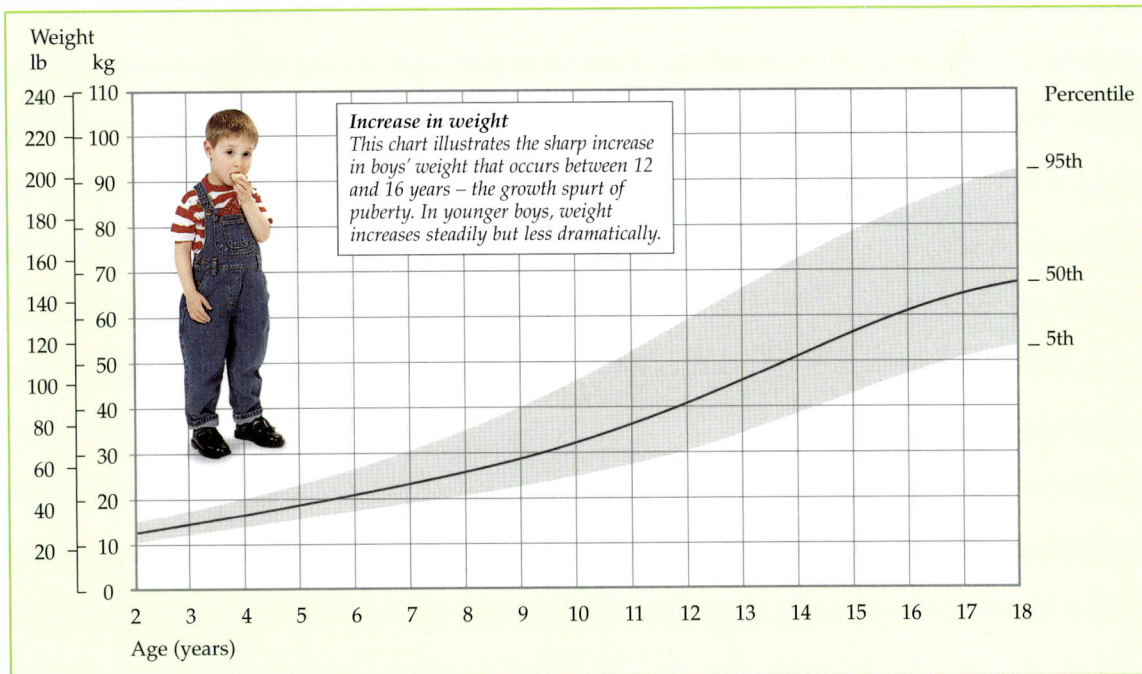

Weight
lb   kg

Increase in weight
*This chart illustrates the sharp increase
in boys' weight that occurs between 12
and 16 years – the growth spurt of
puberty. In younger boys, weight
increases steadily but less dramatically.*

Percentile

— 95th

— 50th

— 5th

Age (years)

GIRLS' GROWTH CHARTS

GIRLS' HEAD CIRCUMFERENCE FROM BIRTH TO 2 YEARS

Head circumference
in   cm

Percentile

— 95th

— 50th

— 5th

Increase in head circumference
*This chart shows the normal range of
growth in the head circumference of
girls. This measurement is an effective
substitute for height in assessing rate
of growth up to 2 years of age.*

Age (months)

GIRLS' WEIGHT FROM BIRTH TO 2 YEARS

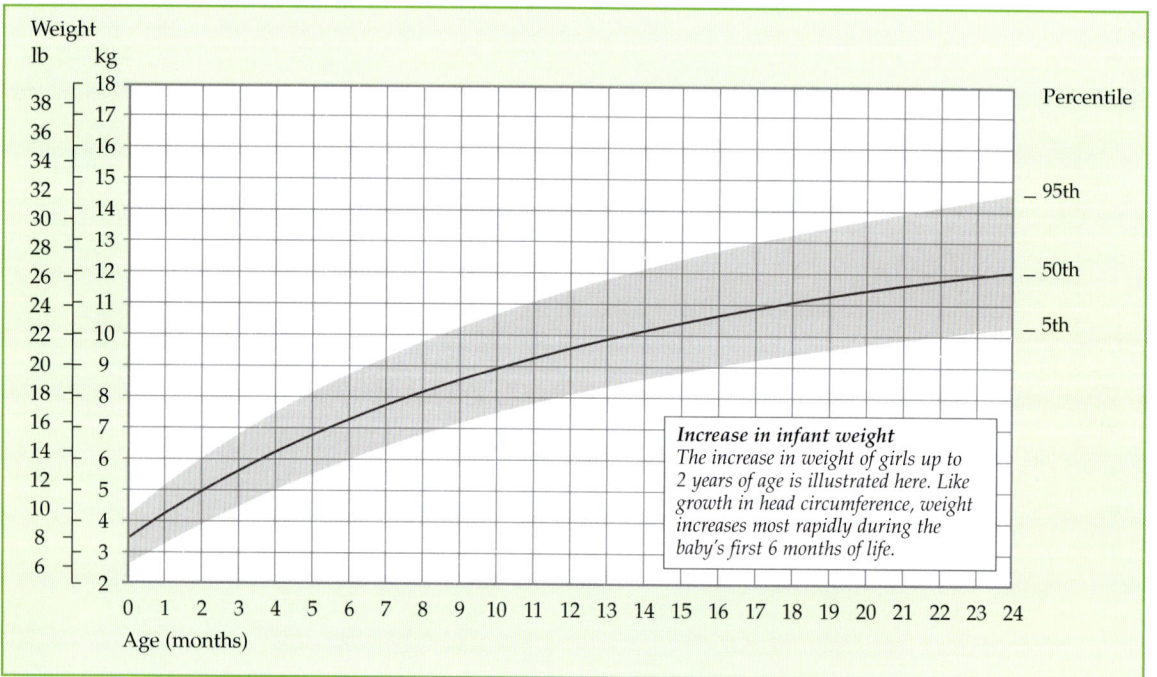

Weight
lb   kg

Percentile

— 95th

— 50th

— 5th

Increase in infant weight
*The increase in weight of girls up to
2 years of age is illustrated here. Like
growth in head circumference, weight
increases most rapidly during the
baby's first 6 months of life.*

Age (months)

GIRLS' HEIGHT FROM 2 TO 18 YEARS

Height
in   cm

Percentile

Increase in height
*This chart shows that the increase in
height in girls tails off after the age of
14 years. Most girls reach an adult
height that is 7 cm less than the
average of their parents' heights.*

95th

50th

5th

Age (years)

GIRLS' WEIGHT FROM 2 TO 18 YEARS

Weight
lb   kg

Percentile

Increase in weight
*This chart illustrates that the peak
period for increase in weight in girls is
10 to 14 years. This corresponds to the
growth spurt of puberty, during which
height increases at a similar rate.*

95th

50th

5th

Age (years)

21

THE NEWBORN BABY

A newborn baby is not merely a passive bundle of reflexes and random movements. From birth, a baby is aware of sights, sounds, smells, and touch. An infant only a few hours old can recognize a human face and his or her mother's smell, and reacts to loud, sudden noise and the gentle tones of a human voice. All babies are very responsive to touch and various touch reflexes are present from birth. A newborn baby is a highly receptive human being full of potential.

Asymmetrical head

Puffy, sticky eyes

Wrinkled, greasy skin

Peeling skin on hand

Red patch on skin

Enlarged genitals

Peeling skin on foot

APPEARANCE OF THE NEWBORN BABY

At birth, many babies have a number of variations in appearance, which, while perfectly normal, may cause the parents some concern. Examples of these variations are: an asymmetrical head; puffy, sticky eyes; drooping eyelids; crossed eyes; wrinkled, hairy, red, and greasy skin; dry and peeling skin on hands and feet; spots and small areas of discolored skin; and yellow skin, caused by jaundice. Also common are breast buds, and overly big genitals in both girls and boys. Most of these features disappear in a few weeks.

Rarely, however, there may be a more serious problem, such as an infection, which requires treatment (see INFANT PROBLEMS, p.31).

Newborn peculiarities
All newborn babies have numerous variations in appearance, many of which are caused by the process of birth and the transition from a sterile, liquid environment to air. Although parents may be worried by the apparent imperfections in their child, most of these have gone within a few weeks.

BEHAVIOR OF THE NEWBORN BABY

A baby's behavior in the newborn period is designed to maximize the chances of survival; it ensures that the baby's basic needs – food, cleanliness, warmth, affection, stimulation, and protection – are met. Some of the reflexes present at birth, for example the rooting and sucking reflexes (see opposite), are concerned with feeding. Others, such as the startle reflex, are relics of a more primitive past and these disappear after a few weeks. All the reflexes are eventually replaced by voluntary, controlled movements and actions as the baby's muscles and nervous system mature.

From the moment of birth, a baby communicates by crying. Over the first few weeks of life you will begin to distinguish the different types of crying caused, for example, by hunger, pain, or tiredness.

Gradually, a pattern of behavior emerges and your baby becomes a more predictable individual.

LOCOMOTION REFLEXES

Baby supported in upright position

Baby supported in upright position

Baby steps up

Baby takes deliberate "steps"

Walking reflex
If you hold your baby upright with the feet on a firm surface, he or she will mimic a walking action. This ability quickly disappears.

Placing reflex
If you touch the baby's leg against the edge of a table, the foot will be lifted up. Like the walking reflex, the placing reflex is soon lost.

SURVIVAL REFLEXES

Head jerked
backward

Hand touches
baby's cheek

Head turns
toward
touch

Arm
outstretched

Hands grasp
reflexively

Hand opened

Mouth opens
reflexively

Baby's weight
supported

Leg outstretched

Grasp reflex
If you touch your baby's palm with your finger, his or her hand will close around it. The clenched fist is surprisingly strong and it can even support the baby's entire body weight. This ability, soon lost, is probably a remnant from our evolutionary past.

Startle (or Moro) reflex
Whenever your baby is startled or feels that he or she might fall or be dropped, you can predict that a violent reaction will follow. The arms are flung out as if the baby is clutching for support, the hands open wide, and the head jerks back.

Rooting and sucking reflex
If you stroke or touch your baby's cheek, he or she will turn toward you with an open mouth. Placing a finger, nipple, or pacifier in your baby's mouth will elicit sucking. This behavior is a combination of the most basic reflexes that allows the newborn baby to feed.

STIMULATION OF THE NEWBORN BABY

Visual and sound stimulation is essential for the normal development of sight and hearing. The eye contact that occurs between mother and baby provides the infant's first means of communication; even a few days after birth an infant may mimic gestures, such as sticking out the tongue, opening the mouth, and moving the head. Talk to your baby at every opportunity, and you will eventually be rewarded with gurgles and smiles.

The newborn baby can see clearly objects that are at a distance of about 20–25 cm. Arrangements of lines and shapes can be discriminated from a young age. It has been observed that newborn babies prefer patterns to bright, solid colors, and stripes and angles to circular patterns. Exposure to such visual stimuli can be increased by providing pictures and toys at the optimum distance for focusing.

Physical contact is also essential for healthy development. A newborn baby is accustomed to the noise and feel of a heartbeat and the motion of walking. A baby who is carried in a sling during early life will be less fretful than one who does not have such close physical contact with a parent.

Early communication
Your face will prove irresistible to your baby, and eye contact is an essential part of the bonding process, which, like stimulation, is essential for healthy physical and emotional development. Talking and singing to your baby will elicit a range of responses, such as movements of the head and sticking out the tongue, and he or she will stop feeding or crying if you speak in a soothing voice. Close physical contact while caring for your baby helps to strengthen bonding.

A stimulating environment
Although your newborn baby will spend most of the day asleep, the waking hours provide many opportunities for stimulation. A mobile hanging within focusing range provides an excellent form of visual stimulation. In your baby's crib or carriage, you can place pictures of faces or abstract patterns cut out of magazines for your baby to focus on. Musical toys may calm your baby while you are out of sight. Such early stimulation will help the brain and nervous system to develop.

DEVELOPMENTAL MILESTONES

The ages at which children acquire various physical, mental, and social skills vary from one child to another. The chart below shows when the main skills, or developmental milestones, are achieved. The abilities appear in a specific order that depends on the maturation of the nervous system and the acquisition of preceding skills. Failure to achieve an individual skill in the time span shown on the chart is not in itself a cause for concern.

Your child's development can be assessed using the chart below. The chart can be used in two ways. First, you can check the normal age range for the acquisition of a particular ability. To do this, find the skill in the chart; the red bar indicates the range of ages at which the ability is usually acquired.

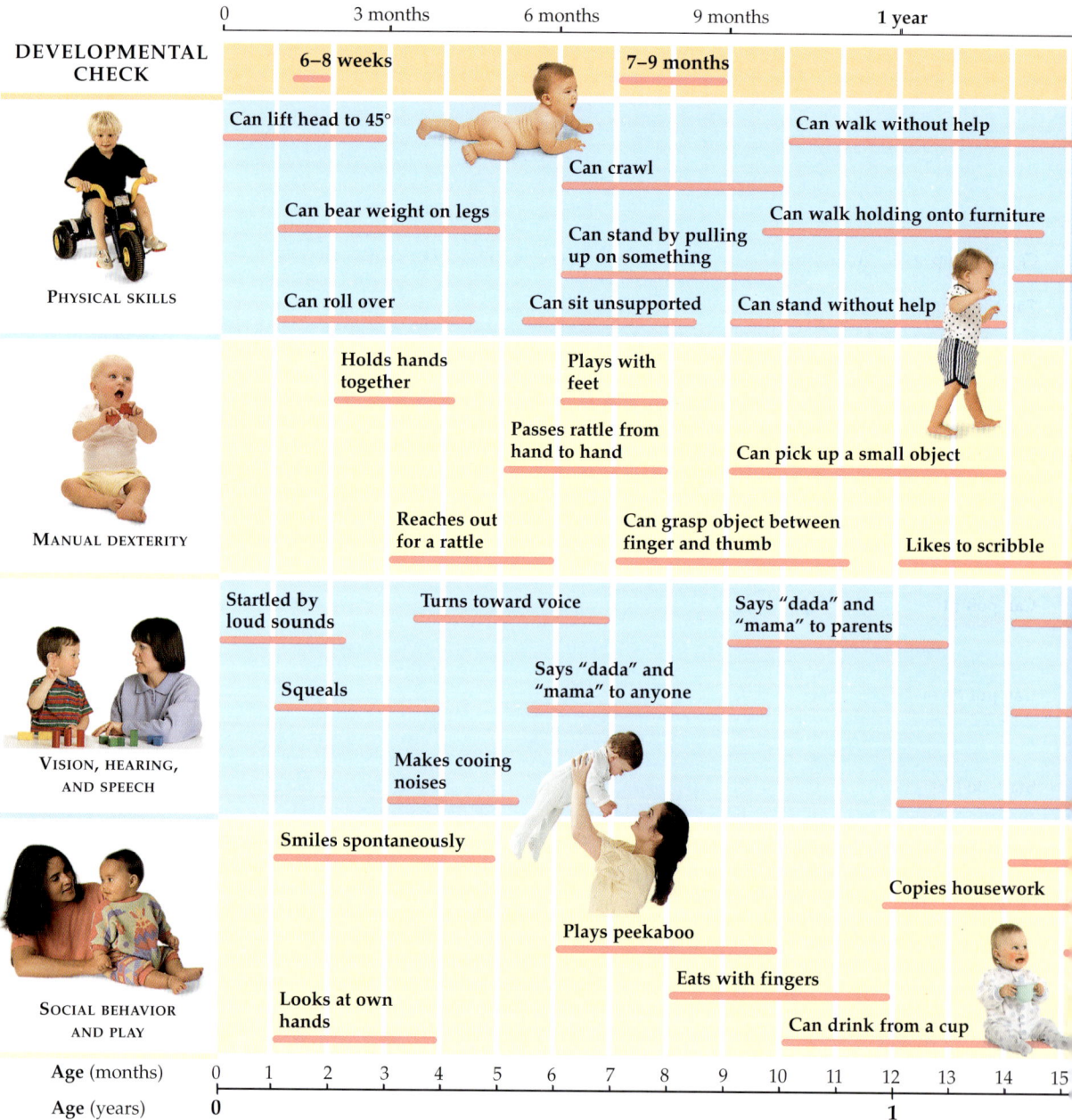

	0	3 months	6 months	9 months	1 year

DEVELOPMENTAL CHECK

6–8 weeks

7–9 months

PHYSICAL SKILLS

Can lift head to 45°

Can crawl

Can walk without help

Can bear weight on legs

Can stand by pulling up on something

Can walk holding onto furniture

Can roll over

Can sit unsupported

Can stand without help

MANUAL DEXTERITY

Holds hands together

Plays with feet

Passes rattle from hand to hand

Can pick up a small object

Reaches out for a rattle

Can grasp object between finger and thumb

Likes to scribble

VISION, HEARING, AND SPEECH

Startled by loud sounds

Turns toward voice

Says "dada" and "mama" to parents

Squeals

Says "dada" and "mama" to anyone

Makes cooing noises

SOCIAL BEHAVIOR AND PLAY

Smiles spontaneously

Copies housework

Plays peekaboo

Eats with fingers

Looks at own hands

Can drink from a cup

Age (months)	0	1	2	3	4	5	6	7	8	9	10	11	12	13	14	15
Age (years)	0												1			

For example, the majority of babies learn to stand unaided between the ages of 9 and 14 months.

Alternatively, the chart can be used to determine the range of skills that might be expected of a baby or child of a particular age. Find your child's age along the bottom of the chart. Then follow that age up the grid to discover which bars cross or end just to the left of that age. For example, in terms of

physical skills, a 4-month-old baby can probably lift his or her head, roll over, and support body weight on his or her legs. A 2-year-old child's verbal skills typically include putting two words together and being able to identify parts of the body by pointing at them.

Although all children acquire skills in much the same order, occasionally a stage is omitted; for example, children may walk without having learned to

crawl. At every well-child examination, your doctor should check your child's development (see top of chart). These checks provide good opportunities to discuss any general or specific concerns you may have about your child's development. The doctor will assess skill acquisition, test your child's sight and hearing, and also check his or her height and weight. The skills and ages shown here are broad guidelines only.

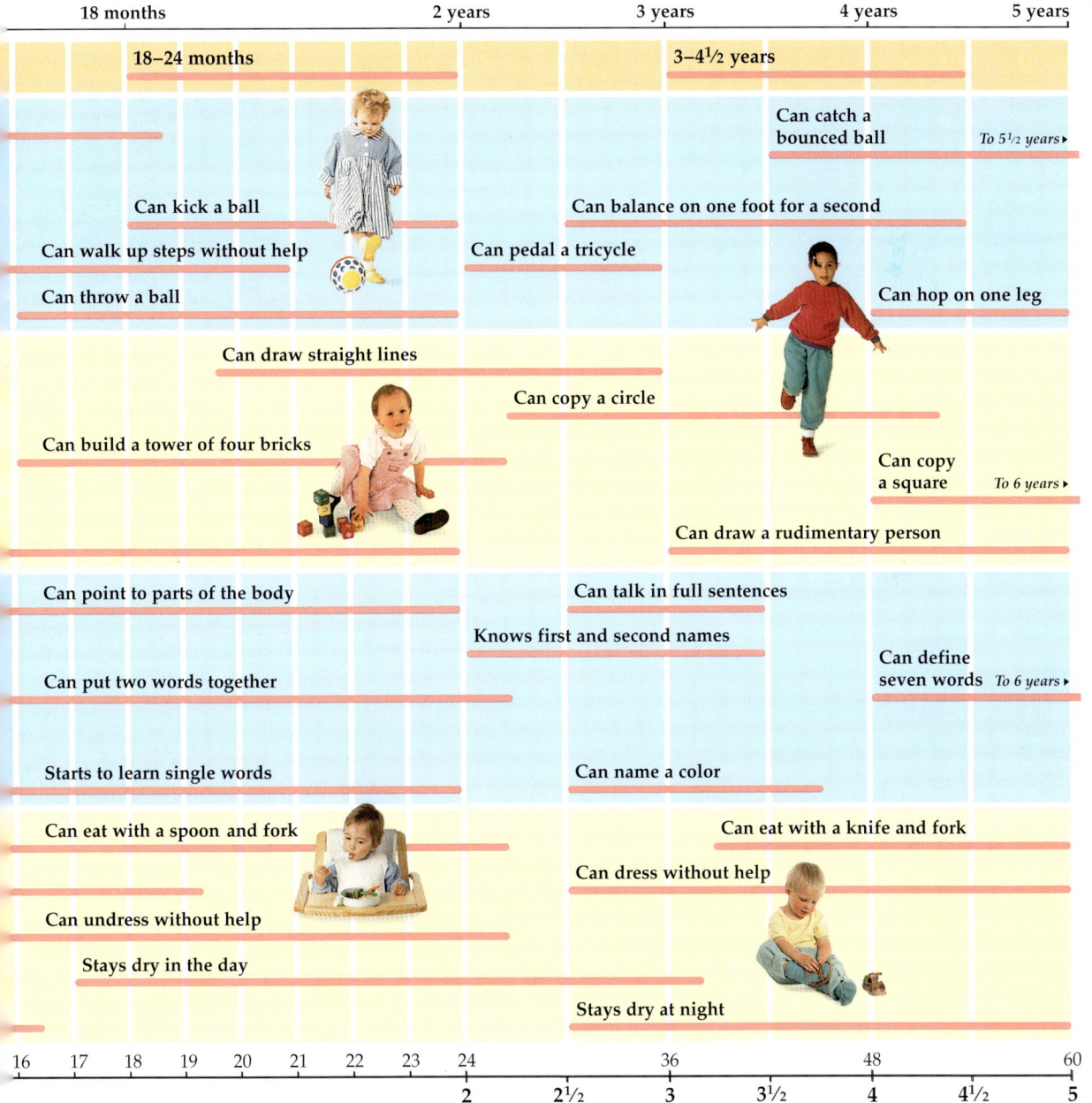

| 18 months | 2 years | 3 years | 4 years | 5 years |

18–24 months **3–4½ years**

Can catch a bounced ball — To 5½ years ▸

Can kick a ball
Can balance on one foot for a second
Can walk up steps without help
Can pedal a tricycle
Can throw a ball
Can hop on one leg

Can draw straight lines
Can copy a circle
Can build a tower of four bricks
Can copy a square — To 6 years ▸
Can draw a rudimentary person

Can point to parts of the body
Can talk in full sentences
Knows first and second names
Can put two words together
Can define seven words — To 6 years ▸

Starts to learn single words
Can name a color

Can eat with a spoon and fork
Can eat with a knife and fork
Can dress without help
Can undress without help
Stays dry in the day
Stays dry at night

| 16 | 17 | 18 | 19 | 20 | 21 | 22 | 23 | 24 | 36 | 48 | 60 |
| | | | | | | | | 2 | 2½ | 3 | 3½ | 4 | 4½ | 5 |

ADOLESCENT DEVELOPMENT

Adolescence marks the change from childhood to adulthood – usually considered the age of 18. The physical changes (puberty) begin in boys at an average age of 12 years, when the testes begin to grow, and in girls at an average age of 11½ years, when the breasts start to develop. Puberty is initiated by hormones, produced by the pituitary and adrenal glands, which stimulate the secretion of estrogen in girls and testosterone in boys. These hormones trigger the physical changes, such as increase in height and weight (known as the growth spurt), and also the emotional changes. The age at which puberty starts varies, but there is no need for concern unless it is before 8 years or after 14 in girls or before 9 years or after 15 in boys.

EMOTIONAL DEVELOPMENT

Adolescence can be a difficult time for both youngsters and parents. It is a period of testing in which your child will try to establish and redefine a sense of identity, both within and outside the family unit. An adolescent may demand independence that is inappropriate for the teenage years. He or she may behave in a manner that is contrary to guidelines and values instilled in childhood, and may seem overly confrontational and critical of you and other adults.

Your child's emotional development will not proceed at the same rate as physical development. Adolescents who look grown up and demand adult privileges may still be emotionally immature, confused, and lacking in confidence. It is important that adults do not have unreasonable expectations of adolescents during this time. The period of maturation should not be viewed too negatively because it is an essential part of growing up, and most adolescents turn into responsible adults.

PHYSICAL CHANGES IN GIRLS

The growth spurt may begin before there are any other signs of physical development. During growth in height, breast buds and pubic hair appear, followed by underarm hair and sweat glands. Menstruation begins between 11 and 14 years, and ovulation follows at varying times afterward.

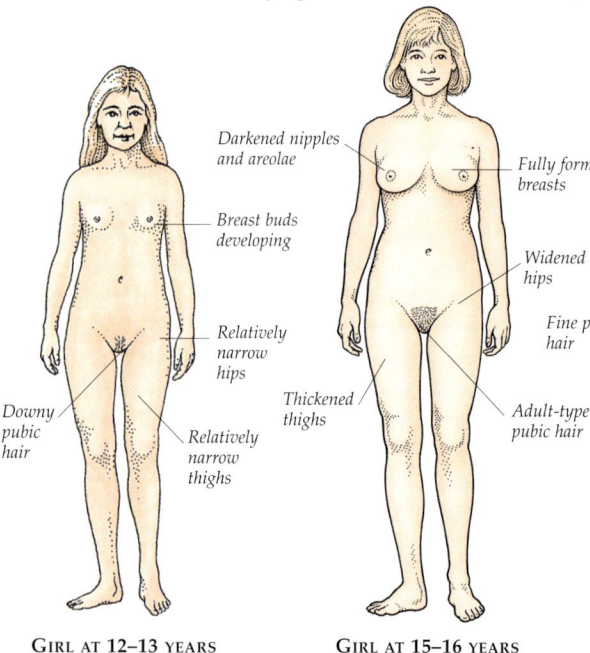

PHYSICAL CHANGES IN BOYS

The growth spurt in boys occurs later than in girls. The first sign of puberty is enlargement of the testes; darkening of the scrotum, appearance of pubic hair, and lengthening of the penis follow. Body hair appears next and the voice deepens when the growth spurt is well established.

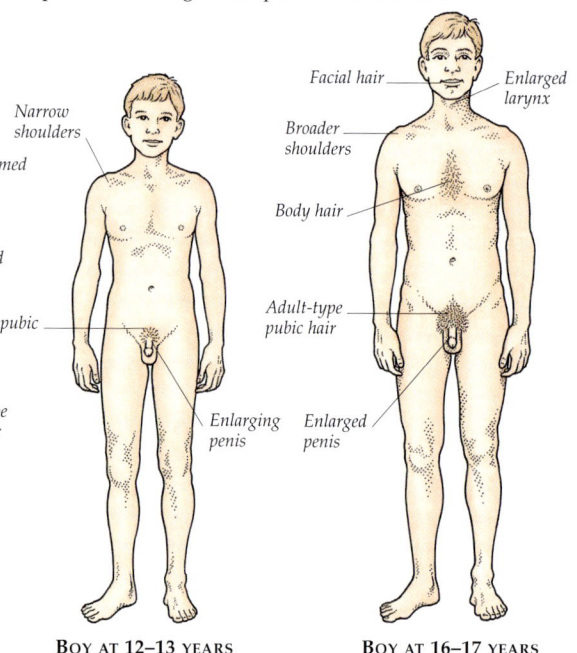

Darkened nipples and areolae
Fully formed breasts
Breast buds developing
Widened hips
Relatively narrow hips
Fine pubic hair
Thickened thighs
Downy pubic hair
Adult-type pubic hair
Relatively narrow thighs

Narrow shoulders
Facial hair
Enlarged larynx
Broader shoulders
Body hair
Adult-type pubic hair
Enlarging penis
Enlarged penis

GIRL AT 12–13 YEARS   GIRL AT 15–16 YEARS   BOY AT 12–13 YEARS   BOY AT 16–17 YEARS

Stages of development in girls
In girls, puberty is heralded by emerging breast buds and growth of downy pubic hair. By 15 or 16 years, a girl will have reached adult proportions, with wider hips, fat deposits in the abdomen and thighs, fully developed breasts, and adult-type pubic and underarm hair.

Stages of development in boys
In early puberty, the testes and scrotum start to enlarge. By the age of about 17 years, a boy's penis will have reached its maximum size, and hair will have grown under the arms and on the face, legs, chest, and abdomen. The voice deepens as the larynx and vocal cords enlarge.

HEALTHY LIVING

THE FOUNDATIONS OF A HEALTHY LIFE are laid down in childhood by sensible eating, immunization against the major childhood illnesses, adequate mental and physical stimulation, and taking precautions against accidents at home, school, and on the road.

INFANT FEEDING

How you decide to feed your baby is your choice entirely, but breast-feeding has many advantages over bottle-feeding: human milk provides the correct proportion of nutrients for a growing infant and antibodies to boost the immune system. However, some women cannot or choose not to breast-feed, and for their babies formula milk in a bottle is an acceptable alternative.

BREAST-FEEDING

If you decide to breast-feed, you can be sure you are giving your baby the best start in life. Breast milk contains the right proportions of nutrients essential for early growth and development; it is also readily available, easily digested, virtually sterile, cheap, comes at the right temperature, and contains the mother's antibodies, which offer some protection against disease. Breast-feeding can be a very rewarding experience for both mother and baby.

Breast-feeding your baby
Sitting in a comfortable upright position, you should maintain eye contact as your baby feeds. This is part of the bonding process.

Most newborns nurse every two hours or so, both day and night. This frequency helps bring in mother's milk shortly after birth. To best evaluate your success with nursing, check these two outcomes. The baby should have at least one wet diaper per day of age of life, so that on the third day there should be a minimum of three wet diapers, until there are four or five wet diapers per day and then adequate hydration has been established. The second sign of successful nursing is when you see your baby's bowel movements change in color from black to mustard yellow.

Some women experience problems, particularly when trying to establish breast-feeding, but with perseverance, help, and time, such early difficulties can usually be overcome. Common problems are latching-on difficulty, engorged or infected breasts or sore nipples, and inadequate milk supply (see FEEDING PROBLEMS, p.32).

Breast-feeding works by supply and demand, so the more a baby sucks, the more milk is produced. After the first few days of feeding, a pattern will emerge that ensures that the baby receives enough milk. Supplementary bottles can upset this balance and should only be given with advice from a professional; a breast pump and a feeding tube may help this problem. Breast-feeding can be difficult, so get as much advice and support as you need from a lactation consultant.

To maintain a good supply of milk, you should eat a well-balanced diet and drink plenty of fluids. Make sure that the extra energy you need in order to feed your baby is obtained from healthy foods, such as fruit, vegetables, and dairy products, rather than sugary carbohydrates.

Bottle-feeding your baby
With your baby cradled in one arm, use the other to hold the bottle firmly and at an angle so that no air is allowed to enter the nipple and milk is delivered at a constant rate.

BOTTLE-FEEDING

Bottle-feeding has the advantage of being less physically demanding on the mother; also, other adults can help with feedings. There may be different FEEDING PROBLEMS (p.32), including an allergic reaction to the protein in cow's milk (see REACTIONS TO FOOD, p.182).

Different brands of milk formula are available, although all are of similar composition. Infants who are allergic to cow's milk can be given an alternative.

Use water from a safe supply for mixing feedings, and carefully follow manufacturer's instructions regarding proportions of powder to water. All bottles, nipples, and other feeding equipment should be washed before every use to prevent infection.

ADDING SOLID FOOD

Babies make the gradual transition from a diet of milk to mixed foods. Before the age of 4 months, milk provides all of the nutrients required by a baby. Between 4 and 6 months your baby's digestive system will have developed sufficiently to cope with more complex food, and there will be signs, such as still being hungry after a feeding or demanding more frequent feedings, that he or she is ready to try solid food.

FIRST FOODS

Adding solid food to your baby's diet is a gradual process that can take 3 or 4 weeks or longer to complete. Some babies take to solids immediately while others are fussy and take longer to adapt. The chart (below) is one way to approach adding solids to the diet, but this can be adapted to suit your needs and your way of life. There are no hard and fast rules about when to start, how long the process should take, or which foods to offer; more important is a positive and flexible attitude.

During the first week that you are making the change, your job is to introduce the idea of solid food and eating from a spoon. Your baby will not be receiving any nourishment from the small amount of food you offer in the initial stages.

Choose a time to start when both you and your baby are relaxed. Often, lunchtime is the best time of day to introduce solids. Your baby may be more willing to try something new then than at breakfast, when hunger may be acute, or dinner, when he or she may be tired. Start with half a milk feeding; with your baby still on your lap, offer a spoon of food, then milk.

Introduce one new food at a time. Baby rice or puréed vegetables or fruit (not citrus) are best to start with; your child is unlikely to react badly to them. If he or she rejects a food or develops diarrhea, vomiting, or a rash, avoid the food for a few weeks. Protein foods should be puréed with a vegetable. Gradually reduce milk intake and use only formula or breast milk until your baby is 1 year old.

NUTRITION

Try to introduce your baby to healthy foods. Offer home-prepared foods using fresh ingredients. Avoid adding salt to your cooking. Sugary foods, such as cakes and cookies, should be restricted to avoid obesity and TOOTH DECAY (p.177) later in life. Try to vary the tastes and textures so that your baby samples a wide range of different foods; this may help make balancing nutritional requirements easier.

suggested weaning schedule					
STAGE	Early morning/ throughout day	Breakfast	Lunch	Dinner	Bedtime
Days 1–4	Milk feeding. Offer cooled, boiled water outside mealtimes.	Milk feeding.	Half a milk feeding. Then 1 to 2 teaspoons of baby rice mixed with milk, or vegetable or fruit purée. Rest of milk feeding.	Milk feeding.	Milk feeding*.
Days 5–8	Milk feeding. Offer cooled, boiled water outside mealtimes.	1 teaspoon of baby rice. Give milk feeding before, during, or after cereal.	3 to 4 teaspoons of baby rice, vegetable, or fruit purée. Give milk feeding before, during, or after solids.	Milk feeding.	Milk feeding*.
Days 9–12	No early milk feeding. Offer cool water or diluted fruit juice outside mealtimes.	1 to 2 teaspoons of cereal. Give milk feeding before, during, or after cereal.	2 to 3 teaspoons of a protein (puréed cheese, vegetable, fish, or meat), then 2 to 3 teaspoons of fruit purée. Give milk feeding before, during, or after solids.	1 to 2 teaspoons of baby cereal, vegetable, or fruit purée. Give milk feeding before, during, or after solids.	Milk feeding*.
Days 13–16	Offer nonmilk drinks in a training cup. You may offer mashed food.	2 to 3 teaspoons of cereal. Give milk feeding before, during, or after cereal.	2 to 3 teaspoons of a protein followed by the same amount of yogurt or mashed fruit. Half a milk feeding.	A protein and fruit. Give milk feeding before, during, or after solids.	Milk feeding*.
Days 17–20	Offer nonmilk drinks in a training cup.	Cereal, with the milk feeding given before, during, or after.	A protein followed by yogurt or fruit purée. Offer milk in a training cup.	A protein followed by yogurt or fruit purée. Half a milk feeding.	Milk feeding*.
Day 21 onward	Your baby should drink about 1 pint (½ liter) of milk each day.	Cereal and milk feeding. From 4 weeks, offer milk at breakfast in a training cup.	A protein followed by yogurt or fruit purée. Offer milk in a training cup.	A protein followed by yogurt or fruit purée. Milk in a training cup.	Milk feeding*. *Remove bottle before sleep.

HEALTHY EATING

By the time your child is 1 year old, he or she should have tried a wide variety of foods. At this stage, definite likes and dislikes in food are common and you may worry that the diet is lacking in variety and nutritional value. You can encourage healthy eating by offering nutritious meals made from fresh ingredients. Processed and convenience foods are not inherently unhealthy provided they are not always given in preference to fresh foods. Sensible eating habits established in childhood will improve your child's chance of a healthy life.

NUTRIENT REQUIREMENTS

Children need more food than adults in proportion to their size because they are more active and need fuel for growth. Food intake peaks in the teenage years – a time of great physical growth and bodily change. Over the age of 5 years, the recommended daily energy requirements should come from the following sources: carbohydrates, 60 percent; fats, 20 percent; proteins, 20 percent. In younger children, especially those uner 1 year, fats should not be kept to adult levels; they provide more concentrated energy than carbohydrates.

Energy requirements
This chart compares daily energy intake for boys and girls of different ages. Over the age of 5 years, most energy should come from starchy foods, such as bread, rice, and pasta.

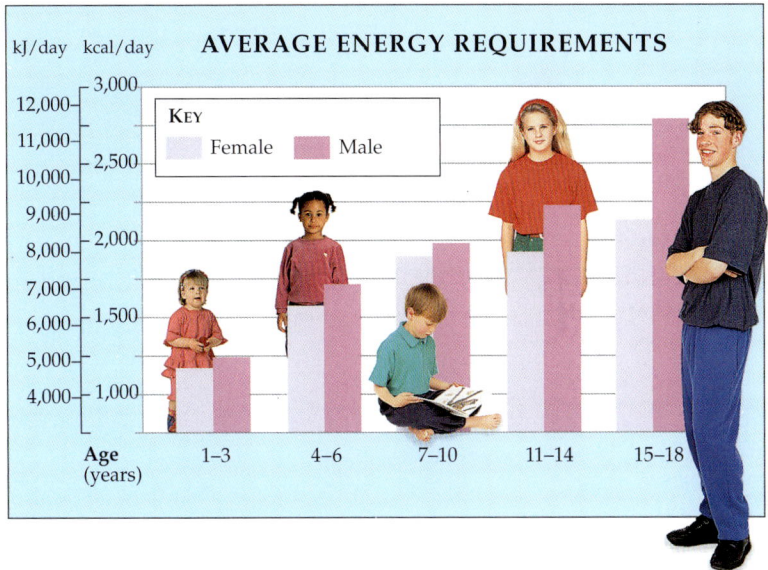

AVERAGE ENERGY REQUIREMENTS

KEY: Female / Male

kJ/day / kcal/day

Age (years): 1–3, 4–6, 7–10, 11–14, 15–18

DIFFERENT PEOPLE NEED DIFFERENT AMOUNTS OF FOOD

The amount of food you need every day from the four food groups and other foods depends on your age, body size, activity level, whether you are male or female, and if you are pregnant or breast-feeding. That's why the Health Canada food guide gives a lower and higher number of servings for each food group. For example, young children can choose the lower number of servings, while male teenagers can go to the higher number. Most other people can choose servings somewhere in between. Keep sugary and fried foods to a minimum. Vitamins and minerals are provided by a balanced diet, but if your child is a fussy eater, a supplement may be required.

The Food Guide
The Health Canada food guide shows sample foods from each food group and the nutrients required each day.

Grain Products 5-12 SERVINGS PER DAY

1 Serving: 1 Slice, Cold Cereal 30 g, Hot Cereal 175 mL 3/4 cup
2 Servings: 1 Bagel, Pita or Bun, Pasta or Rice 250 mL 1 cup

Vegetables & Fruit 5-10 SERVINGS PER DAY

1 Serving: 1 Medium Size Vegetable or Fruit, Fresh, Frozen or Canned Vegetables or Fruit 125 mL 1/2 cup, Salad 250 mL 1 cup, Juice 125 mL 1/2 cup

Milk Products SERVINGS PER DAY
Children 4–9 years: 2–3
Youth 10–16 years: 3–4
Adults: 2–4
Pregnant & Breast-feeding Women: 3–4

1 Serving: Milk 250 mL 1 cup, Cheese 3"x1"x1" 50 g, 2 Slices 50 g, Yogurt 175 g 3/4 cup

Meat & Alternatives 2-3 SERVINGS PER DAY

1 Serving: Meat, Poultry or Fish 50-100 g, Fish 1/3–2/3 Can 50–100 g, 1-2 Eggs, Beans 125-250 mL, Tofu 100 g, Peanut Butter 30 mL 2 tbsp 1/3 cup

Other Foods

Taste and enjoyment can also come from other foods and beverages that are not part of the 4 food groups. Some of these foods are higher in fat or Calories, so use these foods in moderation.

SAFETY AND HEALTH

Although it is not possible to protect your child from every accident or illness, you can take certain precautions to reduce the possibility of a serious illness or life-threatening emergency. Immunization, done as completely and as early as possible, is very effective at preventing a number of childhood diseases, such as measles and pertussis. Protection from sunlight is quite important since a child's skin burns easily, which can lead to skin cancer in adulthood. Use a high-factor sun cream, and make sure that your child wears a hat and other protective clothing; exposure to the sun should be increased gradually day by day. Choking in a small child can be avoided if nuts and toys with small parts are kept out of reach. Keep all hazardous items, including plastic bags, medicines, and garden and household chemicals, locked away. Teach your child what to do in the event of a fire, and install smoke detectors in every room.

IMMUNIZATION

Certain infectious diseases may be prevented by having your child vaccinated according to the schedule below. Serious adverse reactions to vaccines are extremely rare, but please speak to your physician if you are concerned.

AGE	DISEASE
Newborn	Hepatitis B*
1 month	Hepatitis B_2
2 months	Penta (diphtheria, tetanus, acellular pertussis, HIB**, and polio); Prevnar (pneumococcal conjugate)
3 months	Meningococcal C conjugate
4 months	$Penta_2$; $Prevnar_2$
5 months	Meningococcal C $conjugate_2$
6 months	$Penta_3$; $Prevnar_3$; hepatitis B_3
12 months	MMR (measles, mumps, and rubella); varicella (chicken pox)
18 months	$Penta_4$; $Prevnar_4$
4 – 6 years	MMR_2***; DPTP (diphtheria, acellular pertussis, tetanus, and polio)
14 – 16 years	DTP (diphtheria, tetanus, and acellular pertussis)
Yearly	Influenza vaccine (recommended for children 6 months to 2 years; suggested for all other children)

*Given at the Grade 7 level (age 13 years) in some provinces. **HIB is *Haemophilus influenzae* type B. ***Given at 18 months in some provinces.

PREVENTING ACCIDENTS

Between the ages of 1 and 15 years, more children are killed by accidents than by illness. Many accidents can be prevented if you follow certain safety procedures, such as teaching your child how to avoid danger on the road and in the playground and by keeping your home as hazard-free as possible.

Traffic accidents are responsible for the majority of deaths. Approved restraints in the car are essential for the prevention of death or serious injury in the event of an accident.

Children are naturally curious. Even the home environment contains many potential sources of danger, such as electric sockets and wires, razors, glass doors, open windows, bathtubs, swimming pools, and do-it-yourself home and garden equipment.

As your child grows up, the safety requirements will change; for example, a toddler must be protected from stairs and sharp table corners while an older child needs to be taught about bicycle and road safety.

Storing medicines
Medicines should be stored in child-proof containers out of your child's reach, preferably in a locked medicine cabinet. Prescribed drugs should not be kept beyond the course of an illness nor over-the-counter drugs after their expiration date. Always discard drugs in a place where they will not be accessible to your child.

Safety in the kitchen
Burns and scalds are the main causes of accidental death in the home. Teach your child to stay away from the stove. Make sure he or she does not climb on a stool or chair near the stove, inviting a fall. Handles should point toward the center or back of the stove. Always keep noxious household chemicals locked away.

Safety in the garden
There are many substances in the garden that are harmful if swallowed. Remove poisonous species, such as fungi or yew. Always store garden chemicals in a locked cupboard or shed. You should warn your child not to eat leaves or berries, but if accidental ingestion occurs, see FIRST AID: Swallowed poisons (p.211).

Safety in the playground
Teach your child to play safely. Only allow him or her to use a slide that is on a soft surface, such as grass. Turnarounds are a potential source of danger since hands and feet can get caught underneath. Swings should be used only by the age group for which they were designed, and by only one child at a time.

Riding a bicycle or scooter
When your child is riding a bicycle, make sure that he or she wears a protective helmet and fluorescent clothing and reflectors to make him or her easily visible. Make sure that the bicycle is maintained in good working order. Children using a scooter or in-line skates should wear a helmet, knee and elbow pads, and gloves.

Safety in the car
A baby of less than 9 kg or under the age of one year should travel in an approved rear-facing car seat, strapped into the back seat. Do not put a child in the front seat if the car has air bags. Toddlers weighing less than 18 kg should use a molded car seat, and older children should have a booster seat in the back.

INFANCY

MANY INFANTS – NEWBORN AND OLDER – have variations in appearance and behavior patterns that may concern the parents. Crossed eyes or skin discoloration, such as birthmarks, are common in newborn babies and usually disappear in time without treatment. Many difficulties that affect older infants, such as feeding and sleeping problems, can be solved by the parents themselves using self-help measures.

THE NEWBORN BABY

A newborn baby must adapt quickly to a world dramatically different from the uterus out of which he or she has emerged. Many body systems, such as the respiratory and digestive systems, are not fully functional when the baby is born, and take minutes, days, months, or even years to mature.

SKIN PROBLEMS

Many minor problems characteristic of newborn babies affect the skin, and most disappear without treatment.

Birthmarks rarely cause discomfort, but they may be unsightly. Among the most common birthmarks are the flat hemangiomas and nevus. A hemangioma, which is flat and purplish red, does not disappear but it can often be covered with a cream or may be reduced by laser treatment.

A nevus grows rapidly over the first few weeks. Treatment is not required unless it is on an eyelid; most disappear by the age of 7 years.

For the first few days after birth, babies are unable to excrete wastes efficiently; this causes a buildup of yellow pigment in the skin (jaundice). Many newborn babies have a mild form of jaundice that usually clears up without treatment. Some babies require light treatment, also called phototherapy.

OTHER PROBLEMS

Newborn babies may have other minor problems, such as an umbilical HERNIA (p.187), STRABISMUS (p.166), or infections. Some disappear spontaneously.

An umbilical hernia forms when a gap in the muscles of the abdominal wall allows a loop of intestine to bulge out near the navel. The hernia usually disappears before the age of 2 years.

Babies often appear cross-eyed because eye muscle control is poor. A persistent problem or one existing after the age of 4 months may need treatment.

During birth, infections such as ORAL THRUSH (p.176) or PINK EYE (p.165), may be picked up from the mother. Other minor infections of the mouth, eyes, skin, and navel are also common in the first few weeks of life.

SOME MINOR PROBLEMS OF THE NEWBORN BABY

Hemangioma
This purple-red area does not usually fade, but it can be concealed with a special cream or reduced by laser

Sticky eye
Mild pink eye in a newborn baby may be caused by a blocked tear duct or by bacteria in the birth canal

Strawberry nevus
This bright red raised birthmark is made up of blood vessels that are malformed

Erythema toxicum
This hivelike rash disappears in the first week of life

Jaundice
Yellow skin is caused by a buildup of pigment; the immature liver is unable to excrete wastes at a fast enough rate

Sucking blisters
Vigorous sucking from the breast or bottle can cause one or more large blisters to appear on the upper lip

Milia
These are small white spots that occur mainly around the nose; they clear up without any special treatment

THE OLDER INFANT

Infants commonly suffer from a range of minor problems, which include feeding problems and sleeping difficulties. Although most of these problems disappear as the baby grows older, they can cause considerable anxiety and tension in both parents, particularly if several problems occur simultaneously. For most of these problems there are self-help measures that may alleviate them. However, if the difficulties cannot be cured by self-help alone, it is important to seek professional advice from a lactation consultant before resentment or feelings of inadequacy set in.

Burping position
After every feeding, change your baby's position so that any swallowed air will be released from the stomach.

FEEDING PROBLEMS

Before solid food is added to the baby's diet (see p.28), the most common type of feeding problem is the mother's anxiety about whether the baby is getting enough milk. If you are bottle-feeding, it is easy to measure how much milk is being taken, but with breast-feeding this is difficult and you have to rely on the baby's weight gain as a gauge of intake. If you are worried about this, you should discuss it with your doctor.

With bottle-feeding it is important to make up the feedings correctly to avoid overfeeding or underfeeding your baby. Check the size of the nipple opening: one that is too large can cause gas and one that is too small will make feeding difficult. Feeding equipment must always be washed to protect against infection, such as gastroenteritis.

A few feeding problems and possible solutions are shown in the chart below.

GAS

Whether your baby is breast-fed or bottle-fed, gas is distressing and may prevent an adequate intake of nutrients because your baby's stomach will feel full and feeding will stop. During and after a feeding you should help your baby to bring up any air that has been taken in with the milk. The best way to burp your baby is to move him or her from a feeding to a sitting position or to an upright position against your shoulder. Placing your baby stomach-down on your lap also releases gas. Rubbing your baby's back at the same time provides comfort and reassurance.

COLIC

Infants between the ages of about 2 weeks and 3 months are commonly affected by a type of inconsolable crying known as colic. Your baby may

BREAST-FEEDING PROBLEMS			
PROBLEM	SOLUTION	PROBLEM	SOLUTION
Mastitis (infected, blocked milk duct)	Continue to breast-feed. Get medical advice within 24 hours.	**Latching-on difficulty**	Make sure baby takes nipple and areola into mouth. If breasts are full, express a little milk.
Sore nipples	Be sure that baby latches on correctly. Prevent breasts from becoming overfull. Keep nipples dry. Use a nipple cream.	**"Evening colic"**	Offer more frequent feedings in the evening. Try to rest during the day to avoid becoming overtired in the evening.
Engorged breasts	Feed frequently. Express milk if baby is not ready to feed. Place warm flannel cloths on breasts.	**Inadequate milk supply**	Eat a healthy diet (800 kcal/3,345 kJ a day more than usual). Do not get overtired. Offer a feeding when your baby wants one.

BOTTLE-FEEDING PROBLEMS	
PROBLEM	SOLUTION
Infection	Wash hands before giving feedings. Store madeup milk in refrigerator. Throw away any milk left after a feeding.
Formula preparation	Never add more powder or less water than the instructions state. Never add cereal to the bottle, unless directed.
Nipple opening too small	Use a sterilized needle or knife to make a bigger opening in nipple.

draw up his or her legs as if in extreme pain and become very red in the face. A possible cause is failure to bring up gas that enters the stomach during feeding or crying, with the result that air passes into the small intestine and causes pain and excessive contractions.

In "evening colic," the baby cries as if in great pain for a few hours in the early evening. This condition affects breast-fed babies more often than bottle-fed babies, and hunger may be a factor. Even if you fed your baby recently, it is worth offering another feeding. If you breast-feed, your milk supply may be reduced in the evening when you are tired and your baby will need to feed more often; tension, such as that caused by the baby's incessant crying, may further reduce the milk and perpetuate the problem.

Rocking or walking with your baby, going for a ride in the car, or rubbing his or her abdomen, may calm and comfort your baby temporarily. If you are breast-feeding, try to rest during the day so that your evening milk supply is plentiful. Although many products are available that claim to alleviate evening colic, no medical evidence supports these claims.

FAILURE TO THRIVE

Gaining insufficient weight according to the standardized baby growth charts (see pp.17–21) is called failure to thrive. However, most babies who put on weight slowly are perfectly healthy, and you should not be anxious if your baby is putting on weight slowly. Parents' expectations about weight gain may be unrealistic and not take into account factors such as birth weight or parental size.

You should go to a baby clinic or doctor's office on a regular basis to have your baby weighed so that the actual weight change can be plotted and monitored by an expert. If it is established that your baby's weight gain is abnormal, the doctor will look for a physical cause, such as feeding problems or MALABSORPTION (p.183) or an emotional or social problem.

TEETHING

You can expect your baby's first teeth to appear around the age of 6 months and the last of the primary teeth to come through by about 3 years (see DEVELOPMENT OF TEETH, p.14). The incisors often arrive with little upset to the baby, but eruption of the canines and molars can cause some discomfort. The first signs of teething are dribbling, redness of the gum at the site of the new tooth, and a flushed cheek; your baby may be fretful and have problems feeding. While teething, some babies enjoy biting on a hard object, such as a hard biscuit or teething ring. Liquid acetaminophen can be given if there is pain.

You should not attribute symptoms such as fever or diarrhea to teething since there is no medical evidence of any connection.

SLEEPING PROBLEMS

Like adults, babies vary widely in sleep requirements so do not conclude that there is a problem if your infant sleeps less or more than another baby of the same age. Sleeping problems include not settling down at bedtime to waking in the night, or not sleeping during the day. A sleep pattern only becomes a problem if it is unduly disruptive to the parents or child.

By the age of 3 or 4 months, most babies no longer need frequent night feedings and may not wake up at night. If your baby wakes and cries, wait a little while before responding. Establish a routine with a consistent bedtime and a definite order of events leading up to this, such as a bath and a feeding.

Temporary sleeping problems often occur with illness or any disruption to the routine, such as a weekend away.

Teething aids
Various hard or cold objects, such as hard biscuits or teething rings, sometimes have special appeal to teething babies.

FLEXIBLE TEETHING RING

SUGAR-FREE HARD BISCUITS

TEETHING BISCUITS

COOLED TEETHING RING

PREVENTION OF SUDDEN INFANT DEATH

Although sudden infant death is very rare, it is important to follow the latest guidelines for prevention. These are:
- Put your baby to sleep on his or her back.
- Do not smoke; keep your baby out of smoky atmospheres.
- Do not let your baby get too warm (see below).
- Put your baby at the foot of the crib.
- Contact your doctor if you think your baby is sick.
- Do not use lots of soft bedding.

Temperature and bedding
This diagram shows the amount of bedding that is required for a range of room temperatures in order to keep your baby's body temperature at the optimum level.

ROOM	°F	°C	BEDDING
	80	27	Sheet only
Too hot	75	24	Sheet + 1 blanket*
	70	21	Sheet + 2 blankets*
Just right	65	18	Sheet + 3 blankets*
	60	15	
Too cold	55	13	Sheet + 4 blankets*
	50	10	

A double layer of blankets counts as two blankets.

Correct sleeping position
A baby should sleep on his or her back, with the feet at the bottom of the crib.

Incorrect sleeping position
A baby put to sleep at the head of the crib is at risk of moving down under the covers and either overheating or suffocating.

SYMPTOM CHARTS

CHILDREN OFTEN SUFFER from minor ailments, most of which are not serious and disappear within a few days. Sometimes, however, a symptom might indicate a more serious

BOTTLE-FEEDING A BABY

problem. The charts in this section aim to help parents and other caregivers decide whether a child's symptom or set of symptoms require medical assessment and, if so, the urgency with which a diagnosis should be sought. By following the questions and answers you will arrive at one or more possible causes of your child's symptoms. The causes refer you to DISEASES AND DISORDERS (p.116) where the problems are discussed in greater detail. Also included are measures that can be taken at home to help relieve the symptoms. For instructions on using the charts, see HOW TO USE THE CHARTS (p.9).

RELIEF FOR A HEADACHE

1 FEVER IN INFANTS

For children over 1 year, see chart 8

Fever is a raised temperature; it is usually caused by infection. If your baby feels hot or seems listless or unusually irritable, take his or her temperature (see NURSING A SICK CHILD, p.212). Normal body temperature is between 36 and 38°C; a child with a temperature above 38°C has a fever.

DANGER SIGNS
Phone your doctor at once if your baby has a raised temperature and any of the following symptoms:
- Rapid breathing.
- Noisy or difficult breathing.
- Unexplained drowsiness.
- Irritability.
- Unwillingness to drink.
- Decreased urination.
- Persistent vomiting.

START HERE

How old is your baby?

- UNDER 6 MONTHS
- 6 MONTHS OR OVER

Does your baby have a rash?

- RASH
- NO RASH

Go to chart
22 RASH WITH FEVER

POSSIBLE CAUSE
Fever in babies younger than 6 months is important; it may indicate a serious illness.

ACTION NEEDED
MEDICAL HELP
✛ URGENT! Phone or see a doctor immediately!

SELF-HELP
See panel: *Bringing down a high temperature* (opposite).

Does your baby cry and pull at one ear or wake up screaming?

- CRIES AND PULLS AT ONE EAR
- WAKES UP IN THE NIGHT SCREAMING
- NEITHER

POSSIBLE CAUSE
OTITIS MEDIA (p. 162).

ACTION NEEDED
MEDICAL HELP
Get medical advice within 24 hours.

SELF-HELP
See panels: *Bringing down a high temperature* (opposite) and *Relieving earache* (p.101).

POSSIBLE CAUSES
An upper respiratory tract infection (see COMMON COLD, p.148 or INFLUENZA, p.151).

ACTION NEEDED
MEDICAL HELP
If there is no improvement within 48 hours, or if breathing problems develop or a rash appears, phone your doctor immediately.

POSSIBLE CAUSES
PNEUMONIA (p.155) or BRONCHIOLITIS (p.155).

ACTION NEEDED
MEDICAL HELP
✛ URGENT! Phone your doctor immediately!

SELF-HELP
See panel: *Bringing down a high temperature* (opposite).

Is your baby's breathing rate normal (see panel: *Checking breathing rates*, p.90)?

- NORMAL
- FASTER THAN NORMAL

Does your baby have a cough or a runny nose?

- COUGH OR A RUNNY NOSE
- NEITHER

POSSIBLE CAUSES

ROSEOLA INFANTUM (p.121), MENINGITIS (p.158), or URINARY TRACT INFECTION (p.193).

ACTION NEEDED

MEDICAL HELP
✚ URGENT! Phone or see a doctor immediately!

:

Is your baby suffering from any of the following symptoms?

- VOMITING WITHOUT DIARRHEA
- DROWSINESS
- IRRITABILITY
- NONE OF THE ABOVE

POSSIBLE CAUSES

A throat infection, such as tonsillitis (see SORE THROAT, p.151) or a mouth infection, such as GINGIVOSTOMATITIS (p.176).

ACTION NEEDED

MEDICAL HELP
If there is no improvement within 24 hours, phone your doctor immediately.

SELF-HELP
See panels: *Relieving a sore throat* (p.91) and *Bringing down a high temperature* (below).

Does your baby have either of the following symptoms?

- RELUCTANCE TO EAT SOLID FOOD
- VOMITING WITH DIARRHEA
- NEITHER

POSSIBLE CAUSE

GASTROENTERITIS (p.180).

ACTION NEEDED

MEDICAL HELP
Get medical advice within 24 hours.

SELF-HELP
See panel: *Preventing dehydration in babies* (p.38).

POSSIBLE CAUSE

Your baby may have become overheated.

ACTION NEEDED

SELF-HELP
A baby does not usually need to be much more warmly dressed than an adult in a similar environment. If overheating could be the problem, remove some of your baby's clothing and reduce the temperature of the room. If temperature does not return to normal within 1 hour, or if your baby exhibits any of the DANGER SIGNS (opposite), consult your doctor.

Is your baby wearing a lot of clothing or is the room very warm?

- WARM CLOTHING
- WARM ROOM
- NEITHER

If you cannot identify your baby's problem from this chart, talk to your doctor within 24 hours.

SELF-HELP: BRINGING DOWN A HIGH TEMPERATURE

Reducing a high temperature makes a child feel more comfortable, and decreases the possibility of a febrile seizure (in children 3 months to 6 years old; see p.156). The following steps can be taken to lower the temperature in a child of any age:

- Unwrap your child and remove their clothing.
- Give liquid or rectal acetaminophen if your child is over 3 months old, using a dose of 15 mgm per kg every four hours as needed.
- Maintain the temperature of your child's room at between 18 and 20°C.
- Never use rubbing alcohol to sponge your child.

Cooling your child
Uncovering your child and removing his or her clothing can help to bring down a high temperature.

2 DIARRHEA IN INFANTS

For children over 1 year, see chart 9

Diarrhea is the passage of runny stool more frequently than normal. However, babies who are entirely breast-fed pass semifluid stool that should not be confused with diarrhea. Any baby who has diarrhea must be given plenty of fluids in order to prevent dehydration.

DANGER SIGNS
Reasons to phone a doctor at once:
- Vomiting for 6 hours.
- Sunken fontanelle.
- Passing very small amounts of dark, concentrated urine, or dry diapers.
- Sunken eyes and not tearing.
- Loose skin.
- Lethargy, unexplained drowsiness, or irritability.
- Dry mucous membranes.

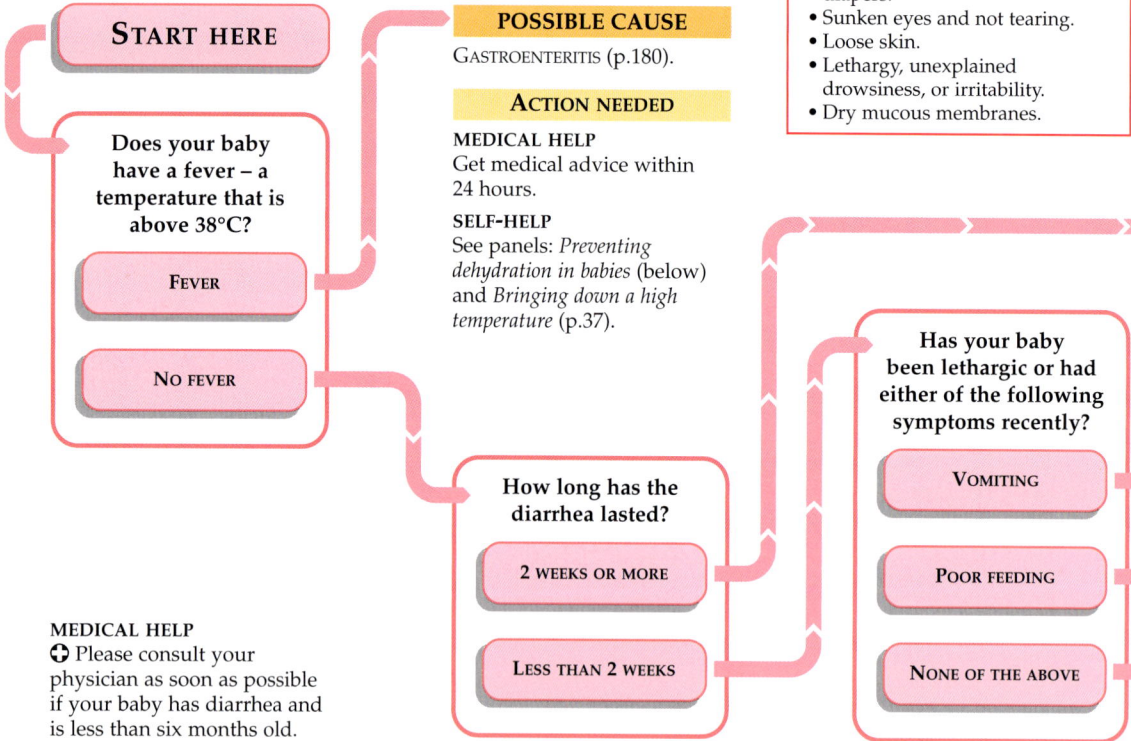

START HERE

Does your baby have a fever – a temperature that is above 38°C?

FEVER

NO FEVER

POSSIBLE CAUSE
GASTROENTERITIS (p.180).

ACTION NEEDED
MEDICAL HELP
Get medical advice within 24 hours.

SELF-HELP
See panels: *Preventing dehydration in babies* (below) and *Bringing down a high temperature* (p.37).

How long has the diarrhea lasted?

2 WEEKS OR MORE

LESS THAN 2 WEEKS

Has your baby been lethargic or had either of the following symptoms recently?

VOMITING

POOR FEEDING

NONE OF THE ABOVE

MEDICAL HELP
✚ Please consult your physician as soon as possible if your baby has diarrhea and is less than six months old.

SELF-HELP: PREVENTING DEHYDRATION IN BABIES

If your baby is in danger of becoming dehydrated – which might result from persistent diarrhea, vomiting, or a fever – it is very important to give extra fluids. It is best to offer one of the commercially available oral electrolyte rehydrating solutions, such as Pedialyte or Rehydralyte, for which you do not need a prescription. However, if these preparations are unavailable, other clear fluids, preferably water, may be substituted. You should not, however, attempt to make your own rehydrating solution or give

your child highly concentrated fluids, such as undiluted juices.

All babies should be rehydrated, to replace ongoing losses and maintain fluid requirements. This is best achieved by offering 20 ml of the oral rehydration solution per kg of body weight in the first hour and then 10 to 20 ml per kg of body weight per hour for the next 6 hours until the diarrhea slows. Early oral feeding is recommended, especially if vomiting has subsided. Breast-feeding is an optimal substitute for the oral rehydration solution.

TIME (in hours)	SOLUTION (ml/kg body weight)
Hour 1	20
Hour 2	10-20
Hour 3	10-20
Hour 4	10-20
Hour 5	10-20
Hour 6	10-20
Hour 7 (if required)	10-20

Rehydrating solution program
To rehydrate your child in the event of fluid loss due to diarrhea, fever, or vomiting, give rehydrating solution following this chart.

POSSIBLE CAUSES

A viral infection is the most likely cause of persistent diarrhea in infants. Other possible causes are conditions that impair digestion including REACTIONS TO FOOD (p.182), GIARDIASIS (p.187), CELIAC DISEASE (p.183), and CYSTIC FIBROSIS (p.201), but these disorders are much less common.

ACTION NEEDED

MEDICAL HELP
Make an appointment to see your doctor.

SELF-HELP
See panel: *Preventing dehydration in babies* (opposite).

Is the amount of fruit juice in your baby's diet more or less than usual?

- MORE THAN USUAL
- LESS THAN USUAL
- NO CHANGE

POSSIBLE CAUSE

In large quantities, the sugar in fruit juice can lead to diarrhea.

ACTION NEEDED

SELF-HELP
Always mix fruit juice with an equal quantity of cool water. Try giving your baby cool water instead of fruit juice. Avoid giving him or her carbonated drinks.

POSSIBLE CAUSE

GASTROENTERITIS (p.180).

ACTION NEEDED

MEDICAL HELP
Get medical advice within 24 hours.

SELF-HELP
See panel: *Preventing dehydration in babies* (opposite).

POSSIBLE CAUSE

New foods may cause diarrhea.

ACTION NEEDED

MEDICAL HELP
Such episodes are usually short-lived. However, if your baby's diarrhea persists or if the diarrhea seems to be associated with particular foods, make an appointment to see your doctor.

SELF-HELP
Make sure your baby does not become dehydrated (see panel: *Preventing dehydration in babies*, opposite). If you can identify the food that is causing your baby's diarrhea, stop offering the food until you have seen your doctor.

When was a new solid introduced into your baby's diet?

- LESS THAN 24 HOURS AGO
- MORE THAN 24 HOURS AGO
- BABY HAS NOT YET EATEN SOLID FOOD

POSSIBLE CAUSES

REACTIONS TO FOOD (p.182) or mild GASTROENTERITIS (p.180).

ACTION NEEDED

MEDICAL HELP
Get medical advice within 24 hours.

SELF-HELP
Stop offering any solid food to your baby until you have seen your doctor. Make sure, however, that your baby does not become dehydrated by giving plenty of liquids (see panel: *Preventing dehydration in babies*, opposite).

Is your baby taking prescribed medicine for any other disorder?

- NO MEDICINE
- MEDICINE

POSSIBLE CAUSE

Your baby's diarrhea could possibly be a side effect of the medicine that he or she is taking.

ACTION NEEDED

MEDICAL HELP
Phone your doctor to find out whether the medicine may be causing your baby's symptoms and whether it should be discontinued.

3 VOMITING IN INFANTS

For children over 1 year, see chart 10

In young babies, it is important not to confuse vomiting, which might indicate an illness, with spitting up, which is the effortless regurgitation of small amounts of milk. However, a single episode of vomiting is common in infants and is unlikely to have a serious cause.

DANGER SIGNS
Reasons to phone a doctor at once:
- Vomiting for 6 hours.
- Sunken fontanelle.
- Passing very small amounts of dark, concentrated urine, or dry diapers.
- Sunken eyes and not tearing.
- Greenish-yellow vomit.
- Unexplained drowsiness or irritability.
- Dry mucous membranes.

START HERE

Does your baby seem healthy and is he or she taking feedings normally?

- SEEMS SICK OR VOMIT IS GREENISH YELLOW
- SEEMS HEALTHY AND IS FEEDING NORMALLY
- IS NOT FEEDING NORMALLY

Was milk brought up effortlessly?

- NO
- YES

How much milk did your baby bring up?

- LARGE AMOUNT
- SMALL AMOUNT

How old is your baby?

- UNDER 2 MONTHS
- 2 MONTHS OR OVER

When does your baby vomit?

- AFTER EVERY FEEDING
- AT UNPREDICTABLE TIMES

Does your baby have a fever – a temperature above 38°C?

- FEVER
- NO FEVER

POSSIBLE CAUSES

INTESTINAL OBSTRUCTION (p.185), dehydration, or overwhelming infection.

ACTION NEEDED

MEDICAL HELP
✚ EMERGENCY! Call an ambulance! While waiting, do not give your baby anything to eat or drink.

POSSIBLE CAUSE

PYLORIC STENOSIS (p.186).

ACTION NEEDED

MEDICAL HELP
Get medical advice within 24 hours.

POSSIBLE CAUSE

GASTROESOPHAGEAL REFLUX (p.186).

ACTION NEEDED

MEDICAL HELP
Get medical advice within 24 hours.

POSSIBLE CAUSES

ROSEOLA INFANTUM (p.121), MENINGITIS (p.158), or URINARY TRACT INFECTION (p.193).

ACTION NEEDED

MEDICAL HELP
✚ URGENT! Phone your doctor immediately!

POSSIBLE CAUSE

GASTROENTERITIS (p.180).

ACTION NEEDED

MEDICAL HELP
✚ URGENT! Phone your doctor immediately!

SELF-HELP
See panel: *Preventing dehydration in babies* (p.38).

POSSIBLE CAUSE

GASTROESOPHAGEAL REFLUX (p.186), which is normal in infants, is the most likely cause.

ACTION NEEDED

SELF-HELP
Have the baby rest on his or her side with the head slightly raised.

Does your baby have any of the following symptoms?

- ABNORMAL DROWSINESS
- REFUSING TO EAT OR DRINK
- DIARRHEA
- COUGH
- NONE OF THE ABOVE

POSSIBLE CAUSES

BRONCHIOLITIS (p.155) or PERTUSSIS (p.123).

ACTION NEEDED

MEDICAL HELP
Get medical advice within 24 hours.

SELF-HELP
See panels: *Bringing down a high temperature* (p.37) and *Relieving a cough* (p.90).

Go to chart
1 FEVER IN INFANTS

POSSIBLE CAUSE

GASTROENTERITIS (p.180).

ACTION NEEDED

MEDICAL HELP
✚ URGENT! Phone your doctor immediately!

SELF-HELP
See panel: *Preventing dehydration in babies* (p.38).

Does your baby have any of the following symptoms?

- DIARRHEA
- COUGH
- NONE OF THE ABOVE

If your baby has vomited only once and otherwise seems quite healthy, he or she is unlikely to be seriously ill. However, if your baby vomits again or if any other symptoms develop, talk to your doctor.

4 FEEDING PROBLEMS

For children over 1 year, see chart 11

Problems with feeding can be distressing for the parents and the child. Breast-feeding problems are common, especially in the first few weeks after birth. However, if your baby is gaining weight at the expected rate and otherwise seems well, there is usually no need to be concerned.

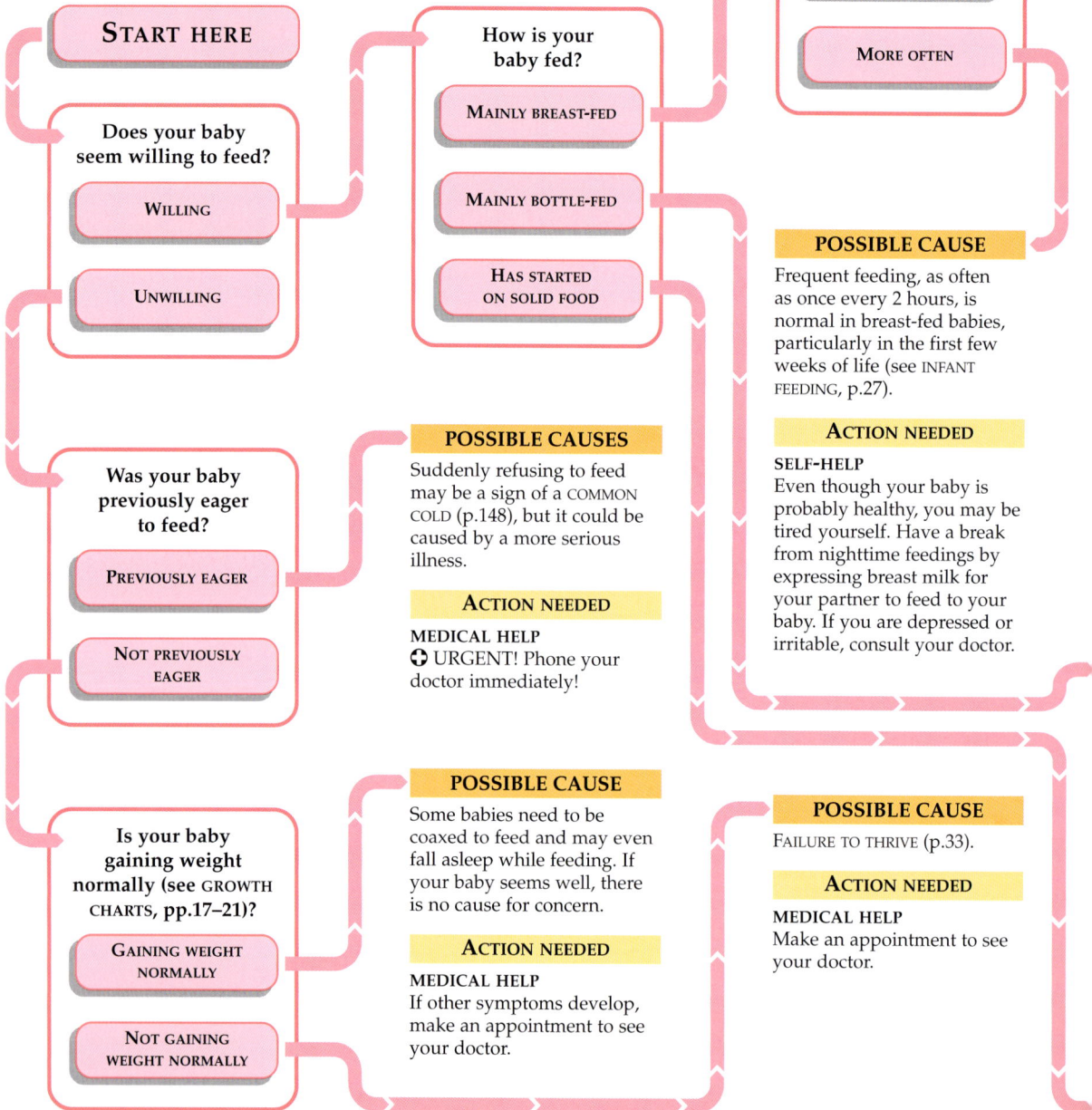

START HERE

Does your baby seem willing to feed?

WILLING

UNWILLING

How is your baby fed?

MAINLY BREAST-FED

MAINLY BOTTLE-FED

HAS STARTED ON SOLID FOOD

Does your baby feed more often than other babies?

ABOUT THE SAME

MORE OFTEN

Was your baby previously eager to feed?

PREVIOUSLY EAGER

NOT PREVIOUSLY EAGER

Is your baby gaining weight normally (see GROWTH CHARTS, pp.17–21)?

GAINING WEIGHT NORMALLY

NOT GAINING WEIGHT NORMALLY

POSSIBLE CAUSE

Frequent feeding, as often as once every 2 hours, is normal in breast-fed babies, particularly in the first few weeks of life (see INFANT FEEDING, p.27).

ACTION NEEDED

SELF-HELP
Even though your baby is probably healthy, you may be tired yourself. Have a break from nighttime feedings by expressing breast milk for your partner to feed to your baby. If you are depressed or irritable, consult your doctor.

POSSIBLE CAUSES

Suddenly refusing to feed may be a sign of a COMMON COLD (p.148), but it could be caused by a more serious illness.

ACTION NEEDED

MEDICAL HELP
✚ URGENT! Phone your doctor immediately!

POSSIBLE CAUSE

Some babies need to be coaxed to feed and may even fall asleep while feeding. If your baby seems well, there is no cause for concern.

ACTION NEEDED

MEDICAL HELP
If other symptoms develop, make an appointment to see your doctor.

POSSIBLE CAUSE

FAILURE TO THRIVE (p.33).

ACTION NEEDED

MEDICAL HELP
Make an appointment to see your doctor.

Are you worried that you are not producing sufficient milk for your baby?

- WORRIED
- NOT WORRIED

Is your baby gaining weight normally (see GROWTH CHARTS, pp.17–21)?

- NOT GAINING WEIGHT NORMALLY
- GAINING WEIGHT NORMALLY

POSSIBLE CAUSE

FAILURE TO THRIVE (p.33).

ACTION NEEDED

MEDICAL HELP
Make an appointment to see your doctor.

POSSIBLE CAUSE

Mothers quite commonly feel that they are not producing sufficient milk if their baby cries a lot and seems difficult to satisfy. However, if your baby is gaining weight at the normal rate, there is no doubt that he or she is receiving enough milk.

ACTION NEEDED

MEDICAL HELP
If your baby continues to cry and you are concerned, consult your doctor.
See also chart 6, EXCESSIVE CRYING.

Does your baby often cry during or after a feeding?

- CRIES AT THE START OF A FEEDING
- CRIES AFTER A FEEDING
- DOES NOT CRY

Go to chart
6 EXCESSIVE CRYING

POSSIBLE CAUSE

The breasts may not release milk immediately, or the flow may be too forceful.

ACTION NEEDED

SELF-HELP
If milk is not released at once, try to be more relaxed when you feed your baby. If the flow is too forceful, express some milk before your baby starts to feed.

POSSIBLE CAUSE

Children have strong likes and dislikes in food from a very young age. Unfamiliar foods and textures may be rejected, and even foods that were accepted initially may later be refused.

ACTION NEEDED

SELF-HELP
During your baby's first year, food and eating are new experiences. If he or she rejects foods, appears not to be interested, or likes only sweet foods, continue to offer a varied diet so that your baby has the best chance of receiving sufficient healthy nutrients (see ADDING SOLID FOOD, p.28).

Does your baby often cry after being fed?

- DOES NOT CRY
- CRIES

Go to chart
6 EXCESSIVE CRYING

If you cannot identify your baby's problem from this chart, talk to your doctor within 48 hours.

Does your baby often reject certain foods that you offer?

- REJECTS CERTAIN FOODS
- EATS MOST FOODS READILY

If you cannot identify your baby's problem from this chart, talk to your doctor within 48 hours.

5 SLOW WEIGHT GAIN

For growth problems in children over 1 year, see chart 12

A close check can be kept on your baby's weight gain by regular attendance at a baby clinic and by using the charts on pp.17–21. If you are concerned about your baby's failure to put on weight as expected and there is no obvious reason for it, you should consult this symptom chart.

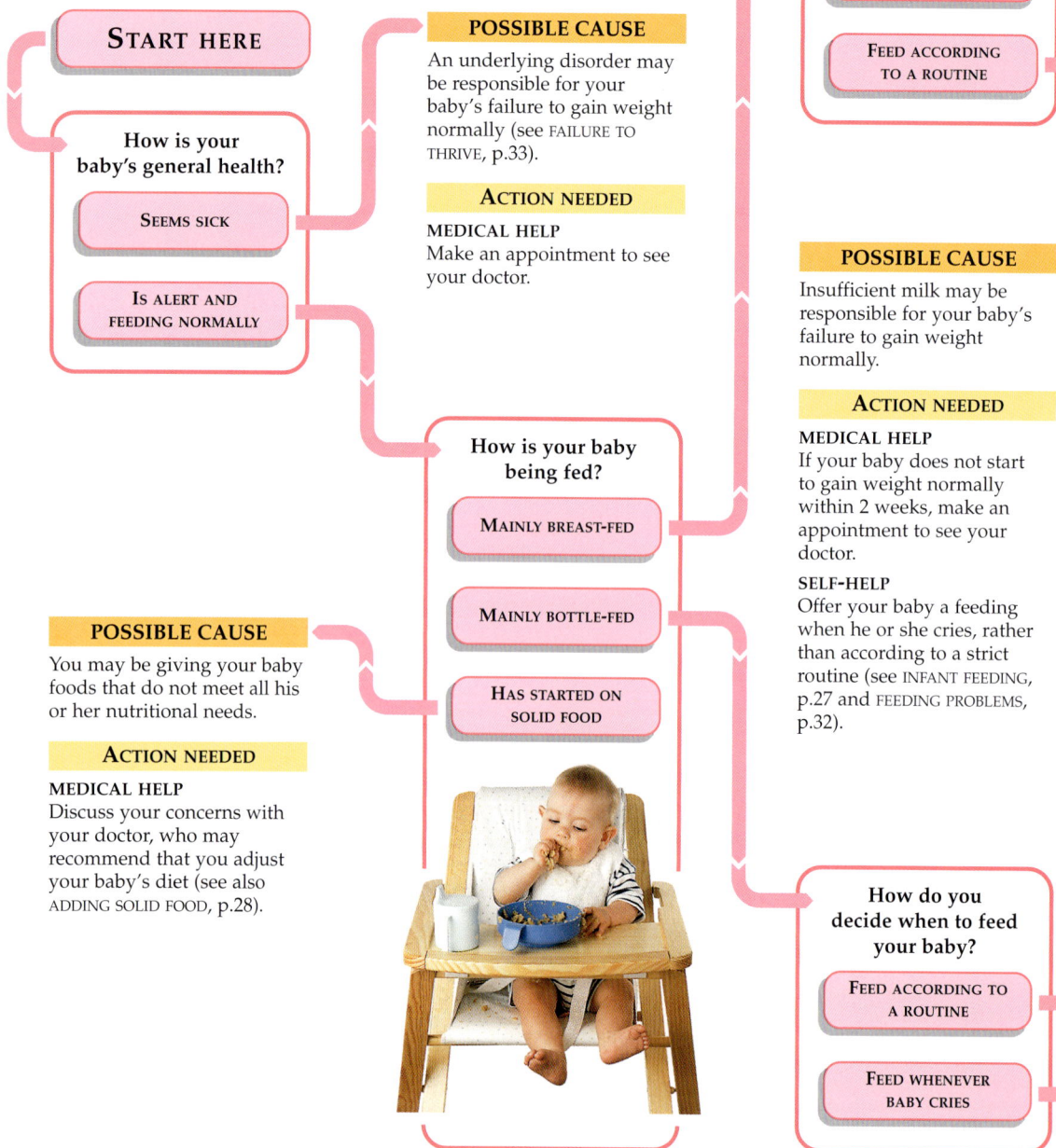

START HERE

How is your baby's general health?

- SEEMS SICK
- IS ALERT AND FEEDING NORMALLY

POSSIBLE CAUSE

An underlying disorder may be responsible for your baby's failure to gain weight normally (see FAILURE TO THRIVE, p.33).

ACTION NEEDED

MEDICAL HELP
Make an appointment to see your doctor.

How is your baby being fed?

- MAINLY BREAST-FED
- MAINLY BOTTLE-FED
- HAS STARTED ON SOLID FOOD

POSSIBLE CAUSE

You may be giving your baby foods that do not meet all his or her nutritional needs.

ACTION NEEDED

MEDICAL HELP
Discuss your concerns with your doctor, who may recommend that you adjust your baby's diet (see also ADDING SOLID FOOD, p.28).

How do you decide when to feed your baby?

- FEED WHENEVER BABY CRIES
- FEED ACCORDING TO A ROUTINE

POSSIBLE CAUSE

Insufficient milk may be responsible for your baby's failure to gain weight normally.

ACTION NEEDED

MEDICAL HELP
If your baby does not start to gain weight normally within 2 weeks, make an appointment to see your doctor.

SELF-HELP
Offer your baby a feeding when he or she cries, rather than according to a strict routine (see INFANT FEEDING, p.27 and FEEDING PROBLEMS, p.32).

How do you decide when to feed your baby?

- FEED ACCORDING TO A ROUTINE
- FEED WHENEVER BABY CRIES

POSSIBLE CAUSE

You may not be producing enough milk to provide your baby with all the nutrients he or she needs. If your baby is over 4 months old, he or she may be ready to start on solid food.

ACTION NEEDED

MEDICAL HELP
Talk to your doctor, who may recommend that you offer supplementary bottles to your baby or start him or her on solid food (see ADDING SOLID FOOD, p.28).

Does your baby always finish the entire contents of the bottle?

ALWAYS DRINKS EVERY DROP

SOMETIMES LEAVES SOME OF THE FEEDING

POSSIBLE CAUSE

Your baby may need more food than the amount you have been offering.

ACTION NEEDED

MEDICAL HELP
If your baby does not start to gain weight normally within 2 weeks, make an appointment to see your doctor.

SELF-HELP
Let your baby have as much milk as he or she wants. If your baby is over 4 months old, it may be time to start him or her on solid food (see ADDING SOLID FOOD, p.28).

POSSIBLE CAUSE

If feedings are too diluted, your baby may not be receiving enough nutrients.

ACTION NEEDED

MEDICAL HELP
If your baby does not start to gain weight normally within 2 weeks, make an appointment to see your doctor.

SELF-HELP
Always follow instructions for making up feedings. You can offer additional cool water if the weather is warm or if your baby has a fever.

Could you possibly be making up your baby's formula in the wrong proportions?

UNLIKELY

COULD BE ADDING TOO MUCH WATER

COULD BE ADDING TOO LITTLE MILK FORMULA

If you cannot identify your baby's problem from this chart, talk to your doctor within 48 hours.

ASSESSMENT: GROWTH PATTERNS IN INFANCY

Most babies follow the standard growth curves, but there may be variations that give the impression that a baby's growth is abnormal:
• If a parent is shorter than average, the baby may also be small.
• Breast-fed babies have a dramatic weight gain in their first few months, which then tapers off.
• The baby of a diabetic mother is heavy at birth but then fails to gain weight for a few months.
• Premature babies appear light for their age.

A small baby
These hypothetical growth charts show a growth pattern for a baby whose parents are small. The starting points on both the head size and weight charts are near the bottom of the normal range. This trend continues as the baby grows, indicating that the baby's growth, as recorded by head circumference, is in proportion to his or her weight gain.

6 EXCESSIVE CRYING

All babies cry because it is the only way in which they can communicate. Crying usually indicates hunger, thirst, tiredness, or discomfort. However, if your baby's crying is inconsolable, more persistent than usual, or sounds different than normal, he or she may require medical attention.

START HERE

Is your baby crying in a way that is unusual for him or her?

UNUSUAL

NO DIFFERENT

Was your baby reluctant to take the last feeding?

RELUCTANT

WILLING

POSSIBLE CAUSE

Your baby may be in pain as a result of a disorder, such as OTITIS MEDIA (p.162).

ACTION NEEDED

MEDICAL HELP
✚ URGENT! Phone your doctor immediately!

POSSIBLE CAUSES

COLIC (p.32), TEETHING (p.33), or, rarely, DIAPER RASH (p.136).

ACTION NEEDED

MEDICAL HELP
If your baby develops further symptoms or is still distressed after 24 hours, make an appointment to see your doctor.

Does feeding your baby stop the crying?

BABY STOPS CRYING

BABY CONTINUES CRYING

POSSIBLE CAUSE

Hunger is one of the most common causes of crying in a young baby.

ACTION NEEDED

SELF-HELP
If your baby stops crying after a feeding, you may need to reduce the intervals between feedings to keep up with the demand.

When you burp your baby, does he or she stop crying?

CONTINUES CRYING

STOPS CRYING

Is your baby comforted by a drink of cool water?

BABY NOT COMFORTED

BABY COMFORTED

POSSIBLE CAUSE

Thirst may be causing your baby to cry, especially if he or she is bottle-fed or if the weather is particularly hot.

ACTION NEEDED

SELF-HELP
Give your baby extra drinks of cool water from a bottle or spoon.

How old is your baby?

- UNDER 3 MONTHS
- 3 MONTHS OR OVER

When does the crying occur?

- LATE AFTERNOON OR EARLY EVENING
- AT OTHER TIMES

POSSIBLE CAUSE

Evening COLIC (p.32).

ACTION NEEDED

SELF-HELP
Feed your baby first. You can then try to calm him or her by rocking, by patting his or her back, or by massaging his or her abdomen.

If you pick up your baby and give your full attention, does this have any effect on the crying?

- STOPS THE CRYING
- NO EFFECT

Has there been a change in household routine or increased tension at home ?

- CHANGE IN HOUSEHOLD ROUTINE
- TENSION AT HOME
- NEITHER

POSSIBLE CAUSE

Your baby may be unsettled because of the change in routine or increased tension.

ACTION NEEDED

SELF-HELP
During a period of domestic upheaval, give your baby extra attention. If your own tension could be upsetting your baby, try to eliminate the cause. Having more time to yourself, using relaxation techniques, or talking over problems with friends or relatives may be helpful. If you are feeling angry or resentful at your baby's crying, consult your doctor.

If you cannot identify your baby's problem from this chart, talk to your doctor within 48 hours.

POSSIBLE CAUSE

Your baby may need more comforting and parental reassurance than other babies of the same age.

ACTION NEEDED

SELF-HELP
Cuddle your baby as often as he or she wants; there is no risk of "spoiling" your child at such a young age.

POSSIBLE CAUSE

GAS (p.32).

ACTION NEEDED

SELF-HELP
See panel: *Dealing with gas* (right).

SELF-HELP: DEALING WITH GAS

A baby who cries just before a feeding or who feeds greedily is likely to swallow air, which gets trapped in the baby's intestine and causes discomfort. The following tips may stop gas from occurring or may help to release the gas:
- Make sure the nipple's hole is the right size and is not blocked.
- Feed your baby in a semiupright position so that the milk falls to the bottom of the stomach.
- Try burping your baby after each feeding. Help release trapped air by holding him or her against your shoulder, or seated or lying face down on your lap. Rub or pat the back to calm your baby.

Burping position
After every feeding, put your baby into a position such as that shown above, in which burping is made easy.

7 SKIN PROBLEMS IN INFANTS

For other spots and rashes, see chart 23

Young babies have very sensitive skin that can be irritated easily. Rashes confined to the diaper area are particularly common and can be distressing for your baby. If the skin inflammation or irritation is persistent or accompanied by other symptoms, your baby should be seen by a doctor.

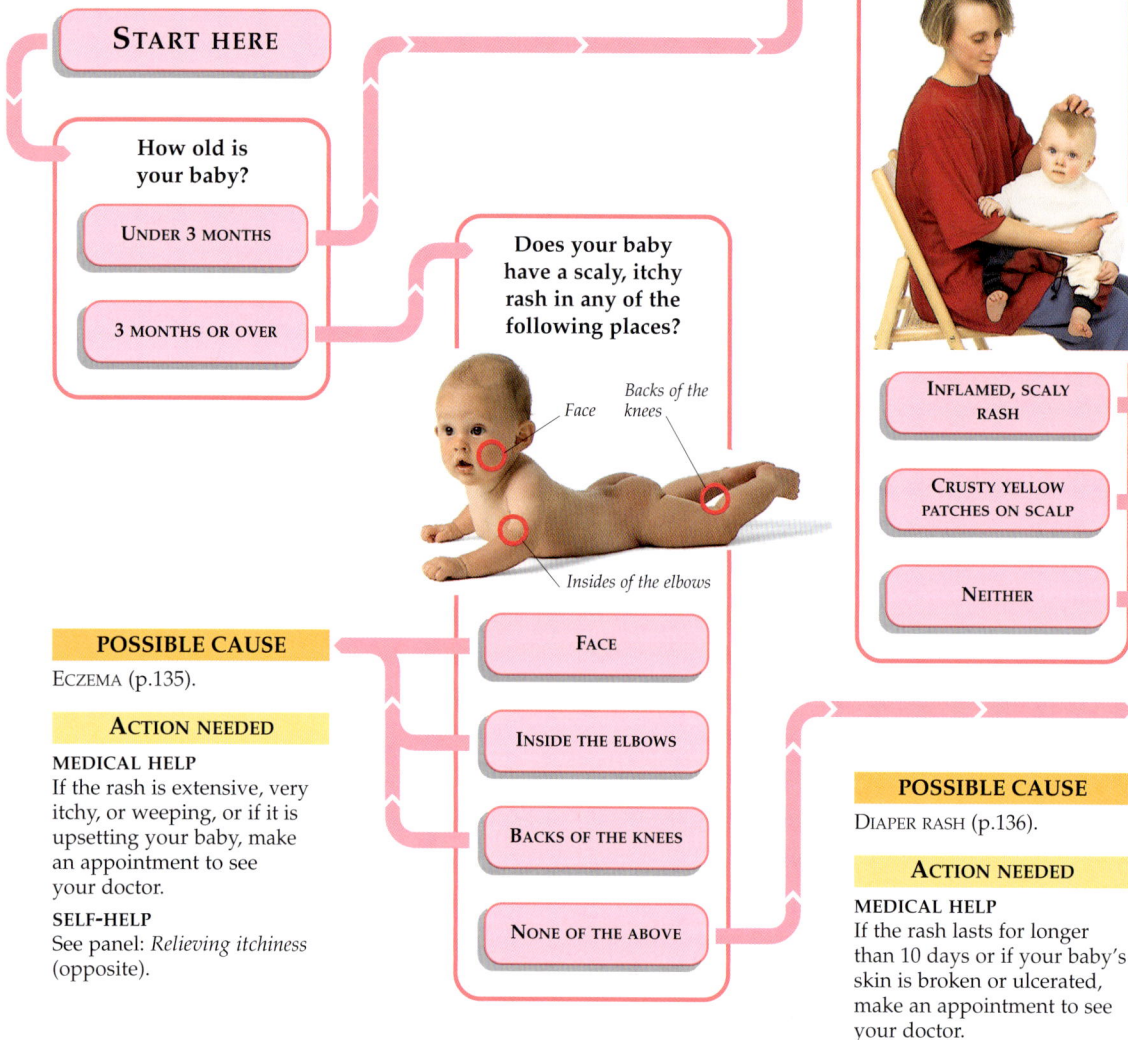

START HERE

How old is your baby?

- UNDER 3 MONTHS
- 3 MONTHS OR OVER

Does your baby have a scaly, itchy rash in any of the following places?

Face
Backs of the knees
Insides of the elbows

- FACE
- INSIDE THE ELBOWS
- BACKS OF THE KNEES
- NONE OF THE ABOVE

POSSIBLE CAUSE

ECZEMA (p.135).

ACTION NEEDED

MEDICAL HELP
If the rash is extensive, very itchy, or weeping, or if it is upsetting your baby, make an appointment to see your doctor.

SELF-HELP
See panel: *Relieving itchiness* (opposite).

Does your baby have either of the following skin problems?

- INFLAMED, SCALY RASH
- CRUSTY YELLOW PATCHES ON SCALP
- NEITHER

POSSIBLE CAUSE

DIAPER RASH (p.136).

ACTION NEEDED

MEDICAL HELP
If the rash lasts for longer than 10 days or if your baby's skin is broken or ulcerated, make an appointment to see your doctor.

If you cannot identify your baby's problem from this chart, talk to your doctor within 48 hours.

Is the rash in any of the following places?

NECK

BEHIND THE EARS

FACE

GROIN

ARMPITS

TWO OR MORE

ONE OR NONE

How is your baby's general health?

BABY IS HEALTHY AND FEEDING NORMALLY

BABY SEEMS SICK WITH A FEVER

BABY SEEMS SICK WITHOUT A FEVER

POSSIBLE CAUSE

SEBORRHEIC DERMATITIS (p.134).

ACTION NEEDED

MEDICAL HELP
If the rash does not clear up within a few weeks or if it is extensive or weeping, make an appointment to see your doctor.

POSSIBLE CAUSE

A minor skin irritation.

ACTION NEEDED

MEDICAL HELP
If the rash lasts for more than a day or if your baby becomes generally sick, make an appointment to see your doctor.

SELF-HELP
See panel: *Relieving itchiness* (below).

Go to chart
22 RASH WITH FEVER

Go to chart
23 SPOTS AND RASHES

POSSIBLE CAUSE

Cradle cap (see SEBORRHEIC DERMATITIS, p.134).

ACTION NEEDED

MEDICAL HELP
If the crusts are extensive or if your baby develops any other symptoms, make an appointment to see your doctor.

Does your baby have either of the following symptoms?

INFLAMED SPOTS ON THE GENITALS OR ANUS

SPOTS OR BLOTCHES ANYWHERE ON THE BODY

NEITHER

SELF-HELP: RELIEVING ITCHINESS

Try to discourage your child from scratching since this may lead to infection. The following tips may help:
• Bath your child briefly every day, using a nonirritating substance, such as a water-based cream or a baby soap. Make sure that the water is not too hot.
• If your child's skin is very dry, itchiness may be more severe. Try to keep the skin moisturized by using petroleum jelly or a water-based cream several times a day.

Bathing a baby
You can use a mild cleanser such as baby soap or a water-based cream, or add a specially formulated oil to the bath.

8 FEVER IN CHILDREN

For children under 1 year, see chart 1

Fever – a temperature above 38°C – is usually an indication of viral or bacterial infection; however, fever can also be caused by overheating. If your child seems sick, take his or her temperature and note any other symptoms that might help the doctor to make a diagnosis.

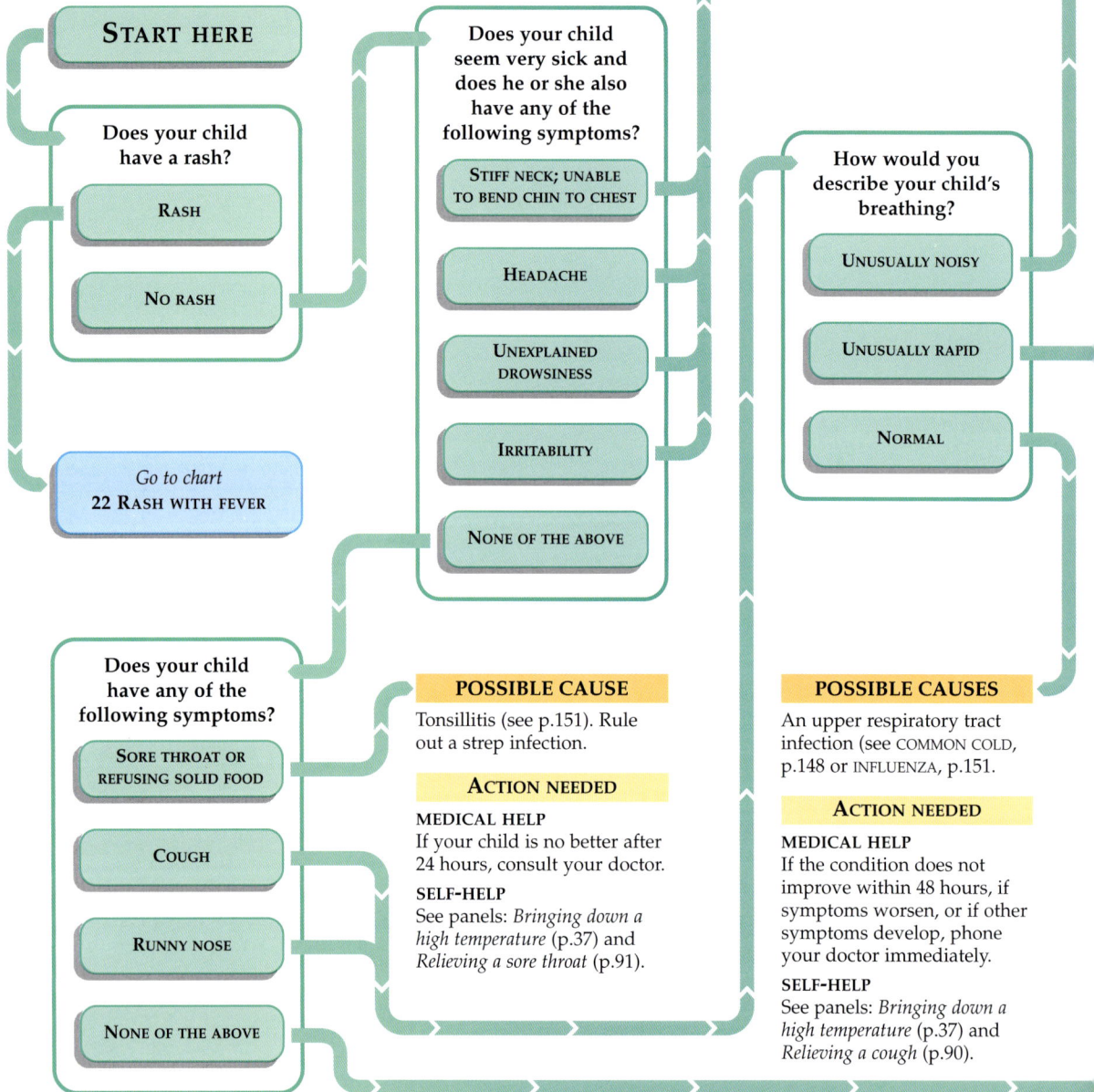

START HERE

Does your child have a rash?

RASH

NO RASH

Go to chart
22 RASH WITH FEVER

Does your child seem very sick and does he or she also have any of the following symptoms?

STIFF NECK; UNABLE TO BEND CHIN TO CHEST

HEADACHE

UNEXPLAINED DROWSINESS

IRRITABILITY

NONE OF THE ABOVE

POSSIBLE CAUSE

MENINGITIS (p.158).

ACTION NEEDED

MEDICAL HELP
✚ **EMERGENCY!** Call an ambulance!

How would you describe your child's breathing?

UNUSUALLY NOISY

UNUSUALLY RAPID

NORMAL

Does your child have any of the following symptoms?

SORE THROAT OR REFUSING SOLID FOOD

COUGH

RUNNY NOSE

NONE OF THE ABOVE

POSSIBLE CAUSE

Tonsillitis (see p.151). Rule out a strep infection.

ACTION NEEDED

MEDICAL HELP
If your child is no better after 24 hours, consult your doctor.

SELF-HELP
See panels: *Bringing down a high temperature* (p.37) and *Relieving a sore throat* (p.91).

POSSIBLE CAUSES

An upper respiratory tract infection (see COMMON COLD, p.148 or INFLUENZA, p.151.

ACTION NEEDED

MEDICAL HELP
If the condition does not improve within 48 hours, if symptoms worsen, or if other symptoms develop, phone your doctor immediately.

SELF-HELP
See panels: *Bringing down a high temperature* (p.37) and *Relieving a cough* (p.90).

POSSIBLE CAUSES

CROUP (p.150), ASTHMA (p.153), or BRONCHIOLITIS (p.155).

ACTION NEEDED

MEDICAL HELP
✚ URGENT! Phone your doctor immediately!

SELF-HELP
See panel: *Easing breathing in an asthma attack* (p.87).

POSSIBLE CAUSE

PNEUMONIA (p.155).

ACTION NEEDED

MEDICAL HELP
✚ URGENT! Phone your doctor immediately!

SELF-HELP
See panels: *Bringing down a high temperature* (p.37) and *Relieving a cough* (p.90).

POSSIBLE CAUSE

MUMPS (p.122) or parotitis.

ACTION NEEDED

MEDICAL HELP
Make an appointment to see your doctor.

SELF-HELP
See panel: *Bringing down a high temperature* (p.37).

Does your child have a swelling between the ear and the angle of the jaw on one or both sides?

- SWELLING
- NO SWELLING

Does your child have any of the following symptoms?

- URINATES MORE FREQUENTLY THAN USUAL
- PAIN OR BURNING SENSATION WHEN URINATING
- VOMITING WITH OR WITHOUT DIARRHEA
- NONE OF THE ABOVE

Does your child have any of the following problems?

- EARACHE OR EAR TUGGING
- WAKES UP SCREAMING DURING THE NIGHT
- NONE OF THE ABOVE

Has your child been outside in the sun or in a hot room for several hours?

- OUT IN THE SUN
- IN A HOT ROOM
- NEITHER

POSSIBLE CAUSE

URINARY TRACT INFECTION (p.193).

ACTION NEEDED

MEDICAL HELP
Get medical advice within 24 hours.

SELF-HELP
See panel: *Bringing down a high temperature* (p.37).

POSSIBLE CAUSE

GASTROENTERITIS (p.180).

ACTION NEEDED

MEDICAL HELP
Get medical advice within 24 hours.

SELF-HELP
See panel: *Preventing dehydration in children* (p.53).

POSSIBLE CAUSE

OTITIS MEDIA (p.162).

ACTION NEEDED

MEDICAL HELP
Get medical advice within 24 hours.

SELF-HELP
See panels: *Bringing down a high temperature* (p.37) and *Relieving earache* (p.101).

POSSIBLE CAUSE

Your child may have become overheated.

ACTION NEEDED

MEDICAL HELP
If the self-help measures do not succeed in lowering your child's temperature within 1 hour, phone your doctor immediately.

SELF-HELP
See panel: *Bringing down a high temperature* (p.37).

If you cannot identify your child's problem from this chart, phone your doctor at once.

9 DIARRHEA IN CHILDREN

For children under 1 year, see chart 2

Frequent, loose stool is usually caused by infection and does not normally continue for more than a few days. If your child drinks plenty of clear fluids while the diarrhea lasts, there should be no ill effects. If the diarrhea recurs or lasts for over a week, your child should see a doctor.

DANGER SIGNS
Phone your doctor at once if your child has any of the following symptoms:
- Abdominal pain for 3 hours.
- Vomiting for 12 hours.
- Refusing to drink for 6 hours.
- Sunken eyes.
- Abnormal drowsiness.
- Not urinating for more than 6 hours during the day.

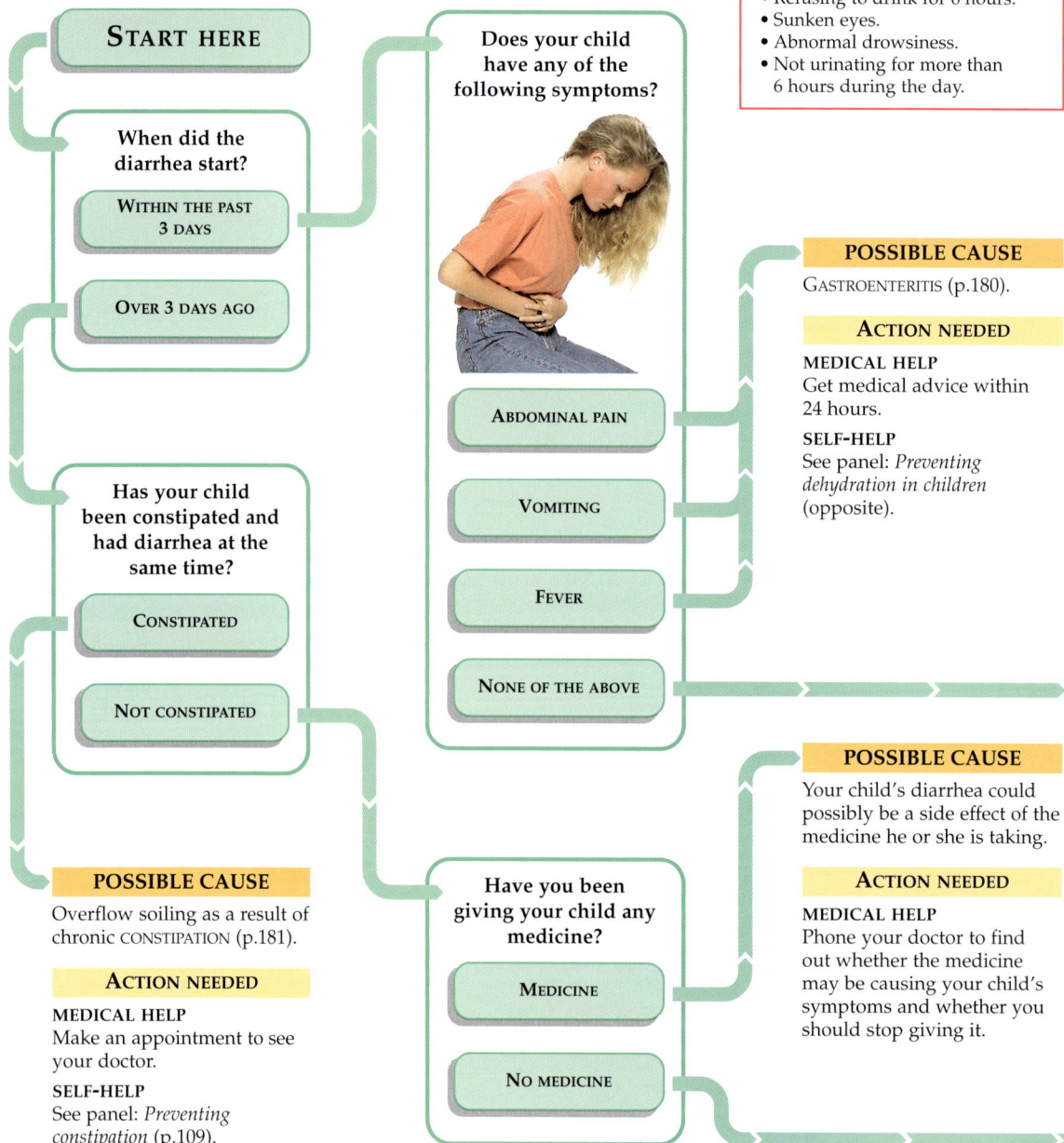

START HERE

When did the diarrhea start?

WITHIN THE PAST 3 DAYS

OVER 3 DAYS AGO

Does your child have any of the following symptoms?

ABDOMINAL PAIN

VOMITING

FEVER

NONE OF THE ABOVE

Has your child been constipated and had diarrhea at the same time?

CONSTIPATED

NOT CONSTIPATED

POSSIBLE CAUSE
GASTROENTERITIS (p.180).

ACTION NEEDED
MEDICAL HELP
Get medical advice within 24 hours.

SELF-HELP
See panel: *Preventing dehydration in children* (opposite).

POSSIBLE CAUSE
Your child's diarrhea could possibly be a side effect of the medicine he or she is taking.

ACTION NEEDED
MEDICAL HELP
Phone your doctor to find out whether the medicine may be causing your child's symptoms and whether you should stop giving it.

POSSIBLE CAUSE
Overflow soiling as a result of chronic CONSTIPATION (p.181).

ACTION NEEDED
MEDICAL HELP
Make an appointment to see your doctor.

SELF-HELP
See panel: *Preventing constipation* (p.109).

Have you been giving your child any medicine?

MEDICINE

NO MEDICINE

Did the diarrhea start just before an exciting or stressful event or period of time?

- EXCITING EVENT OR PERIOD OF TIME
- STRESSFUL EVENT OR PERIOD OF TIME
- NEITHER

POSSIBLE CAUSE

Children may suffer from diarrhea in response to excitement or emotional stress. The diarrhea is likely to clear up quickly.

ACTION NEEDED

MEDICAL HELP
If the diarrhea continues or is distressing to your child, consult your doctor.

POSSIBLE CAUSE

GASTROENTERITIS (p.180).

ACTION NEEDED

MEDICAL HELP
Get medical advice within 24 hours.

SELF-HELP
See panel: *Preventing dehydration in children* (below).

POSSIBLE CAUSE

TODDLER'S DIARRHEA (p.181).

ACTION NEEDED

MEDICAL HELP
Make an appointment to see your doctor.

How old is your child?

- UNDER 3 YEARS
- 3 YEARS OR OVER

What are the features of your child's stool?

- CONTAINS RECOGNIZABLE MORSELS OF FOOD
- WATERY

SELF-HELP: PREVENTING DEHYDRATION IN CHILDREN

If your child has persistent diarrhea, vomiting, or a fever, it is very important to give them extra fluids to replace ongoing losses and maintain fluid requirements. It is best to offer one of the commercially available oral electrolyte rehydrating solutions, such as Pedialyte or Rehydralyte, for which you do not need a prescription. If these preparations are unavailable, other clear fluids, such as water, may be substituted. Do not, however, attempt to make your own rehydrating solution or give highly concentrated fluids such as undiluted juices.

Rehydration is best achieved by offering 20 ml of the oral rehydrating solution per kg of body weight in the first hour and then 10 to 20 ml per kg of body weight for the next 6 hours until the diarrhea or vomiting slows. Early oral feeding is recommended, especially if vomiting has subsided.

Rehydrating solution
Encourage your child to stay hydrated by offering small amounts of clear fluids every few hours through day and night.

POSSIBLE CAUSES

In children, chronic (long-lasting) diarrhea is most likely to be caused by either REACTIONS TO FOOD (p.182) or GIARDIASIS (p.187). Some other possibilities include CELIAC DISEASE (p.183) and CYSTIC FIBROSIS (p.201) but these are rare. Crohn's disease (see INFLAMMATORY BOWEL DISEASE, p.184) is a less likely cause because it is very rare for this disease to affect children under the age of about 7 years.

ACTION NEEDED

MEDICAL HELP
Make an appointment to see your doctor.

SELF-HELP
See panel: *Preventing dehydration in children* (at left).

10 VOMITING IN CHILDREN

For children under 1 year, see chart 3

In children, an episode of vomiting without other symptoms is unlikely to indicate a serious disorder; it may be a result of overeating or excitement. Repeated vomiting is often caused by infection of the digestive tract, but infection anywhere else in the body can also be responsible.

DANGER SIGNS

Call an ambulance at once if your child has any of the following symptoms:
- Greenish yellow vomit.
- Abdominal pain for 6 hours.
- Flat pink or purple spots that do not disappear when pressed.

Phone your doctor at once if your child has any of the following symptoms:
- Vomiting for 12 hours.
- Abnormal drowsiness.
- Refusing to drink for 6 hours.
- Sunken eyes.
- Dry tongue.
- Not urinating for more than 6 hours during the day.

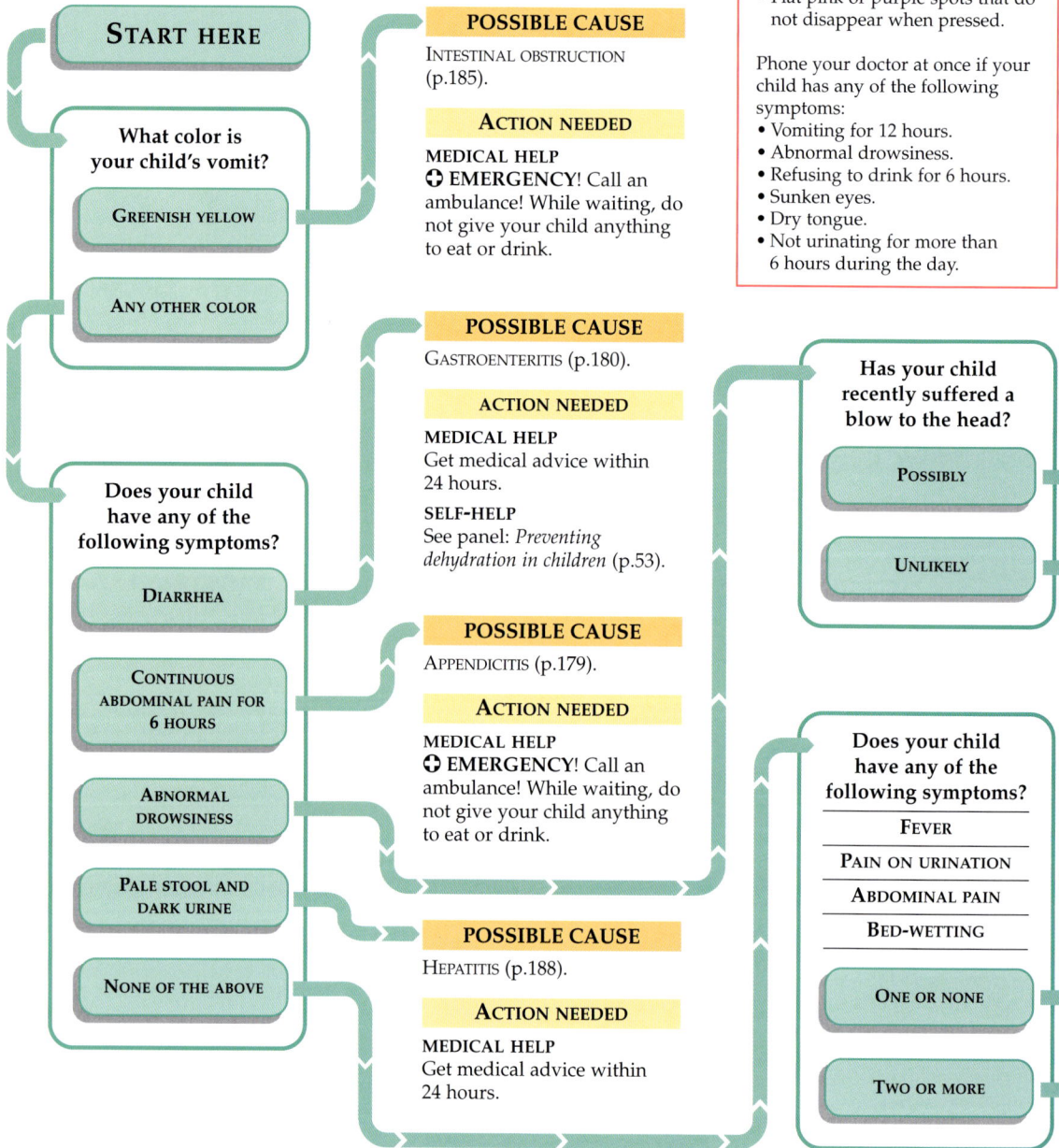

START HERE

What color is your child's vomit?
- GREENISH YELLOW
- ANY OTHER COLOR

Does your child have any of the following symptoms?
- DIARRHEA
- CONTINUOUS ABDOMINAL PAIN FOR 6 HOURS
- ABNORMAL DROWSINESS
- PALE STOOL AND DARK URINE
- NONE OF THE ABOVE

POSSIBLE CAUSE

INTESTINAL OBSTRUCTION (p.185).

ACTION NEEDED

MEDICAL HELP
✚ EMERGENCY! Call an ambulance! While waiting, do not give your child anything to eat or drink.

POSSIBLE CAUSE

GASTROENTERITIS (p.180).

ACTION NEEDED

MEDICAL HELP
Get medical advice within 24 hours.

SELF-HELP
See panel: *Preventing dehydration in children* (p.53).

POSSIBLE CAUSE

APPENDICITIS (p.179).

ACTION NEEDED

MEDICAL HELP
✚ EMERGENCY! Call an ambulance! While waiting, do not give your child anything to eat or drink.

POSSIBLE CAUSE

HEPATITIS (p.188).

ACTION NEEDED

MEDICAL HELP
Get medical advice within 24 hours.

Has your child recently suffered a blow to the head?
- POSSIBLY
- UNLIKELY

Does your child have any of the following symptoms?
- FEVER
- PAIN ON URINATION
- ABDOMINAL PAIN
- BED-WETTING
- ONE OR NONE
- TWO OR MORE

POSSIBLE CAUSE

HEAD INJURY (p.159).

ACTION NEEDED

MEDICAL HELP
✚ **EMERGENCY!** Call an ambulance! While waiting, do not give your child anything to eat or drink.

SELF-HELP: DEALING WITH VOMITING

When your child vomits, the following suggestions may help:
• Support your child's head during vomiting. When the vomiting has stopped, sponge your child's face and give sips of water to rinse out his or her mouth.
• Reassure your child, who might be upset or frightened.
• Offer your child small drinks of water or rehydrating solution every hour to replace fluids lost by vomiting (see panel: *Preventing dehydration in children*, p.53).
• Encourage your child to lie down and rest. Put a bowl by the bed in case the vomiting starts again.

Preventing dehydration
Encourage your child to drink plenty of water or rehydrating solution to avoid the danger of dehydration.

Does your child have any of the following symptoms?

- HEADACHE
- STIFF NECK
- FLAT SPOTS THAT DO NOT DISAPPEAR WHEN PRESSED
- NONE OF THE ABOVE

POSSIBLE CAUSE

MENINGITIS (p.158).

ACTION NEEDED

MEDICAL HELP
✚ **EMERGENCY!** Call an ambulance!

POSSIBLE CAUSE

PERTUSSIS (p.123), rarely.

ACTION NEEDED

MEDICAL HELP
Get medical advice if child becomes dehydrated.

SELF-HELP
See panels: *Dealing with vomiting* (above) and *Relieving a cough* (p.90).

If you cannot identify your child's problem from this chart, talk to your doctor within 48 hours.

Did the vomiting occur in any of the following situations?

- FOLLOWING A BOUT OF COUGHING
- BEFORE OR AFTER AN EXCITING OR STRESSFUL EVENT
- DURING A JOURNEY
- NONE OF THE ABOVE

POSSIBLE CAUSE

Children often vomit in reaction to an exciting event or to stress.

ACTION NEEDED

MEDICAL HELP
If the vomiting persists, consult your doctor.

POSSIBLE CAUSE

URINARY TRACT INFECTION (p.193).

ACTION NEEDED

MEDICAL HELP
Get medical advice within 24 hours.

SELF-HELP
See panel: *Bringing down a high temperature* (p.37).

If you cannot identify your child's problem from this chart, talk to your doctor within 48 hours.

POSSIBLE CAUSE

Motion sickness.

ACTION NEEDED

SELF-HELP
In a car, try to avoid driving in stop-and-go traffic. Open car windows to improve ventilation. Giving a motion sickness remedy to a child of this age is not recommended.

11 POOR APPETITE

For children under 1 year, see chart 4

A child's appetite increases or decreases according to energy requirements and periods of growth. Provided that there are no other symptoms and growth is in the normal range for your child's age (see GROWTH CHARTS, pp.17–21), you need not be concerned about any temporary loss of appetite.

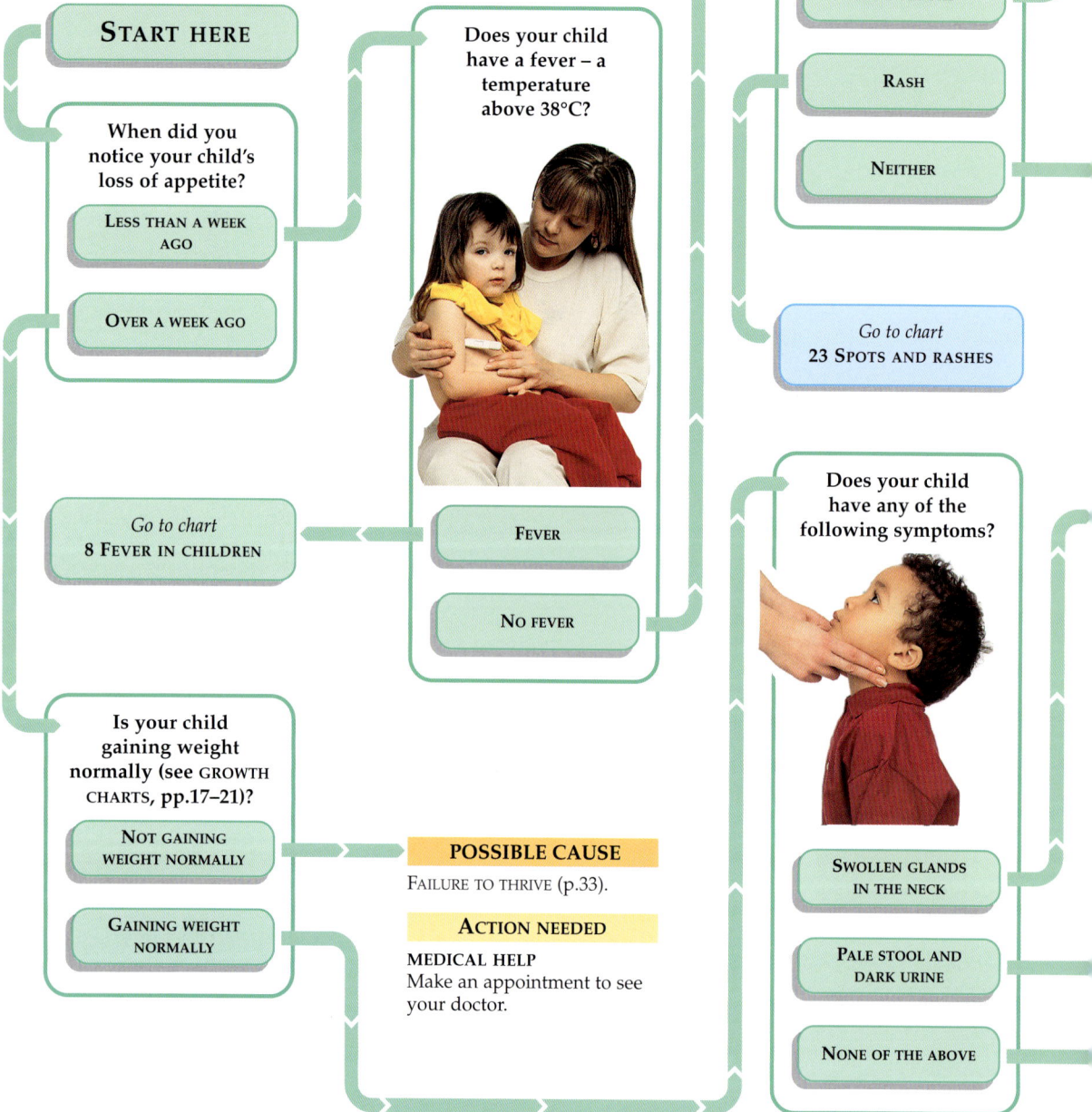

START HERE

When did you notice your child's loss of appetite?

LESS THAN A WEEK AGO

OVER A WEEK AGO

Go to chart
8 FEVER IN CHILDREN

Is your child gaining weight normally (see GROWTH CHARTS, pp.17–21)?

NOT GAINING WEIGHT NORMALLY

GAINING WEIGHT NORMALLY

Does your child have a fever – a temperature above 38°C?

FEVER

NO FEVER

POSSIBLE CAUSE

FAILURE TO THRIVE (p.33).

ACTION NEEDED

MEDICAL HELP
Make an appointment to see your doctor.

Is your child also suffering from either of the following symptoms?

SORE THROAT

RASH

NEITHER

Go to chart
23 SPOTS AND RASHES

Does your child have any of the following symptoms?

SWOLLEN GLANDS IN THE NECK

PALE STOOL AND DARK URINE

NONE OF THE ABOVE

Go to chart
28 SORE THROAT

POSSIBLE CAUSES

Your child may be eating between meals or exercising less than usual, resulting in reduced energy requirements. As long as your child seems healthy otherwise, there is no cause for concern.

ACTION NEEDED

MEDICAL HELP
If your child complains of feeling sick, get medical advice within 24 hours.

SELF-HELP
See HEALTHY EATING (p.29) and panel: *Stimulating your child's appetite* (at right).

POSSIBLE CAUSE

INFECTIOUS MONONUCLEOSIS (p.124).

ACTION NEEDED

MEDICAL HELP
Make an appointment to see your doctor.

POSSIBLE CAUSE

Viral HEPATITIS (p.188).

ACTION NEEDED

MEDICAL HELP
Make an appointment to see your doctor.

SELF-HELP: STIMULATING YOUR CHILD'S APPETITE

A child who is reluctant to eat or who has lost his or her appetite may need some encouragement.
- If the loss of appetite is caused by illness, do not force your child to eat. A sick child may only want liquids; ice cream and yogurt will soothe a painful throat and provide some nutrients.
- You can make eating fun for a young child by playing an eating game like "trains" or "planes."
- Do not expect your child to eat as much as you do at mealtimes; five or six smaller meals or snacks may be more suitable for a child's immature digestive system and active metabolism.
- You may be able to tempt a fussy eater by offering small portions of a wide range of foods.
- Try to ensure that your child eats the appropriate quantities of food from each of the food groups (see HEALTHY EATING, p.29).
- If fruits and vegetables are tough to encourage, consider a multivitamin supplement.

Tempting a fussy eater
Helpings of favorite foods, particularly if they are nutritious, can be offered to a fussy eater or a child who has lost his or her appetite, whatever the reason.

POSSIBLE CAUSE

URINARY TRACT INFECTION (p.193).

ACTION NEEDED

MEDICAL HELP
Get medical advice within 24 hours.

Does your child have either of the following symptoms?

- URINATING MORE FREQUENTLY
- BED-WETTING (AFTER BEING DRY AT NIGHT)
- NEITHER

POSSIBLE CAUSES

A number of factors could cause a temporary loss of appetite. For instance, your child may be having snacks between meals or exercising less than usual, which results in reduced energy requirements. However, if your child seems healthy, there is no cause for concern.

ACTION NEEDED

MEDICAL HELP
If your child complains of feeling sick, get medical advice within 24 hours.

SELF-HELP
See HEALTHY EATING (p.29) and panel: *Stimulating your child's appetite* (above). Make sure that your child's fluid intake is not filling his or her caloric needs. Encourage greater water intake in place of fruit juices and other drinks containing large amounts of carbohydrate.

12 GROWTH PROBLEMS

For slow weight gain in children under 1 year, see chart 5

Some children are naturally smaller or larger than their peers, and there is wide variation in what is considered normal for height, weight, and rate of growth at any age. In most children, growth occurs in irregular spurts; if you are concerned about your child, consult the charts on pp.17–21.

START HERE

In what way does your child's growth seem abnormal?

- INCREASE IN HEIGHT SEEMS SLOW
- WEIGHT GAIN IS SLOW COMPARED TO INCREASE IN HEIGHT

How is your child's health in general?

- SEEMS SICK OR IS NOT EATING NORMALLY
- SEEMS HEALTHY AND IS EATING NORMALLY

POSSIBLE CAUSES

Loss of appetite because of an underlying disorder such as an infection is the most likely explanation. Rarely, an inability to absorb nutrients as a result of CELIAC DISEASE (p.183), CYSTIC FIBROSIS (p.201), or Crohn's disease (see INFLAMMATORY BOWEL DISEASE, p.184) may be responsible.

ACTION NEEDED

MEDICAL HELP
Make an appointment to see your doctor.

Is your child's height normal for his or her age (see GROWTH CHARTS, pp.17–21)?

- NORMAL
- BELOW NORMAL

POSSIBLE CAUSE

Slow growth during any 6-month period is not abnormal if your child seems healthy and grows normally during the next 6 months.

ACTION NEEDED

MEDICAL HELP
If your child seems sick or grows less than 2.5 cm during the next 6 months, make an appointment to see your doctor.

SELF-HELP
See HEALTHY EATING (p.29) and panel: *Growth patterns in childhood* (opposite).

POSSIBLE CAUSES

Very short stature is usually inherited. A long illness, GROWTH HORMONE DEFICIENCY (p.189), or HYPOTHYROIDISM (p.189) are other possibilities.

ACTION NEEDED

MEDICAL HELP
Make an appointment to see your doctor.

How much has your child grown in height during the last 6 months?

- LESS THAN 2.5 CM
- 2.5 CM OR MORE

Has your child had a prolonged illness since he or she was last measured and weighed?

HAS HAD A PROLONGED ILLNESS

HAS BEEN GENERALLY HEALTHY

POSSIBLE CAUSE

A prolonged period of illness, particularly one in which your child is confined to bed for any length of time or has to undergo extensive hospital treatment, can interrupt normal growth.

ACTION NEEDED

MEDICAL HELP
If your child does not start to put on weight normally within the next 4 weeks, make an appointment to see your doctor.

SELF-HELP
See HEALTHY EATING (p.29) and panel: *Growth patterns in childhood* (below).

POSSIBLE CAUSE

There are certain times in all children's development when either their weight gain or their increase in height is slow. At other times they may have a growth spurt – for instance, during puberty. Such an irregular growth pattern is normal and should not be a cause for concern.

ACTION NEEDED

MEDICAL HELP
If your child does not start to put on weight normally within the next 4 weeks, make an appointment to see your doctor.

SELF-HELP
See HEALTHY EATING (p.29) and panel: *Growth patterns in childhood* (below).

POSSIBLE CAUSE

Many children have irregular growth patterns, but these rarely indicate an underlying problem. Your child may grow relatively slowly at certain times and more rapidly at others. Around puberty, both boys and girls have a growth spurt.

ACTION NEEDED

MEDICAL HELP
If your child seems sick or grows less than 2.5 cm during the next 6 months, make an appointment to see your doctor.

SELF-HELP
See HEALTHY EATING (p.29) and panel: *Growth patterns in childhood* (right).

ASSESSMENT: GROWTH PATTERNS IN CHILDHOOD

Although most children follow the standard growth curves (pp.17–21), there are a number of variations that may give the impression that a child is not growing normally:
- A naturally slim child may appear to gain weight slowly relative to his or her height.
- An overweight child may appear to increase relatively slowly in height compared to his or her weight gain.

- A child whose mother or father is shorter than average may grow slowly and be smaller than his or her classmates.
- An overweight toddler will grow faster in height than in weight as he or she grows older.
- An adolescent who is late reaching puberty may be shorter and lighter than his or her classmates. However, most late developers catch up eventually.

A slender child
These charts show a hypothetical growth pattern for a child who is naturally slim, but fit and healthy. The points plotted for height are near the top of the curve while weight is closer to average (shown by the 50th percentile line). As long as both height and weight increase in proportion, and weight gain is only slightly less than expected, you need not be concerned.

HEIGHT chart: Age (years) 0 1 2 3 4 5 6 7; in / cm axis: 48/120, 44/110, 40/100, 36/90, 32/80, 28/70, 24/60, 20/50

WEIGHT chart: Age (years) 0 1 2 3 4 5 6 7; lb / kg axis: 90/40, 80/35, 70/30, 60/25, 50/20, 40/15, 30/10, 20, 10/5

13 SPEECH PROBLEMS

When your child is learning to talk, it is normal for his or her speech to be hesitant and repetitive. If the stammering persists more than 4 months or if the learning of new words is slow, there may be a physical cause. Individual variation is normal, and boys are often slower than girls at learning verbal skills.

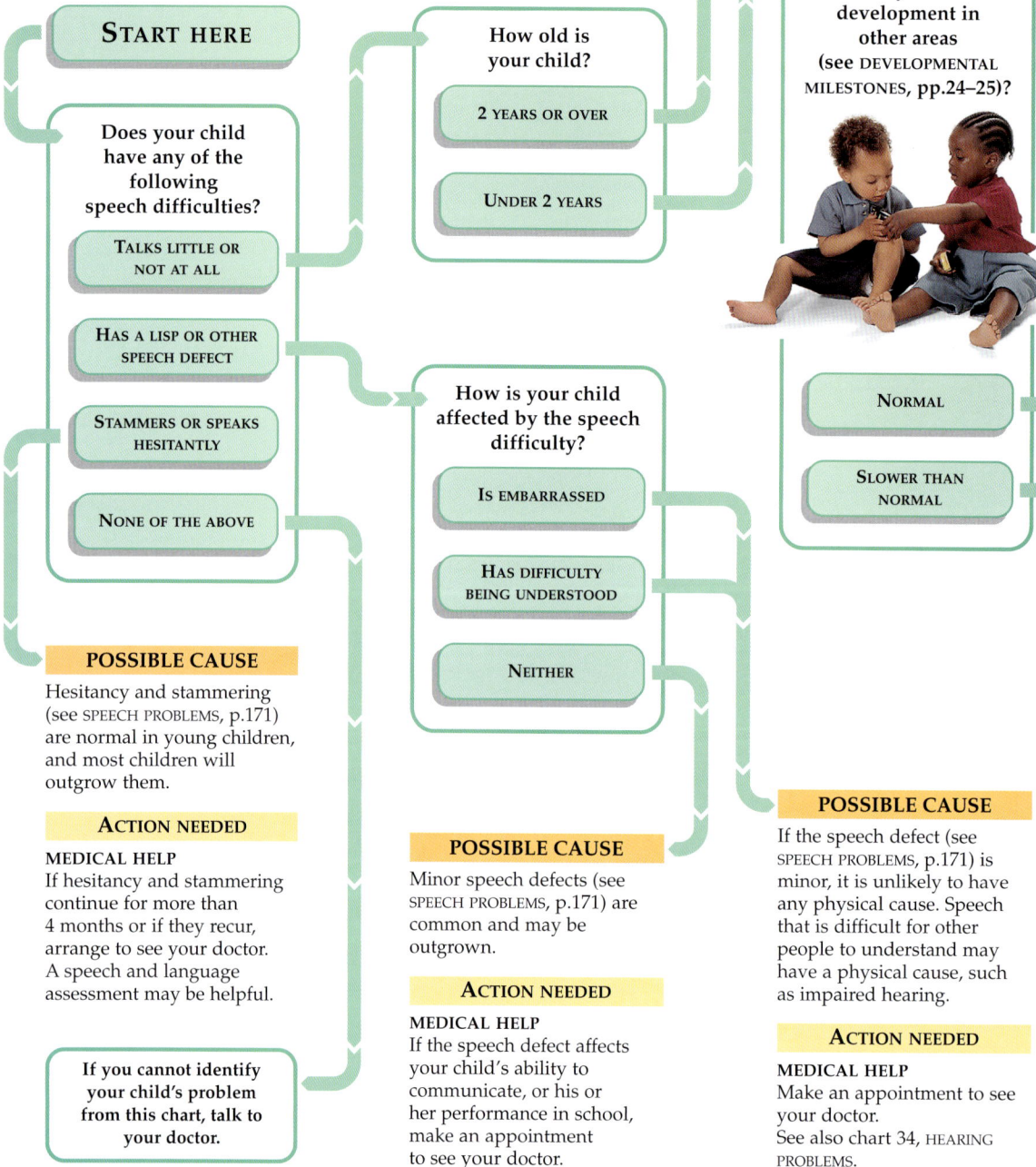

START HERE

Does your child have any of the following speech difficulties?

- TALKS LITTLE OR NOT AT ALL
- HAS A LISP OR OTHER SPEECH DEFECT
- STAMMERS OR SPEAKS HESITANTLY
- NONE OF THE ABOVE

How old is your child?

- 2 YEARS OR OVER
- UNDER 2 YEARS

How is your child affected by the speech difficulty?

- IS EMBARRASSED
- HAS DIFFICULTY BEING UNDERSTOOD
- NEITHER

How would you describe your child's development in other areas (see DEVELOPMENTAL MILESTONES, pp.24–25)?

- NORMAL
- SLOWER THAN NORMAL

POSSIBLE CAUSE

Hesitancy and stammering (see SPEECH PROBLEMS, p.171) are normal in young children, and most children will outgrow them.

ACTION NEEDED

MEDICAL HELP
If hesitancy and stammering continue for more than 4 months or if they recur, arrange to see your doctor. A speech and language assessment may be helpful.

If you cannot identify your child's problem from this chart, talk to your doctor.

POSSIBLE CAUSE

Minor speech defects (see SPEECH PROBLEMS, p.171) are common and may be outgrown.

ACTION NEEDED

MEDICAL HELP
If the speech defect affects your child's ability to communicate, or his or her performance in school, make an appointment to see your doctor.

POSSIBLE CAUSE

If the speech defect (see SPEECH PROBLEMS, p.171) is minor, it is unlikely to have any physical cause. Speech that is difficult for other people to understand may have a physical cause, such as impaired hearing.

ACTION NEEDED

MEDICAL HELP
Make an appointment to see your doctor.
See also chart 34, HEARING PROBLEMS.

How many words can your child say?

MORE THAN FIVE

FIVE OR FEWER

How do the words sound?

CLEAR AND DISTINCT

DIFFICULT TO UNDERSTAND

POSSIBLE CAUSE

Late speech development (see SPEECH PROBLEMS, p.171) is not likely to be a cause for concern if your child is developing normally in most other areas and has normal hearing.

ACTION NEEDED

MEDICAL HELP
Check your child's hearing by having an audiogram. If it is normal, take your child to see a speech therapist.

SELF-HELP
Encourage your child to talk by speaking to him or her often and by providing frequent opportunities to play with other children.

POSSIBLE CAUSE

A child who is reluctant to speak but is capable of pronouncing words clearly and using them meaningfully is unlikely to have a physical defect that affects either speaking or hearing (see SPEECH PROBLEMS, p.171). An emotional problem may be responsible for your child's reluctance to speak.

ACTION NEEDED

MEDICAL HELP
Make an appointment to see your doctor.

POSSIBLE CAUSES

A physical abnormality, slow mental development, or autism spectrum disorder may be the cause.

ACTION NEEDED

MEDICAL HELP
Make an appointment to see your doctor. Ask for an audiogram and speech therapy consultation.

SELF-HELP
Speak to your child often and and encourage him or her to respond to you. Providing frequent opportunities for your child to play with other children may be helpful.

POSSIBLE CAUSES

Delayed speech development (see SPEECH PROBLEMS, p.171) may be caused by a variety of factors, including lack of stimulation, emotional stress, impaired hearing, or slow mental development. It may also result from the normal variation in development.

ACTION NEEDED

MEDICAL HELP
Make an appointment to see your doctor.

SELF-HELP
Encourage your child to talk by speaking to him or her often and by providing frequent opportunities for your child to play with other children.

POSSIBLE CAUSE

Unclearly spoken words are often a result of a physical defect, such as impaired hearing. When a hearing-impaired child learns speech from parents, teachers, and siblings, the words are heard indistinctly and are then pronounced unclearly when repeated by the child.

ACTION NEEDED

MEDICAL HELP
Make an appointment to see your doctor.
See also chart 34, HEARING PROBLEMS.

SELF-HELP
Always try to speak clearly to your child and emphasize the pronunciation of any new words. Make sure your child can see your lips as you talk.

Some provinces offer a preschool speech and language program for children with delayed speech development. Other provinces offer an infant hearing program to rule out hearing defects at birth.

14 TOILET-TRAINING PROBLEMS

Most children achieve bladder and bowel control between the ages of 2 and 5 years, although older children may have the occasional "accident." Unless there is a physical problem, toilet-training occurs naturally and the process cannot be hastened by pressure from parents.

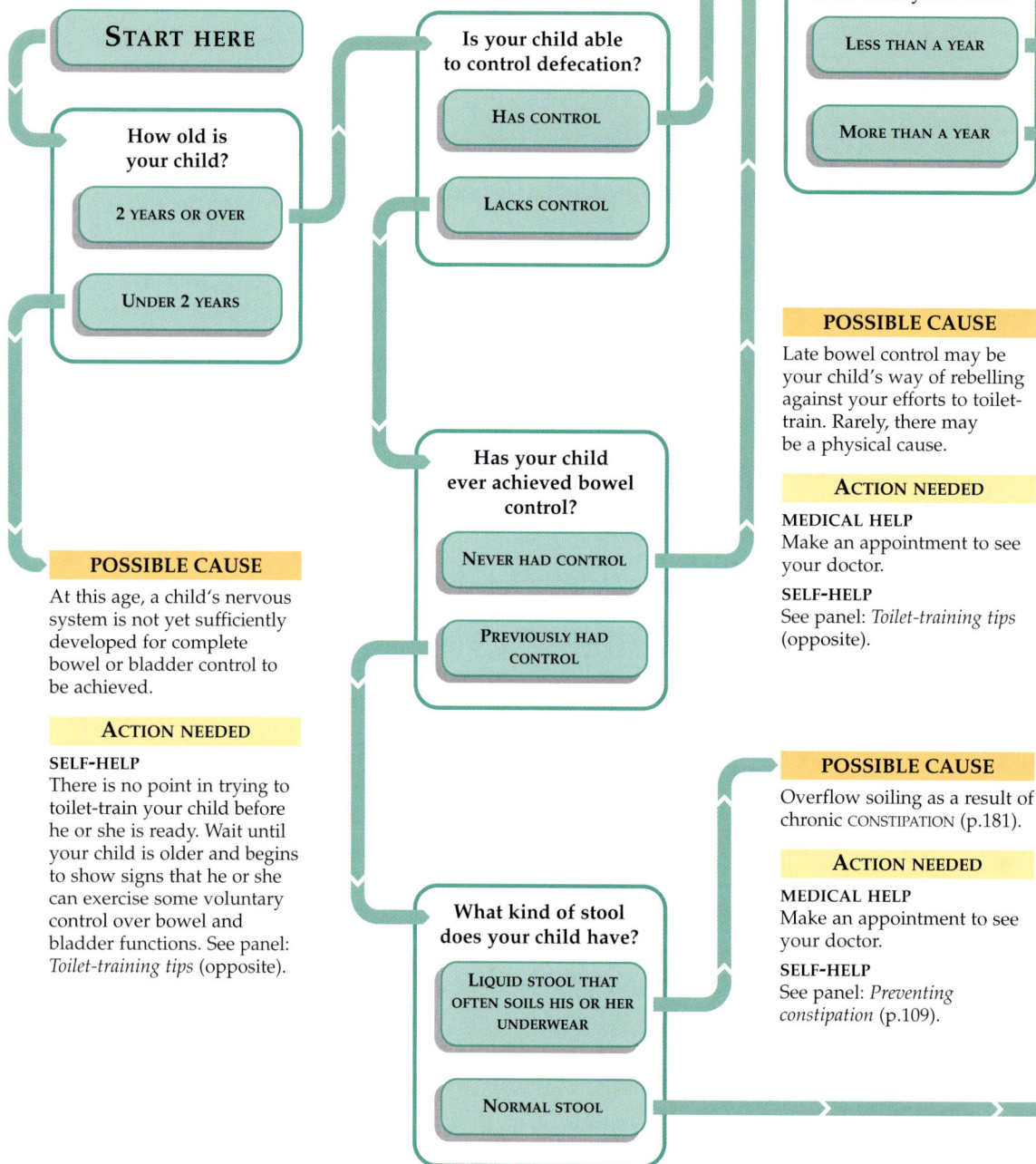

START HERE

How old is your child?

- 2 YEARS OR OVER
- UNDER 2 YEARS

Is your child able to control defecation?

- HAS CONTROL
- LACKS CONTROL

How long have you been trying to toilet-train your child?

- LESS THAN A YEAR
- MORE THAN A YEAR

Has your child ever achieved bowel control?

- NEVER HAD CONTROL
- PREVIOUSLY HAD CONTROL

What kind of stool does your child have?

- LIQUID STOOL THAT OFTEN SOILS HIS OR HER UNDERWEAR
- NORMAL STOOL

POSSIBLE CAUSE

At this age, a child's nervous system is not yet sufficiently developed for complete bowel or bladder control to be achieved.

ACTION NEEDED

SELF-HELP
There is no point in trying to toilet-train your child before he or she is ready. Wait until your child is older and begins to show signs that he or she can exercise some voluntary control over bowel and bladder functions. See panel: *Toilet-training tips* (opposite).

POSSIBLE CAUSE

Late bowel control may be your child's way of rebelling against your efforts to toilet-train. Rarely, there may be a physical cause.

ACTION NEEDED

MEDICAL HELP
Make an appointment to see your doctor.

SELF-HELP
See panel: *Toilet-training tips* (opposite).

POSSIBLE CAUSE

Overflow soiling as a result of chronic CONSTIPATION (p.181).

ACTION NEEDED

MEDICAL HELP
Make an appointment to see your doctor.

SELF-HELP
See panel: *Preventing constipation* (p.109).

Does your child have bladder control?

- No control day or night
- Control during the day but not at night

How old is your child?

- Between 2 and 3 years
- 3 years or over

POSSIBLE CAUSE

Few children have reliable control over their bowel or bladder functions before they are 3 years old. This is normal and is not a cause for concern.

ACTION NEEDED

SELF-HELP
See panel: *Toilet-training tips* (below).

Could your child be worried or anxious about something?

- Possibly
- Unlikely

Has your child ever been dry at night for periods of a week or more?

- No
- Yes

POSSIBLE CAUSE

Delayed maturation of the nervous system, often familial, is the most likely explanation, rather than a physical disorder (see BED-WETTING, p.192).

ACTION NEEDED

MEDICAL HELP
If your child is over 5 years old, make an appointment to see your doctor.

POSSIBLE CAUSE

URINARY TRACT INFECTION (p.193).

ACTION NEEDED

MEDICAL HELP
Get medical advice within 24 hours.

POSSIBLE CAUSES

Emotional stress or anxiety (see ANXIETY AND FEARS, p.170) may sometimes result in your child's temporarily losing bowel or bladder control.

ACTION NEEDED

MEDICAL HELP
If the problem continues or recurs, make an appointment to see your doctor.

SELF-HELP: TOILET-TRAINING TIPS

Achieving bowel and bladder control is as natural a part of a child's development as learning to walk; your role is to make the process as easy and relaxed as possible. Bowel control is usually achieved before bladder control, and nighttime bladder control is the last to occur. It is advisable to leave toilet-training until your child is physiologically and mentally ready, which is unlikely to be before the age of about 18 months. The earlier you start, the longer it will take. The following tips may help:
- Familiarize your child with the potty.
- Help and encourage your child to use the potty but avoid making it a source of tension.
- Sit your child on the potty at specific times of the day when you know success is likely.

Second stage of toilet-training
A child who has mastered the use of the potty can progress to using the toilet with a child seat.

15 HEADACHE

Headaches may accompany any acute infection with fever. They may also occur on their own or, more seriously, with a variety of other symptoms. You should consult your doctor if your child has a headache that is severe, persistent, or recurrent, or of an unusual nature.

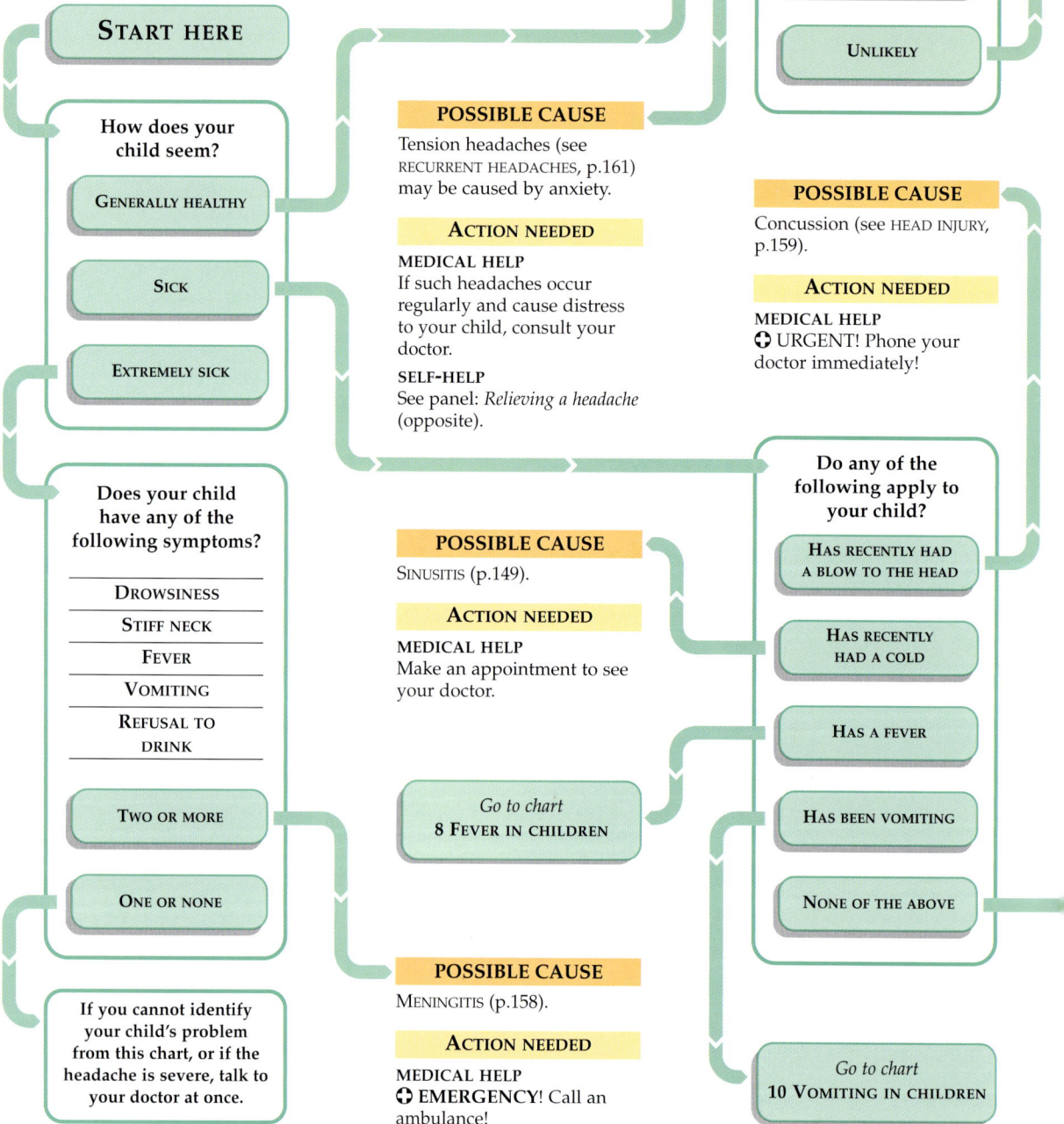

Might your child be worried or anxious about something?

- POSSIBLY
- UNLIKELY

START HERE

How does your child seem?

- GENERALLY HEALTHY
- SICK
- EXTREMELY SICK

POSSIBLE CAUSE

Tension headaches (see RECURRENT HEADACHES, p.161) may be caused by anxiety.

ACTION NEEDED

MEDICAL HELP
If such headaches occur regularly and cause distress to your child, consult your doctor.

SELF-HELP
See panel: *Relieving a headache* (opposite).

POSSIBLE CAUSE

Concussion (see HEAD INJURY, p.159).

ACTION NEEDED

MEDICAL HELP
✚ URGENT! Phone your doctor immediately!

Do any of the following apply to your child?

- HAS RECENTLY HAD A BLOW TO THE HEAD
- HAS RECENTLY HAD A COLD
- HAS A FEVER
- HAS BEEN VOMITING
- NONE OF THE ABOVE

Does your child have any of the following symptoms?

- DROWSINESS
- STIFF NECK
- FEVER
- VOMITING
- REFUSAL TO DRINK

- TWO OR MORE
- ONE OR NONE

POSSIBLE CAUSE

SINUSITIS (p.149).

ACTION NEEDED

MEDICAL HELP
Make an appointment to see your doctor.

Go to chart
8 FEVER IN CHILDREN

If you cannot identify your child's problem from this chart, or if the headache is severe, talk to your doctor at once.

POSSIBLE CAUSE

MENINGITIS (p.158).

ACTION NEEDED

MEDICAL HELP
✚ EMERGENCY! Call an ambulance!

Go to chart
10 VOMITING IN CHILDREN

How often does your child suffer from headaches?

- OCCASIONALLY
- FREQUENTLY

SELF-HELP: RELIEVING A HEADACHE

Most headaches can be treated simply and effectively at home, but if a headache lasts for more than 4 hours, if your child seems very sick, or if other symptoms develop, phone your doctor at once. The following measures might help to relieve the pain:

- Give liquid acetaminophen (dose of 15 mgm per kg) or children's ibuprofen (10 mgm per kg).
- Let your child lie down in a cool, dark room. If he or she can sleep, it might relieve the headache.
- If your child feels hungry, offer milk or a cracker.

A light snack
Hunger is sometimes the cause of a headache. An easily digestible snack, such as a cracker, might relieve it.

When has your child been getting headaches?

- EVERY DAY
- AFTER READING
- AFTER USING A COMPUTER OR WATCHING TELEVISION
- NONE OF THE ABOVE

POSSIBLE CAUSE

An occasional headache is rarely cause for concern.

ACTION NEEDED

SELF-HELP
See panel: *Relieving a headache* (above).

POSSIBLE CAUSE

Frequent headaches (see RECURRENT HEADACHES, p.161), particularly those occurring at night or early in the morning, may be due to a brain abnormality.

ACTION NEEDED

MEDICAL HELP
Make an appointment to see your doctor.

POSSIBLE CAUSE

Migraine (see RECURRENT HEADACHES, p.161).

ACTION NEEDED

MEDICAL HELP
For a first attack, if severe or prolonged, or for frequent attacks, make an appointment to see your doctor.

POSSIBLE CAUSE

Eyesight problems (see REFRACTIVE ERRORS, p.167) can sometimes cause headaches.

ACTION NEEDED

MEDICAL HELP
Make an appointment to see your doctor or optician.

Are the headaches accompanied or preceded by any of the following symptoms?

- ABDOMINAL PAIN
- NAUSEA OR VOMITING
- FLASHING LIGHTS OR OTHER VISUAL DISTURBANCES
- NONE OF THE ABOVE

Does anyone else in the family suffer from recurrent headaches?

- CLOSE RELATIVE, SUCH AS PARENT OR SIBLING
- DISTANT RELATIVE OR NO OTHER FAMILY MEMBER

If you cannot identify your child's problem from this chart, or if the headache is severe, talk to your doctor at once.

16 TOOTHACHE

The most likely cause of toothache in children is tooth decay (dental caries). Any child with pain that affects the teeth or gums should be seen by a dentist without delay. The key to preventing problems is to make sure your child has a healthy diet and takes good care of his or her teeth.

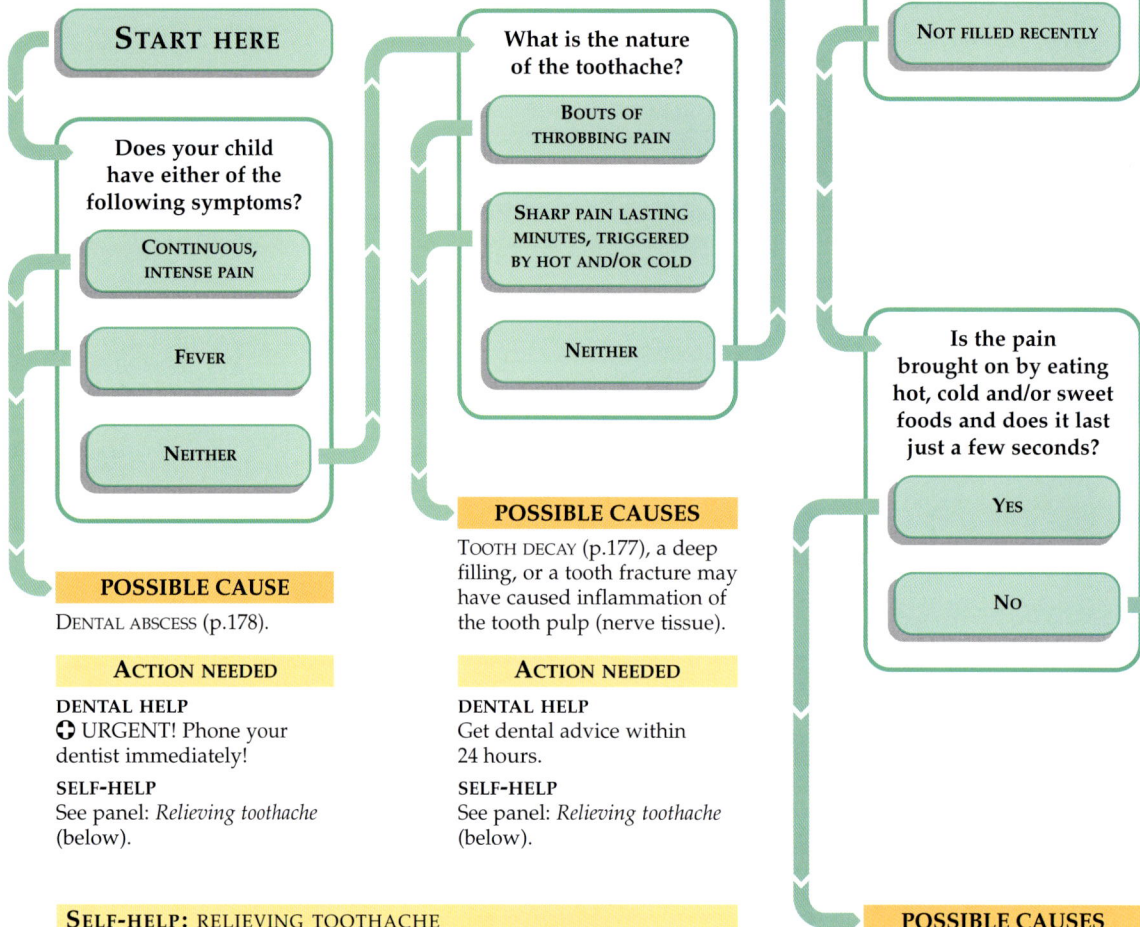

START HERE

Does your child have either of the following symptoms?

- CONTINUOUS, INTENSE PAIN
- FEVER
- NEITHER

What is the nature of the toothache?

- BOUTS OF THROBBING PAIN
- SHARP PAIN LASTING MINUTES, TRIGGERED BY HOT AND/OR COLD
- NEITHER

Has the tooth been filled recently?

- FILLED RECENTLY
- NOT FILLED RECENTLY

Is the pain brought on by eating hot, cold and/or sweet foods and does it last just a few seconds?

- YES
- NO

POSSIBLE CAUSE

DENTAL ABSCESS (p.178).

ACTION NEEDED

DENTAL HELP
✚ URGENT! Phone your dentist immediately!

SELF-HELP
See panel: *Relieving toothache* (below).

POSSIBLE CAUSES

TOOTH DECAY (p.177), a deep filling, or a tooth fracture may have caused inflammation of the tooth pulp (nerve tissue).

ACTION NEEDED

DENTAL HELP
Get dental advice within 24 hours.

SELF-HELP
See panel: *Relieving toothache* (below).

POSSIBLE CAUSES

The pain may be caused by TOOTH DECAY (p.177), a damaged filling, or a cracked or fractured tooth.

ACTION NEEDED

DENTAL HELP
Make an appointment to see your dentist.

SELF-HELP
See panels: *Relieving toothache* (left) and *How can I prevent tooth decay?* (p.177).

SELF-HELP: RELIEVING TOOTHACHE

- Give liquid acetaminophen in the recommended dose of 15 mgm per kg. Do not apply it directly to the tooth since prolonged contact with the gums can result in a chemical burn.
- A young child may feel better if he or she is propped up against several pillows.

Easing toothache
A well-covered hot water bottle, held against the affected side of the face, may relieve your child's toothache.

When is the tooth painful?

ON AND OFF, UNPREDICTABLY

ONLY WHEN BITING OR CHEWING ON IT

SELF-HELP: DEALING WITH A KNOCKED-OUT TOOTH

If a primary tooth is knocked out of your child's mouth, try to find it to ensure that it has not been inhaled or swallowed. A primary tooth cannot be reimplanted. However, a knocked-out secondary tooth can be grafted back into your child's gum by a dentist if this is done soon after the accident.
• Do not attempt to clean the tooth, which may damage the pulp (nerve tissue); put the tooth into a glass of milk, and take it, with your child, to the dentist.
• If a piece of a tooth crown has broken off, take it to the dentist, who may be able to bond it back into place.

Treating a bleeding tooth socket
If the gum at the empty tooth socket is bleeding, place a gauze pad across it and tell your child to bite down hard.

POSSIBLE CAUSE

A filling that is uneven or higher than the level of the tooth's biting surface may cause pain when your child bites down on it.

ACTION NEEDED

DENTAL HELP
Make an appointment to see your dentist.

SELF-HELP
Until your child is able to see a dentist, give a diet of soft and liquid foods, and tell him or her to chew on the other side of the mouth.

Does your child have either of the following symptoms?

TENDER GUMS JUST BEHIND THE SECOND MOLARS

CONTINUOUS, DULL PAIN IN SEVERAL UPPER BACK TEETH

NEITHER

POSSIBLE CAUSE

The wisdom teeth may be starting to emerge.

ACTION NEEDED

DENTAL HELP
Make an appointment to see your dentist.

SELF-HELP
See panel: *Relieving a sore mouth* (p.105).

POSSIBLE CAUSE

TOOTH DECAY (p.177).

ACTION NEEDED

DENTAL HELP
Make an appointment to see your dentist.

SELF-HELP
See panels: *Relieving toothache* (opposite) and *How can I prevent tooth decay?* (p.177).

POSSIBLE CAUSE

A tooth that has been filled very recently is often slightly sensitive, particularly to cold. Sensitivity is especially likely after a deep filling.

ACTION NEEDED

DENTAL HELP
If sensitivity to heat develops or if pain intensifies or lasts for more than a few seconds, make an appointment to see your dentist. Such symptoms may indicate damage to the tooth pulp (nerve tissue).

POSSIBLE CAUSE

SINUSITIS (p.149), rarely.

ACTION NEEDED

MEDICAL HELP
Make an appointment to see your doctor.

67

17 FEELING GENERALLY SICK

If your child complains of feeling sick, you should check his or her temperature and look for a rash. A symptom such as a headache may clear up with self-help measures, or it may be the first sign of an infection, such as influenza. If your child's condition worsens, consult your doctor.

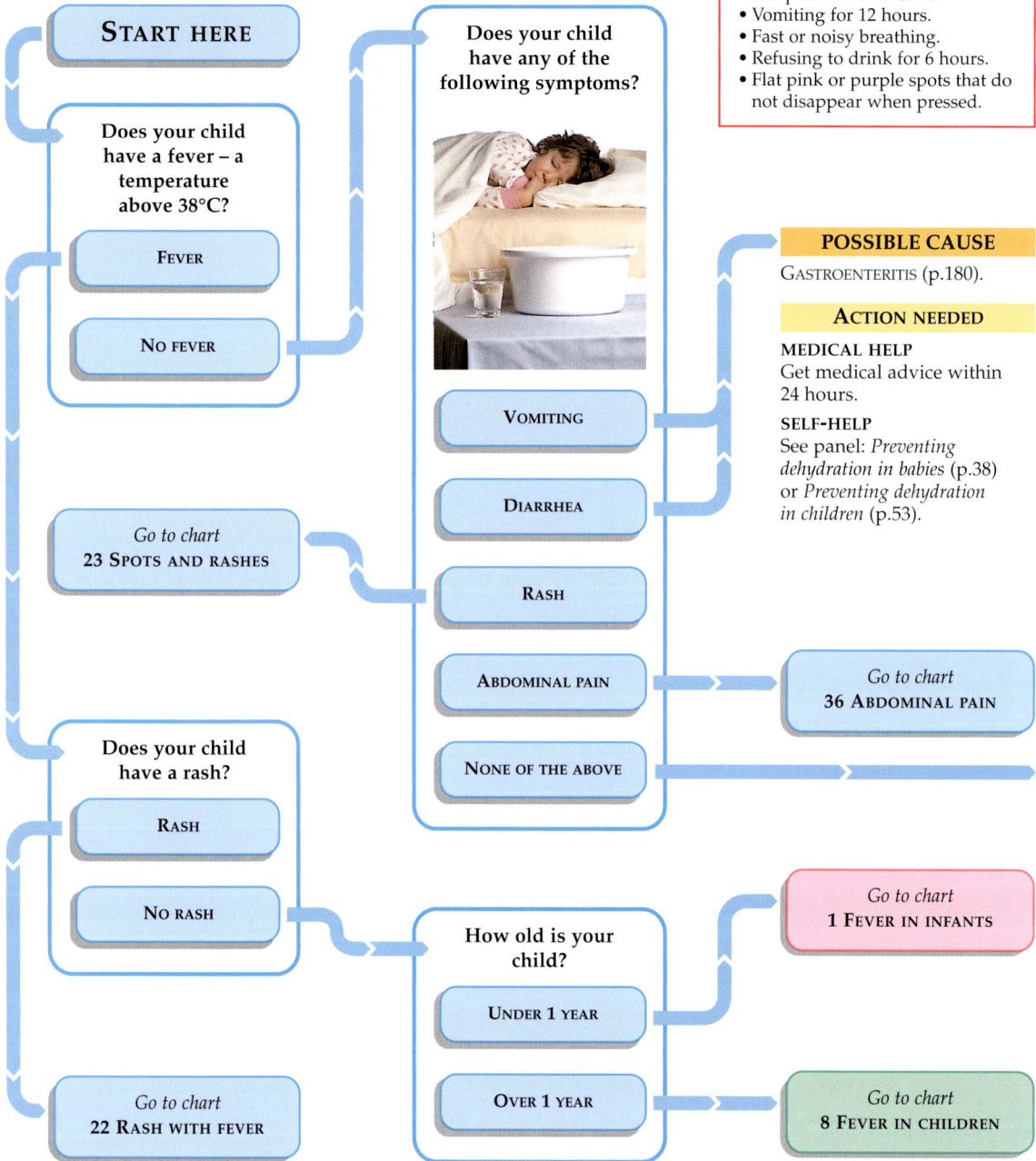

START HERE

Does your child have a fever – a temperature above 38°C?

- FEVER
- NO FEVER

Go to chart
23 SPOTS AND RASHES

Does your child have a rash?

- RASH
- NO RASH

Go to chart
22 RASH WITH FEVER

Does your child have any of the following symptoms?

- VOMITING
- DIARRHEA
- RASH
- ABDOMINAL PAIN
- NONE OF THE ABOVE

How old is your child?

- UNDER 1 YEAR
- OVER 1 YEAR

POSSIBLE CAUSE
GASTROENTERITIS (p.180).

ACTION NEEDED

MEDICAL HELP
Get medical advice within 24 hours.

SELF-HELP
See panel: *Preventing dehydration in babies* (p.38) or *Preventing dehydration in children* (p.53).

Go to chart
36 ABDOMINAL PAIN

Go to chart
1 FEVER IN INFANTS

Go to chart
8 FEVER IN CHILDREN

Is your child interested in food and drink?

REFUSES TO EAT AND DRINK

REFUSES TO EAT

EATS AND DRINKS NORMALLY

POSSIBLE CAUSE

Your child may be developing an infectious disease (see pp.118–125), particularly if he or she is listless or irritable or has other signs of illness.

ACTION NEEDED

MEDICAL HELP
If your child feels no better after 24 hours or develops other symptoms, call your doctor to discuss your child's condition.

SELF-HELP
Encourage your child to drink by offering a favorite beverage. See panel: *Preventing dehydration in babies* (p.38) or *Preventing dehydration in children* (p.53).

Go to chart
28 SORE THROAT

Could your child be worried or anxious about something?

POSSIBLY

UNLIKELY

POSSIBLE CAUSES

Anxiety or problems at school can result in a child feeling sick (see ANXIETY AND FEARS, p.170).

ACTION NEEDED

MEDICAL HELP
If your child still feels sick after a day at home or if he or she regularly refuses to go to school, make an appointment to see your doctor.

In the past 3 weeks could your child have had contact with anyone who has an infectious disease?

NO CONTACT

CONTACT

If you cannot identify your child's problem from this chart, talk to your doctor within 48 hours.

POSSIBLE CAUSE

One of the childhood infectious diseases (see pp.118–125), in its incubation period, might be causing your child to feel sick.

ACTION NEEDED

MEDICAL HELP
If your child feels no better after 24 hours, or he or she develops other symptoms, make an appointment to see your doctor.

18 LUMPS AND SWELLINGS

Lumps and swellings occur on, or just below, the surface of the skin. Swellings may be lymph glands that have swollen to fight infection in a nearby part of the body. Injuries, bites, and stings can also cause lumps and swellings. A persistent or painful lump or swelling should be examined by a doctor.

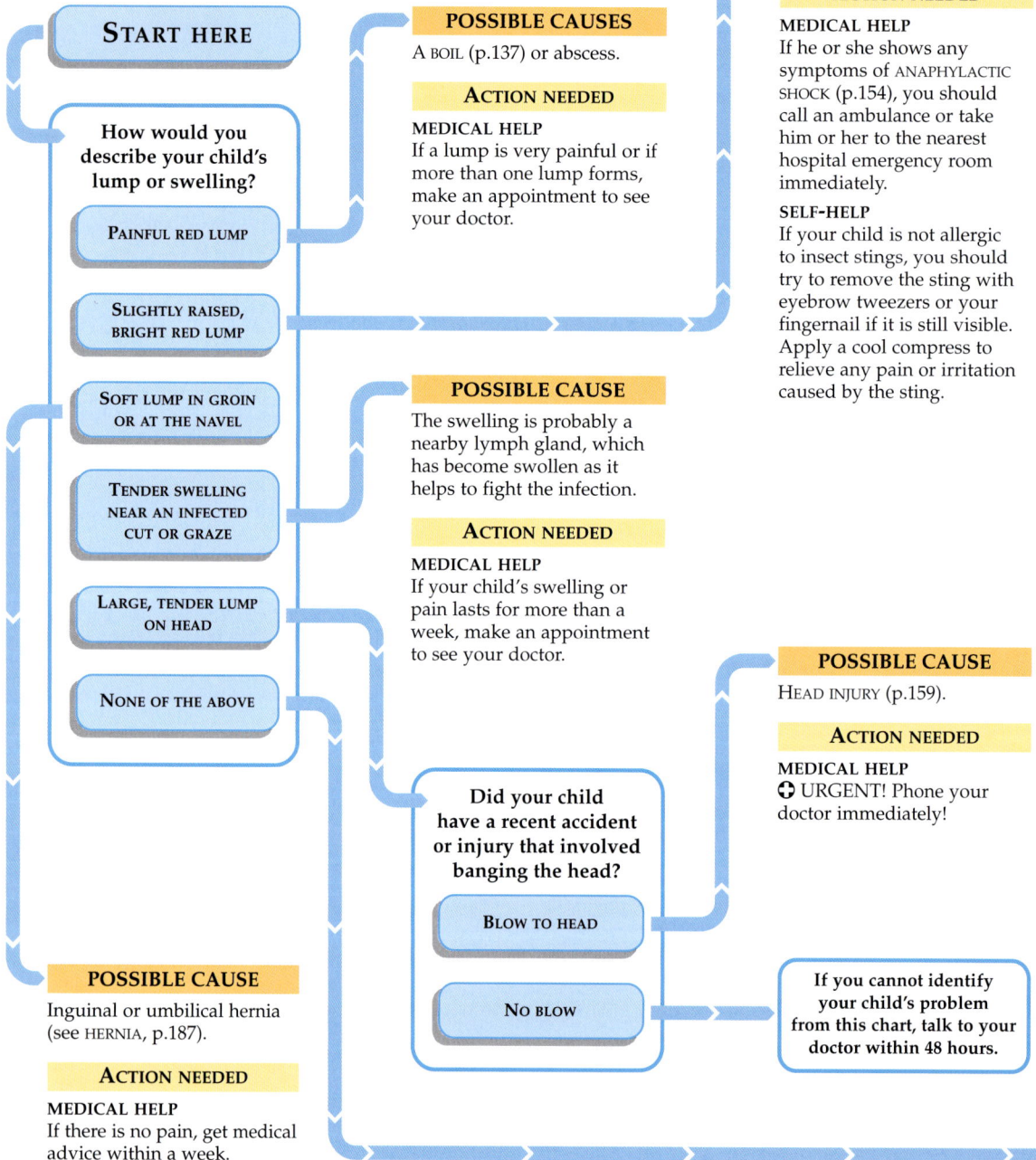

START HERE

How would you describe your child's lump or swelling?

- PAINFUL RED LUMP
- SLIGHTLY RAISED, BRIGHT RED LUMP
- SOFT LUMP IN GROIN OR AT THE NAVEL
- TENDER SWELLING NEAR AN INFECTED CUT OR GRAZE
- LARGE, TENDER LUMP ON HEAD
- NONE OF THE ABOVE

POSSIBLE CAUSES

A BOIL (p.137) or abscess.

ACTION NEEDED

MEDICAL HELP
If a lump is very painful or if more than one lump forms, make an appointment to see your doctor.

POSSIBLE CAUSE

The swelling is probably a nearby lymph gland, which has become swollen as it helps to fight the infection.

ACTION NEEDED

MEDICAL HELP
If your child's swelling or pain lasts for more than a week, make an appointment to see your doctor.

POSSIBLE CAUSE

Your child may have been stung by an insect such as a bee or wasp (see INSECT BITES AND STINGS, p.138).

ACTION NEEDED

MEDICAL HELP
If he or she shows any symptoms of ANAPHYLACTIC SHOCK (p.154), you should call an ambulance or take him or her to the nearest hospital emergency room immediately.

SELF-HELP
If your child is not allergic to insect stings, you should try to remove the sting with eyebrow tweezers or your fingernail if it is still visible. Apply a cool compress to relieve any pain or irritation caused by the sting.

POSSIBLE CAUSE

HEAD INJURY (p.159).

ACTION NEEDED

MEDICAL HELP
✚ URGENT! Phone your doctor immediately!

Did your child have a recent accident or injury that involved banging the head?

- BLOW TO HEAD
- NO BLOW

If you cannot identify your child's problem from this chart, talk to your doctor within 48 hours.

POSSIBLE CAUSE

Inguinal or umbilical hernia (see HERNIA, p.187).

ACTION NEEDED

MEDICAL HELP
If there is no pain, get medical advice within a week.

POSSIBLE CAUSES

ECZEMA (p.135) or a viral infection, such as RUBELLA (p.119).

ACTION NEEDED

MEDICAL HELP
Make an appointment to see your doctor.

Does your child have any of the following symptoms?

- SORE THROAT
- RELUCTANCE TO EAT OR DRINK
- EARACHE
- NONE OF THE ABOVE

POSSIBLE CAUSE

Tonsillitis (see SORE THROAT, p.151).

ACTION NEEDED

MEDICAL HELP
If your child feels no better after 24 hours, consult your doctor.

SELF-HELP
See panel: *Relieving a sore throat* (p.91).

POSSIBLE CAUSE

OTITIS MEDIA (p.162).

ACTION NEEDED

MEDICAL HELP
Get medical advice within 24 hours.

SELF-HELP
See panel: *Relieving earache* (p.101).

What is the location of the lumps or swellings?

- BACK OF NECK
- SIDES OF NECK
- BETWEEN EAR AND JAW
- IN NECK AND ARMPIT AND/OR GROIN
- NONE OF THE ABOVE

If you cannot identify your child's problem from this chart, talk to your doctor within 48 hours.

POSSIBLE CAUSE

Parotitis, e.g. MUMPS (p.122).

ACTION NEEDED

MEDICAL HELP
Make an appointment to see your doctor.

POSSIBLE CAUSE

INFECTIOUS MONONUCLEOSIS (p.124).

ACTION NEEDED

MEDICAL HELP
Make an appointment to see your doctor.

Do any of the following apply?

- ANKLE IS SWOLLEN
- FOOT IS SWOLLEN
- SWELLING IN SCROTUM OR PENIS
- NONE OF THE ABOVE

Go to chart **21 FOOT PROBLEMS**

Go to chart **40 GENITAL PROBLEMS IN BOYS**

POSSIBLE CAUSES

STRAIN OR SPRAIN (p.127).

ACTION NEEDED

MEDICAL HELP
If pain is severe or there is no improvement after 24 hours, consult your doctor.

SELF-HELP
See panel: *Treating strains and sprains* (p.73).

If you cannot identify your child's problem from this chart, talk to your doctor within 48 hours.

19 PAINFUL LIMBS

Many children experience pain in an arm or leg; this pain is usually the result of a minor fall or injury and rarely requires medical attention. Sometimes a bone may be broken or a joint dislocated; these conditions need urgent treatment. Unexplained or persistent pain may also require attention.

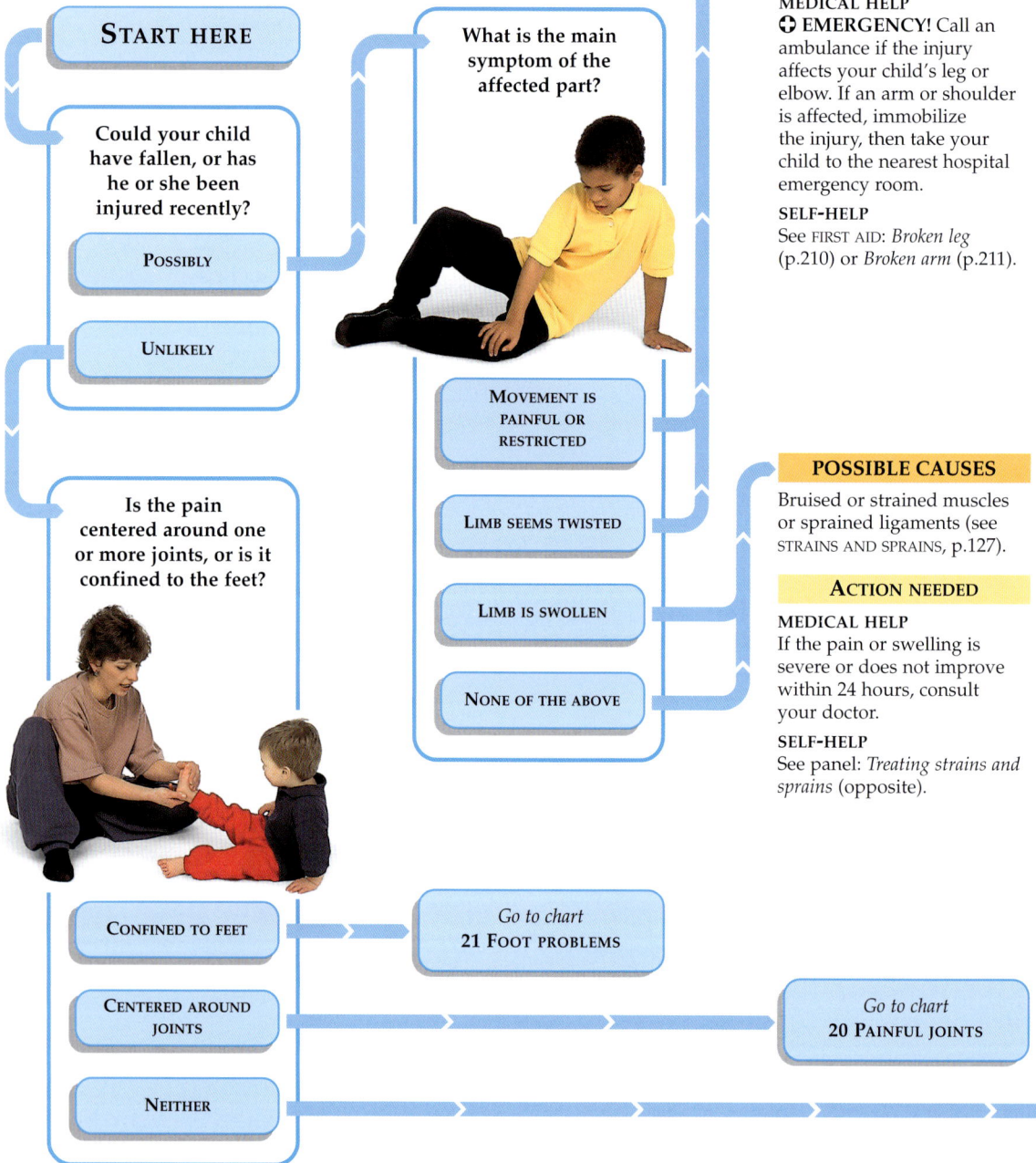

POSSIBLE CAUSES

A broken bone or a dislocated joint (see FRACTURES AND DISLOCATIONS, p.128).

ACTION NEEDED

MEDICAL HELP
✚ **EMERGENCY!** Call an ambulance if the injury affects your child's leg or elbow. If an arm or shoulder is affected, immobilize the injury, then take your child to the nearest hospital emergency room.

SELF-HELP
See FIRST AID: *Broken leg* (p.210) or *Broken arm* (p.211).

START HERE

Could your child have fallen, or has he or she been injured recently?

- **POSSIBLY**
- **UNLIKELY**

Is the pain centered around one or more joints, or is it confined to the feet?

What is the main symptom of the affected part?

- **MOVEMENT IS PAINFUL OR RESTRICTED**
- **LIMB SEEMS TWISTED**
- **LIMB IS SWOLLEN**
- **NONE OF THE ABOVE**

POSSIBLE CAUSES

Bruised or strained muscles or sprained ligaments (see STRAINS AND SPRAINS, p.127).

ACTION NEEDED

MEDICAL HELP
If the pain or swelling is severe or does not improve within 24 hours, consult your doctor.

SELF-HELP
See panel: *Treating strains and sprains* (opposite).

- **CONFINED TO FEET** → *Go to chart* **21 FOOT PROBLEMS**
- **CENTERED AROUND JOINTS** → *Go to chart* **20 PAINFUL JOINTS**
- **NEITHER**

Does your child have a fever – a temperature above 38°C – or does he or she seem sick?

FEVER

SEEMS SICK

NEITHER

Is your child suffering from any of the following symptoms?

HEADACHE

COUGH

SORE THROAT

RED OR TENDER AREA OVER A BONE

NONE OF THE ABOVE

POSSIBLE CAUSE

INFLUENZA (p.151).

ACTION NEEDED

MEDICAL HELP
If there is no improvement within 48 hours, if breathing difficulties develop, or a rash appears, phone your doctor immediately.

SELF-HELP
See panel: *Bringing down a high temperature* (p.37).

POSSIBLE CAUSE

Bone infection (see BONE AND JOINT INFECTION, p.133).

ACTION NEEDED

MEDICAL HELP
✚ URGENT! Phone your doctor immediately!

Has your child been experiencing pain in the lower leg that lasts for a few minutes?

YES

NO

POSSIBLE CAUSE

CRAMPS (p.127).

ACTION NEEDED

MEDICAL HELP
If the problem persists, make an appointment to see your doctor.

SELF-HELP
Gently massage or stretch the affected leg.

If you cannot identify your child's problem from this chart or if the pain lasts for over 24 hours, talk to your doctor.

POSSIBLE CAUSES

Bruised or strained muscles or sprained ligaments, possibly caused by an unnoticed injury (see STRAINS AND SPRAINS, p.127).

ACTION NEEDED

MEDICAL HELP
If your child is in severe pain, or he or she is reluctant to use the affected limb, or if there is no improvement within 24 hours, consult your doctor.

SELF-HELP
See panel: *Treating strains and sprains* (right).

SELF-HELP: TREATING STRAINS AND SPRAINS

If your child suffers a strain or sprain, the appropriate treatment is remembered as RICE – Rest, Ice, Compression, and Elevation. This treatment can also be used for deep bruising.

- Rest: tell your child to rest the affected part.
- Ice: apply a cold compress, such as ice or frozen peas wrapped in cotton, for 10–15 minutes.
- Compression: bandage a thick layer of cotton gauze firmly around the injured area.
- Elevation: raise and support the affected part to minimize further swelling.

Compression
Wrap a pad of cotton gauze around the affected area. Use an elastic bandage to secure the gauze in place.

20 PAINFUL JOINTS

It is uncommon but not rare for a child to be affected by a serious joint disorder. Usually, pain is caused by a minor strain or sprain of the muscles or ligaments around a joint. If your child's pain is persistent or if there are other symptoms, such as a fever, you should consult your doctor.

START HERE

Could your child have fallen or has he or she been injured recently?

POSSIBLY

UNLIKELY

How many joints are affected?

ONLY ONE JOINT

MORE THAN ONE JOINT

What is the main symptom of the affected joint?

RESTRICTED OR PAINFUL MOVEMENT

JOINT SEEMS DEFORMED

JOINT IS SWOLLEN

NONE OF THE ABOVE

Does your child have any of the following symptoms?

FEVER

SEEMS SICK

RED, HOT, OR SWOLLEN JOINT

NONE OF THE ABOVE

POSSIBLE CAUSES

A dislocated joint or a break in a bone near the joint (see FRACTURES AND DISLOCATIONS, p.128).

ACTION NEEDED

MEDICAL HELP
✚ **EMERGENCY!** Call an ambulance if the injury affects your child's leg or elbow. If an arm, finger, or shoulder is affected, take your child to the nearest hospital emergency room.

SELF-HELP
See FIRST AID: *Broken leg* (p.210) or *Broken arm* (p.211).

POSSIBLE CAUSE

Strained muscles or sprained ligaments near the joint (see STRAINS AND SPRAINS, p.127).

ACTION NEEDED

MEDICAL HELP
If the pain or swelling is severe or does not improve within 24 hours, consult your doctor.

SELF-HELP
See panel: *Treating strains and sprains* (p.73).

POSSIBLE CAUSE

Joint infection (see BONE AND JOINT INFECTION, p.133).

ACTION NEEDED

MEDICAL HELP
✚ **URGENT!** Phone your doctor immediately!

Does your child have a painful knee or hip joint or a limp?

- **LIMP**
- **PAINFUL HIP**
- **PAINFUL KNEE**
- **NONE OF THE ABOVE**

POSSIBLE CAUSES

CONGENITAL HIP DISLOCATION (p.130) is a possibility in a child who is just learning to walk. An older child may be suffering from LEGG-PERTHES' DISEASE (p.131) or SLIPPED FEMORAL EPIPHYSIS (p.131). Bone or joint infection (see BONE AND JOINT INFECTION, p.133 or HIP PAIN (p.130) are possibilities in a child of any age. See also LIMPING (p.126).

ACTION NEEDED
MEDICAL HELP
Get medical advice within 24 hours.

POSSIBLE CAUSES

A minor STRAIN OR SPRAIN (p.127) is the most likely cause. Bone or joint infection (see BONE AND JOINT INFECTION, p.133) is also a possibility. If the knee is the joint affected, your child may have either chondromalacia patellae or Osgood-Schlatter disease (see KNEE DISORDERS, p.132). See also LIMPING (p.126).

ACTION NEEDED
MEDICAL HELP
If the pain is severe, is no better after 24 hours, or recurs, consult your doctor.

SELF-HELP
See panel: *Treating strains and sprains (p.73).*

POSSIBLE CAUSES

A short-lasting arthritis, which may occur after an acute infection, or JUVENILE RHEUMATOID ARTHRITIS (p.132).

ACTION NEEDED
MEDICAL HELP
Get medical advice within 24 hours.

Is your child suffering from either of the following symptoms?

- **RED OR HOT JOINTS**
- **SWOLLEN JOINTS**
- **NEITHER**

If you cannot identify your child's problem from this chart or if the affected joint remains painful for more than 24 hours, talk to your doctor.

Does your child have any of the following symptoms?

- **FEVER**
- **SEEMS SICK**
- **PURPLISH RASH ON LIMBS**
- **NONE OF THE ABOVE**

POSSIBLE CAUSE

HENOCH-SCHÖNLEIN PURPURA (p.147).

ACTION NEEDED
MEDICAL HELP
✚ URGENT! Phone your doctor immediately!

POSSIBLE CAUSES

A short-lasting arthritis after an acute infection or JUVENILE RHEUMATOID ARTHRITIS (p.132).

ACTION NEEDED
MEDICAL HELP
Get medical advice within 24 hours.

21 FOOT PROBLEMS

The majority of foot problems in childhood are minor. Most common are those resulting from falls and those that affect the skin of one or both feet. Poorly fitting shoes may also cause foot problems. If the foot is very painful or very swollen, or if walking is difficult, consult your doctor.

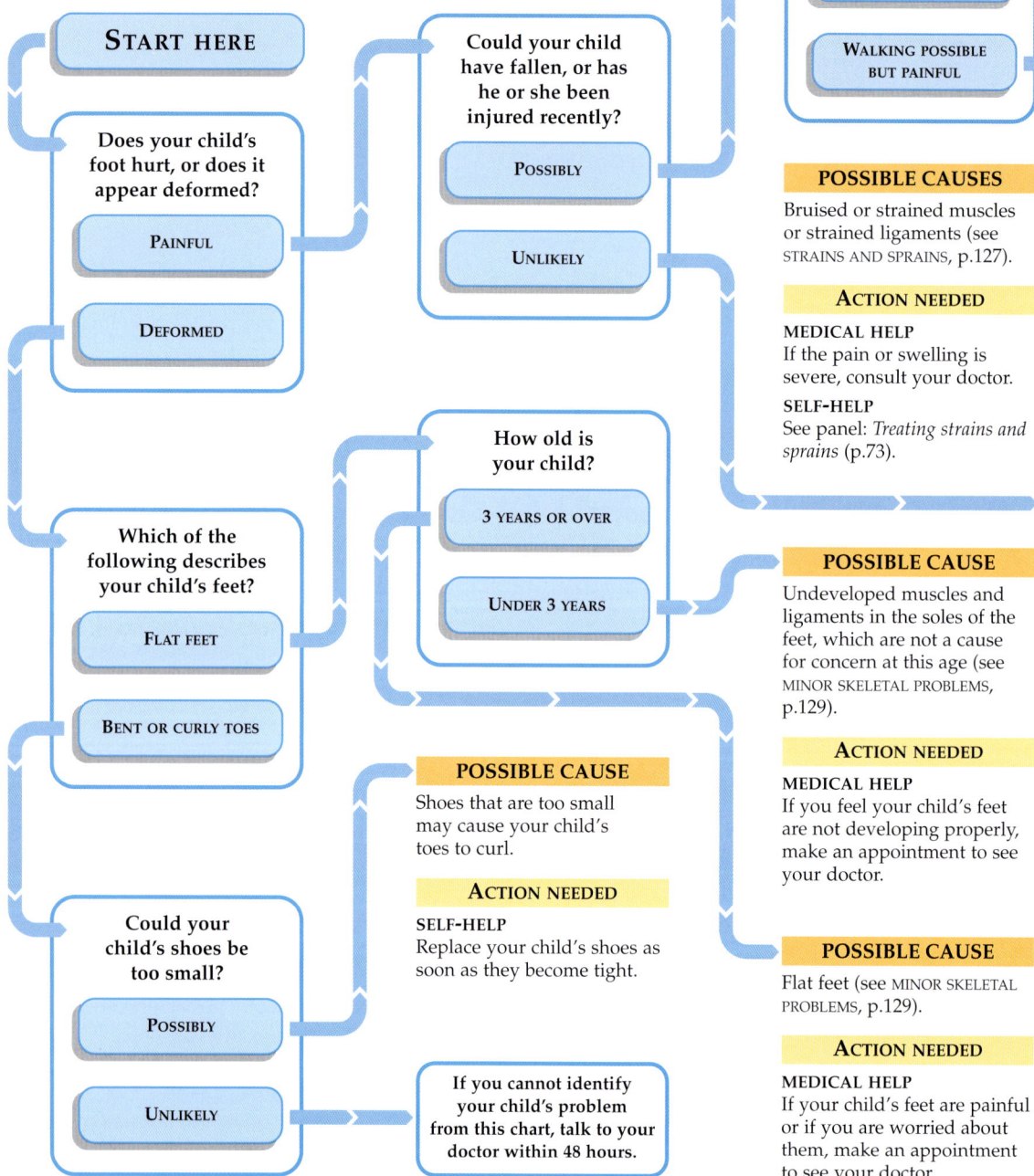

START HERE

Does your child's foot hurt, or does it appear deformed?

- PAINFUL
- DEFORMED

Could your child have fallen, or has he or she been injured recently?

- POSSIBLY
- UNLIKELY

How has the injury affected your child's walking?

- CHILD CANNOT WALK ON AFFECTED FOOT
- WALKING POSSIBLE BUT PAINFUL

POSSIBLE CAUSES

Bruised or strained muscles or strained ligaments (see STRAINS AND SPRAINS, p.127).

ACTION NEEDED

MEDICAL HELP
If the pain or swelling is severe, consult your doctor.

SELF-HELP
See panel: *Treating strains and sprains* (p.73).

Which of the following describes your child's feet?

- FLAT FEET
- BENT OR CURLY TOES

How old is your child?

- 3 YEARS OR OVER
- UNDER 3 YEARS

POSSIBLE CAUSE

Undeveloped muscles and ligaments in the soles of the feet, which are not a cause for concern at this age (see MINOR SKELETAL PROBLEMS, p.129).

ACTION NEEDED

MEDICAL HELP
If you feel your child's feet are not developing properly, make an appointment to see your doctor.

POSSIBLE CAUSE

Shoes that are too small may cause your child's toes to curl.

ACTION NEEDED

SELF-HELP
Replace your child's shoes as soon as they become tight.

Could your child's shoes be too small?

- POSSIBLY
- UNLIKELY

If you cannot identify your child's problem from this chart, talk to your doctor within 48 hours.

POSSIBLE CAUSE

Flat feet (see MINOR SKELETAL PROBLEMS, p.129).

ACTION NEEDED

MEDICAL HELP
If your child's feet are painful or if you are worried about them, make an appointment to see your doctor.

POSSIBLE CAUSE

A bone in your child's foot, toe, or ankle may have been fractured (see FRACTURES AND DISLOCATIONS, p.128).

ACTION NEEDED

MEDICAL HELP
✚ **EMERGENCY**! Take your child to the nearest hospital emergency room. If you are unable to move your child, you should call an ambulance.

POSSIBLE CAUSE

Your child's feet may hurt because his or her shoes do not fit properly.

ACTION NEEDED

SELF-HELP
Replace your child's shoes as soon as they become tight. Make sure new shoes are long and wide enough. Try to buy from stores where the salespeople are trained to fit children's shoes.

POSSIBLE CAUSE

Plantar wart (see WARTS, p.141).

ACTION NEEDED

MEDICAL HELP
Make an appointment to see your doctor.

POSSIBLE CAUSE

Athlete's foot (see p.142) or ECZEMA (see p.135).

ACTION NEEDED

MEDICAL HELP
If the rash does not clear up within 2 weeks of starting self-help treatment, or if your child's toenails are affected, make an appointment to see your doctor.

SELF-HELP
Apply an antifungal powder, cream, or spray to the rash. Make sure your child's feet are dried well after bathing, and then moisturize them.

When does your child feel pain?

- ONLY WHEN WEARING SHOES
- ONLY WHEN WEIGHT IS PUT ON THE FOOT
- AT ALL TIMES

Is there anything abnormal on the sole of your child's foot?

- FLATTENED, HARD LUMP OF SKIN
- ITCHY, PEELING RASH
- NOTHING

Can you see any redness or swelling on one of your child's feet or toes?

- REDNESS OR SWELLING
- NEITHER

If you cannot identify your child's problem from this chart, talk to your doctor within 48 hours.

POSSIBLE CAUSE

Infection from a cut or a foreign body, such as a splinter, may cause redness or swelling.

ACTION NEEDED

MEDICAL HELP
Get medical advice within 24 hours.

SELF-HELP
Remove a foreign body with sterilized tweezers. Cover the affected area with a clean, sterile bandage, then elevate and support the foot to reduce swelling.

22 RASH WITH FEVER

The combination of rash and fever – a temperature above 38°C – is usually caused by an infectious disease. Most of these diseases are caused by viruses and usually clear up quickly without special treatment. You should, however, consult your doctor for a diagnosis.

START HERE

What are the features of your child's rash?

- FLAT SPOTS THAT DO NOT DISAPPEAR WHEN PRESSED
- FINE RED RASH THAT TURNS WHITE WHEN PRESSED
- BLOTCHY, RAISED RED RASH
- CROPS OF ITCHY SPOTS THAT BLISTER AND DRY INTO SCABS
- FLAT PINK SPOTS STARTING ON THE FACE (HAIRLINE) OR TRUNK
- BRIGHT RED RASH CONFINED TO THE CHEEKS
- NONE OF THE ABOVE

If you cannot identify your child's problem from this chart, talk to your doctor within 24 hours.

POSSIBLE CAUSE

Blood infection with meningococcus, a bacterium that causes MENINGITIS (p.158).

ACTION NEEDED

MEDICAL HELP
✚ EMERGENCY! Call an ambulance!

POSSIBLE CAUSE

CHICKENPOX (p.120).

ACTION NEEDED

MEDICAL HELP
If the spots become infected, make an appointment to see your doctor.

SELF-HELP
See panel: *Bringing down a high temperature* (p.37).

POSSIBLE CAUSE

FIFTH DISEASE (p.119).

ACTION NEEDED

MEDICAL HELP
If you are concerned about your child's condition or if your child has SICKLE-CELL ANEMIA (p.199), make an appointment to see your doctor.

SELF-HELP
See panel: *Bringing down a high temperature* (p.37).

How high was your child's temperature during the 3 to 4 days before the rash appeared?

- 38.5°C OR ABOVE
- BELOW 38.5°C

POSSIBLE CAUSE

RUBELLA (p.119), rarely.

ACTION NEEDED

MEDICAL HELP
Make an appointment to see your doctor.

SELF-HELP
See panel: *Bringing down a high temperature* (p.37).

DANGER SIGNS

Phone your doctor at once if your child has any of the following symptoms during, or after apparent recovery from, any of the common childhood infectious diseases:
- Abnormal drowsiness.
- Seizures.
- Fever higher than 40°C.
- Abnormally fast breathing.
- Noisy or difficult breathing.
- Severe headache.
- Refusing to drink for over 6 hours.
- Rash that does not fade with pressure.

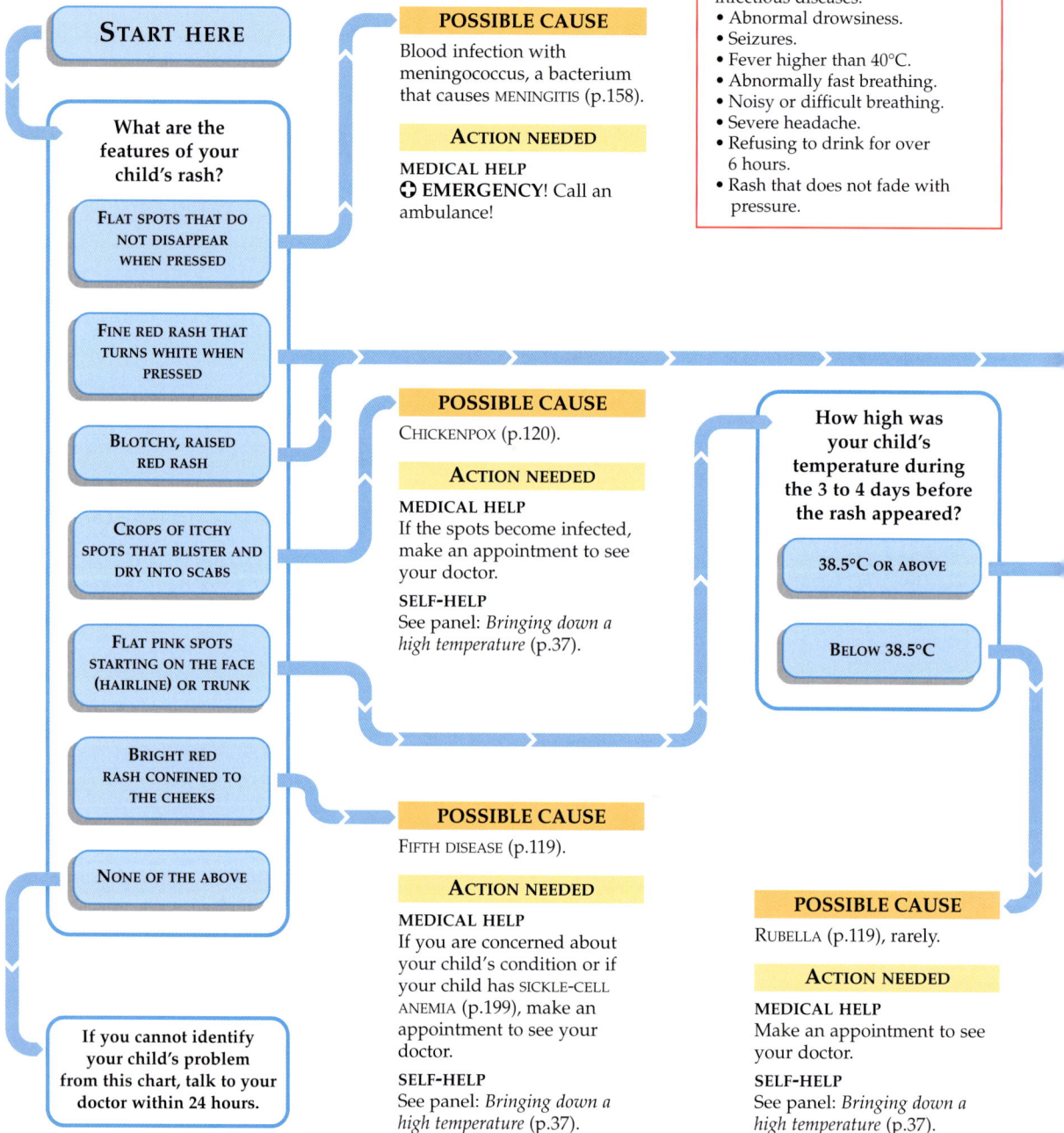

POSSIBLE CAUSE

MEASLES (p.118) or, rarely, KAWASAKI DISEASE (p.125).

ACTION NEEDED

MEDICAL HELP
Get medical advice within 24 hours.

SELF-HELP
See panel: *Bringing down a high temperature* (p.37).

COMMON RASHES

This is an identification guide to some of the childhood rashes. However, rashes may differ in appearance depending on how severely your child is affected and the color of the skin, so a firm diagnosis should always be made by a doctor. Call an ambulance if your child's rash resembles the meningitis rash.

MENINGOCOCCUS

SCARLET FEVER

MEASLES

CHICKENPOX

RUBELLA

ROSEOLA INFANTUM

Before the rash appeared, did your child also have any of the following symptoms?

- RUNNY NOSE
- COUGH
- RED EYES
- SORE THROAT
- VOMITING
- NONE OF THE ABOVE

POSSIBLE CAUSE

SCARLET FEVER (p.121).

ACTION NEEDED

MEDICAL HELP
Get medical advice within 24 hours.

SELF-HELP
See panels: *Bringing down a high temperature* (p.37) and *Relieving a sore throat* (p.91).

POSSIBLE CAUSE

Drug allergy (see ALLERGIES, p.152).

ACTION NEEDED

MEDICAL HELP
✚ URGENT! Phone your doctor immediately to find out whether the medicine may be causing your child's symptoms and whether you should stop giving it.

Has your child taken any medicine in the past week?

- MEDICINE
- NO MEDICINE

POSSIBLE CAUSE

ROSEOLA INFANTUM (p.121).

ACTION NEEDED

MEDICAL HELP
If you are concerned about your child's condition, make an appointment to see your doctor.

SELF-HELP
See panel: *Bringing down a high temperature* (p.37).

If you cannot identify your child's problem from this chart, talk to your doctor within 24 hours.

23 SPOTS AND RASHES

For other skin problems in infants, see chart 7

Most spots and rashes are a response to a local or general infection or a symptom of an allergic reaction. The spots or rashes are probably not serious if there are no other signs of being sick. However, if the skin is very itchy or sore or if your child is upset, you should consult your doctor.

DANGER SIGNS
Call an ambulance at once if your child develops any of the following symptoms:
• Swelling of face or mouth.
• Noisy or difficult breathing.
• Difficulty in swallowing.
• Abnormal drowsiness.

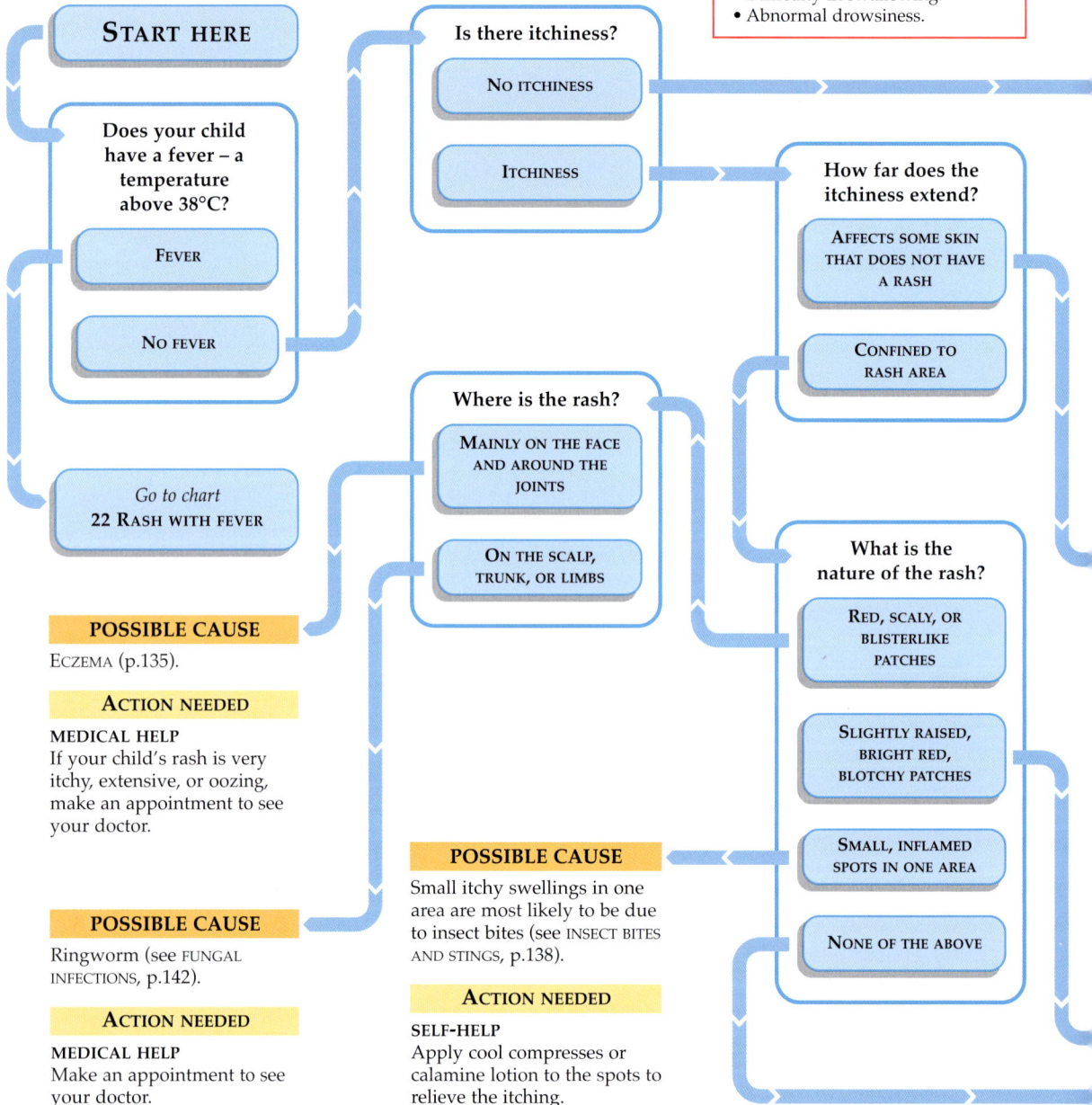

START HERE

Does your child have a fever – a temperature above 38°C?

FEVER

NO FEVER

Go to chart
22 RASH WITH FEVER

Is there itchiness?

NO ITCHINESS

ITCHINESS

How far does the itchiness extend?

AFFECTS SOME SKIN THAT DOES NOT HAVE A RASH

CONFINED TO RASH AREA

Where is the rash?

MAINLY ON THE FACE AND AROUND THE JOINTS

ON THE SCALP, TRUNK, OR LIMBS

What is the nature of the rash?

RED, SCALY, OR BLISTERLIKE PATCHES

SLIGHTLY RAISED, BRIGHT RED, BLOTCHY PATCHES

SMALL, INFLAMED SPOTS IN ONE AREA

NONE OF THE ABOVE

POSSIBLE CAUSE

ECZEMA (p.135).

ACTION NEEDED

MEDICAL HELP
If your child's rash is very itchy, extensive, or oozing, make an appointment to see your doctor.

POSSIBLE CAUSE

Ringworm (see FUNGAL INFECTIONS, p.142).

ACTION NEEDED

MEDICAL HELP
Make an appointment to see your doctor.

POSSIBLE CAUSE

Small itchy swellings in one area are most likely to be due to insect bites (see INSECT BITES AND STINGS, p.138).

ACTION NEEDED

SELF-HELP
Apply cool compresses or calamine lotion to the spots to relieve the itching.

**What does the
rash or spot look like?**

- GROUPS OF LUMPS, EACH WITH A CENTRAL DEPRESSION
- PUS-FILLED AREAS OR GOLDEN CRUSTS, OFTEN ON THE FACE
- ONE OR MORE FIRM, ROUGH LUMPS
- A PAINFUL RED LUMP, POSSIBLY WITH A YELLOW TOP
- TINY, RED, ITCHY SPOTS OR FLUID-FILLED BLISTERS
- NONE OF THE ABOVE

POSSIBLE CAUSE

MOLLUSCUM CONTAGIOSUM (p.141).

ACTION NEEDED

MEDICAL HELP
Make an appointment to see your doctor.

POSSIBLE CAUSE

IMPETIGO (p.139).

ACTION NEEDED

MEDICAL HELP
Get medical advice within 24 hours.

POSSIBLE CAUSE

WARTS (p.141).

ACTION NEEDED

MEDICAL HELP
If the warts are troublesome, make an appointment to see your doctor.

continued on p.82, top

POSSIBLE CAUSE

HIVES (p.138).

ACTION NEEDED

MEDICAL HELP
If the rash does not disappear within 24 to 48 hours, or if your child has repeated attacks, make an appointment to see your doctor.

SELF-HELP
Apply cool compresses or calamine lotion to the spots to relieve the itchiness.

POSSIBLE CAUSE

A BOIL (p.137).

ACTION NEEDED

MEDICAL HELP
If a boil is very painful or if more than one boil forms, make an appointment to see your doctor.

POSSIBLE CAUSE

Prickly heat, a rash caused by unevaporated sweat.

ACTION NEEDED

SELF-HELP
Apply cool compresses as often as needed to relieve the itchiness. Do not use soap on the affected areas.

POSSIBLE CAUSE

SCABIES (p.143).

ACTION NEEDED

MEDICAL HELP
Make an appointment to see your doctor.

**Is your child's
face or mouth swollen?**

- NOT SWOLLEN
- SWOLLEN

POSSIBLE CAUSE

An allergic reaction, which may be caused by insect stings, peanuts, or other factors, and can lead to ANAPHYLACTIC SHOCK (p.154).

ACTION NEEDED

MEDICAL HELP
✚ EMERGENCY! Call an ambulance!

continued on p.82, bottom

23 Spots and rashes (continued)

continued from p.81, top

Has your child reached puberty?

HAS REACHED PUBERTY

HAS NOT REACHED PUBERTY

continued from p.81, bottom

Have you noticed any of the following types of spots?

ROUND, SCALY SPOTS ON THE TRUNK, UPPER ARMS, OR THIGHS

TINY BLACK SPOTS (BLACKHEADS)

WHITE-CENTERED, INFLAMED SPOTS (WHITEHEADS)

SMALL, SOLID, TENDER SWELLINGS UNDER THE SKIN

NONE OF THE ABOVE

Does your child have small, oval pink spots arranged along the lines of the ribs?

YES

NO

Are you giving your child any medicine?

MEDICINE

NO MEDICINE

POSSIBLE CAUSE
ECZEMA (p.135).

ACTION NEEDED
MEDICAL HELP
Make an appointment to see your doctor.

POSSIBLE CAUSE
ACNE (p.140).

ACTION NEEDED
MEDICAL HELP
If the acne is severe, make an appointment to see your doctor.

POSSIBLE CAUSE
An allergic reaction to certain medicines can cause a rash (see ALLERGIES, p.152).

ACTION NEEDED
MEDICAL HELP
✚ URGENT! Phone your doctor immediately to find out whether the medicine may be causing your child's symptoms and whether you should stop giving it.

POSSIBLE CAUSE
PITYRIASIS ROSEA (p.140).

ACTION NEEDED
MEDICAL HELP
Make an appointment to see your doctor.
SELF-HELP
See panel: *Relieving itchiness* (p.49).

If you cannot identify your child's problem from this chart, talk to your doctor within 48 hours.

24 ITCHINESS

Itchiness may affect your child's entire body or just one area. The causes of itchiness are varied and range from allergic reactions to infestation by parasites. Intense itchiness can be very upsetting and scratching may lead to infection, so prompt treatment of any underlying disorder is essential.

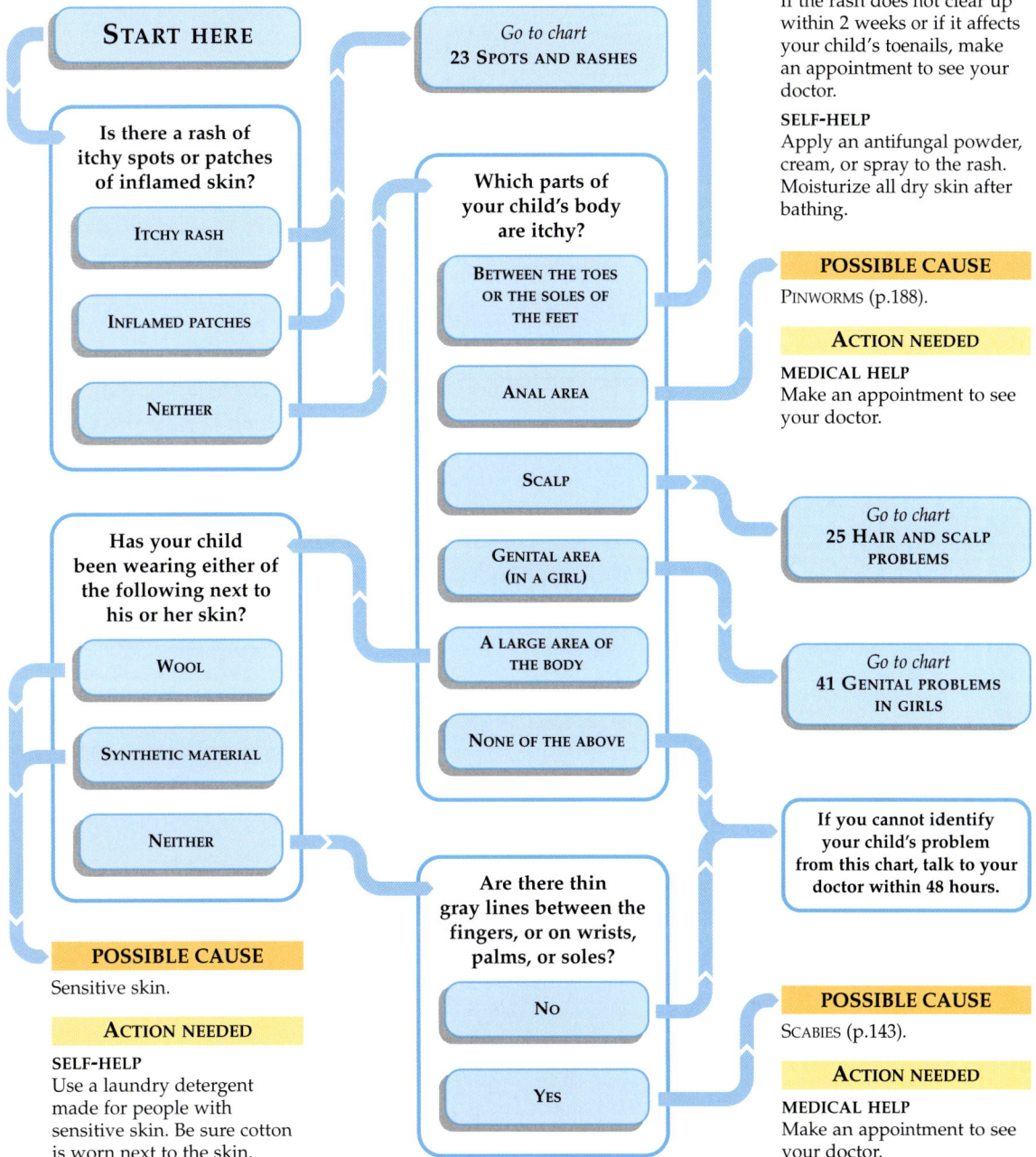

START HERE

**Go to chart
23 SPOTS AND RASHES**

Is there a rash of itchy spots or patches of inflamed skin?

- ITCHY RASH
- INFLAMED PATCHES
- NEITHER

Which parts of your child's body are itchy?

- BETWEEN THE TOES OR THE SOLES OF THE FEET
- ANAL AREA
- SCALP
- GENITAL AREA (IN A GIRL)
- A LARGE AREA OF THE BODY
- NONE OF THE ABOVE

Has your child been wearing either of the following next to his or her skin?

- WOOL
- SYNTHETIC MATERIAL
- NEITHER

Are there thin gray lines between the fingers, or on wrists, palms, or soles?

- NO
- YES

POSSIBLE CAUSE

Athlete's foot (see p.142) or ECZEMA (see p.135).

ACTION NEEDED

MEDICAL HELP
If the rash does not clear up within 2 weeks or if it affects your child's toenails, make an appointment to see your doctor.

SELF-HELP
Apply an antifungal powder, cream, or spray to the rash. Moisturize all dry skin after bathing.

POSSIBLE CAUSE

PINWORMS (p.188).

ACTION NEEDED

MEDICAL HELP
Make an appointment to see your doctor.

**Go to chart
25 HAIR AND SCALP PROBLEMS**

**Go to chart
41 GENITAL PROBLEMS IN GIRLS**

If you cannot identify your child's problem from this chart, talk to your doctor within 48 hours.

POSSIBLE CAUSE

Sensitive skin.

ACTION NEEDED

SELF-HELP
Use a laundry detergent made for people with sensitive skin. Be sure cotton is worn next to the skin.

POSSIBLE CAUSE

SCABIES (p.143).

ACTION NEEDED

MEDICAL HELP
Make an appointment to see your doctor.

25 HAIR AND SCALP PROBLEMS

Although problems with the hair and scalp are fairly common in children, they are rarely serious. Skin conditions, infections, or infestations by parasites are the most likely causes of scalp problems, while pulling on the hair or having the hair tied back tightly are the most probable reasons for hair loss.

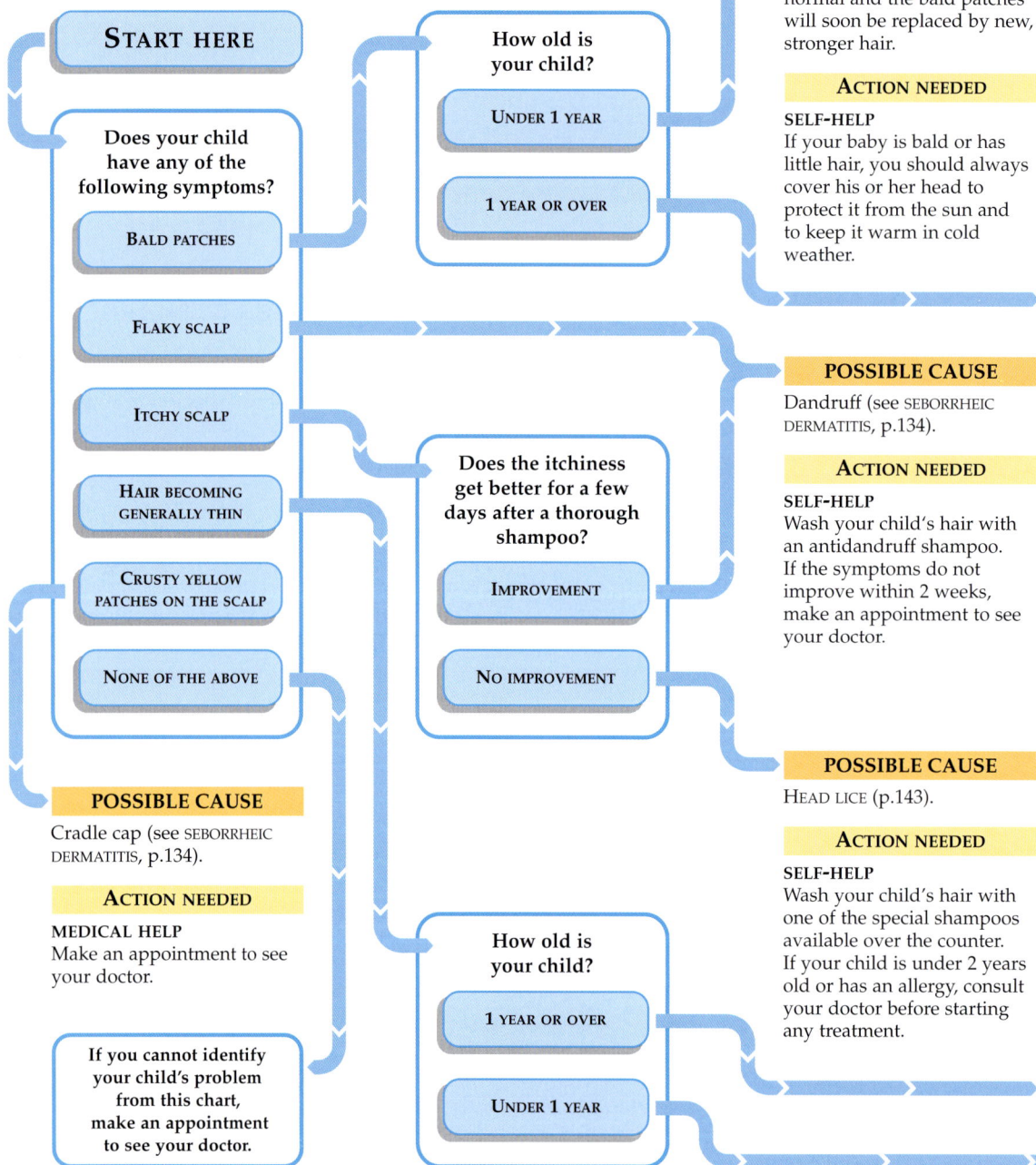

START HERE

Does your child have any of the following symptoms?

- BALD PATCHES
- FLAKY SCALP
- ITCHY SCALP
- HAIR BECOMING GENERALLY THIN
- CRUSTY YELLOW PATCHES ON THE SCALP
- NONE OF THE ABOVE

How old is your child?

- UNDER 1 YEAR
- 1 YEAR OR OVER

Does the itchiness get better for a few days after a thorough shampoo?

- IMPROVEMENT
- NO IMPROVEMENT

How old is your child?

- 1 YEAR OR OVER
- UNDER 1 YEAR

POSSIBLE CAUSE

If your infant often rubs his or her head on the crib or baby seat, bald patches may develop as the delicate first hair falls out. This hair loss is normal and the bald patches will soon be replaced by new, stronger hair.

ACTION NEEDED

SELF-HELP
If your baby is bald or has little hair, you should always cover his or her head to protect it from the sun and to keep it warm in cold weather.

POSSIBLE CAUSE

Dandruff (see SEBORRHEIC DERMATITIS, p.134).

ACTION NEEDED

SELF-HELP
Wash your child's hair with an antidandruff shampoo. If the symptoms do not improve within 2 weeks, make an appointment to see your doctor.

POSSIBLE CAUSE

HEAD LICE (p.143).

ACTION NEEDED

SELF-HELP
Wash your child's hair with one of the special shampoos available over the counter. If your child is under 2 years old or has an allergy, consult your doctor before starting any treatment.

POSSIBLE CAUSE

Cradle cap (see SEBORRHEIC DERMATITIS, p.134).

ACTION NEEDED

MEDICAL HELP
Make an appointment to see your doctor.

If you cannot identify your child's problem from this chart, make an appointment to see your doctor.

How does the skin in the bald areas look?

NORMAL

SCALY AND INFLAMED

POSSIBLE CAUSE

A form of localized baldness, which often may have no apparent cause.

ACTION NEEDED

MEDICAL HELP
Make an appointment to see your doctor.

POSSIBLE CAUSE

Ringworm (see FUNGAL INFECTIONS, p.142)

ACTION NEEDED

MEDICAL HELP
Make an appointment to see your doctor.

Do either of the following apply to your child?

HAS RECENTLY HAD AN ILLNESS

IS TAKING MEDICINE

NEITHER

POSSIBLE CAUSE

General thinning of the hair could be a result of a recent illness. The hair will probably return to its normal thickness over the next few months.

ACTION NEEDED

MEDICAL HELP
If you are worried, consult your doctor.

POSSIBLE CAUSE

The thinning of your child's hair could be a side effect of the medicine that he or she is taking.

ACTION NEEDED

MEDICAL HELP
Phone your doctor to find out whether the medicine may be causing your child's symptoms and whether you should stop giving it.

Does your child play with his or her hair or is it tied back?

HABITUALLY PULLS OR TWISTS HAIR

WEARS HAIR IN TIGHT PONYTAILS OR BRAIDS

NEITHER

POSSIBLE CAUSE

As the baby hair falls out, your infant's hair will be noticeably thinner until the new, stronger hair grows in. This process is normal and is not a cause for concern.

ACTION NEEDED

SELF-HELP
Cover your baby's head to protect it from the sun and to keep it warm in cold weather.

POSSIBLE CAUSE

Habitual hair pulling may indicate an underlying psychological problem (see HABITUAL BEHAVIOR, p.169).

ACTION NEEDED

MEDICAL HELP
If your child is losing a lot of hair or if he or she has other behavioral problems, make an appointment to see your doctor.

POSSIBLE CAUSE

Damage to the hair roots, caused by excessive pulling of the hair, can result in temporary hair loss.

ACTION NEEDED

SELF-HELP
Change your child's hairstyle or have his or her hair cut.

If you cannot identify your child's problem from this chart, make an appointment to see your doctor.

26 BREATHING PROBLEMS

Breathing problems range from noisy or fast breathing to difficulty in breathing. Many babies and children wheeze slightly when they have a minor respiratory infection. However, breathing problems that are accompanied by danger signs (see right) constitute a medical emergency.

DANGER SIGNS
If your child's breathing problems are accompanied by any of the following symptoms, you should call an ambulance at once:
• Blue-tinged lips or tongue.
• Abnormal drowsiness.
• Inability to talk or produce sounds normally.

START HERE

How long has your child had breathing problems?
- STARTED SUDDENLY A FEW MINUTES AGO
- STARTED MORE THAN A FEW MINUTES AGO

Are any of the following danger signs present?
- BLUE-TINGED LIPS OR TONGUE
- ABNORMAL DROWSINESS
- INABILITY TO TALK OR PRODUCE SOUNDS NORMALLY
- NONE OF THE ABOVE

How old is your child?
- 18 MONTHS OR OVER
- UNDER 18 MONTHS

Could your child be choking on a small object?
- POSSIBLY
- UNLIKELY

Has your child had an asthma attack in the past or is he or she being treated for asthma?

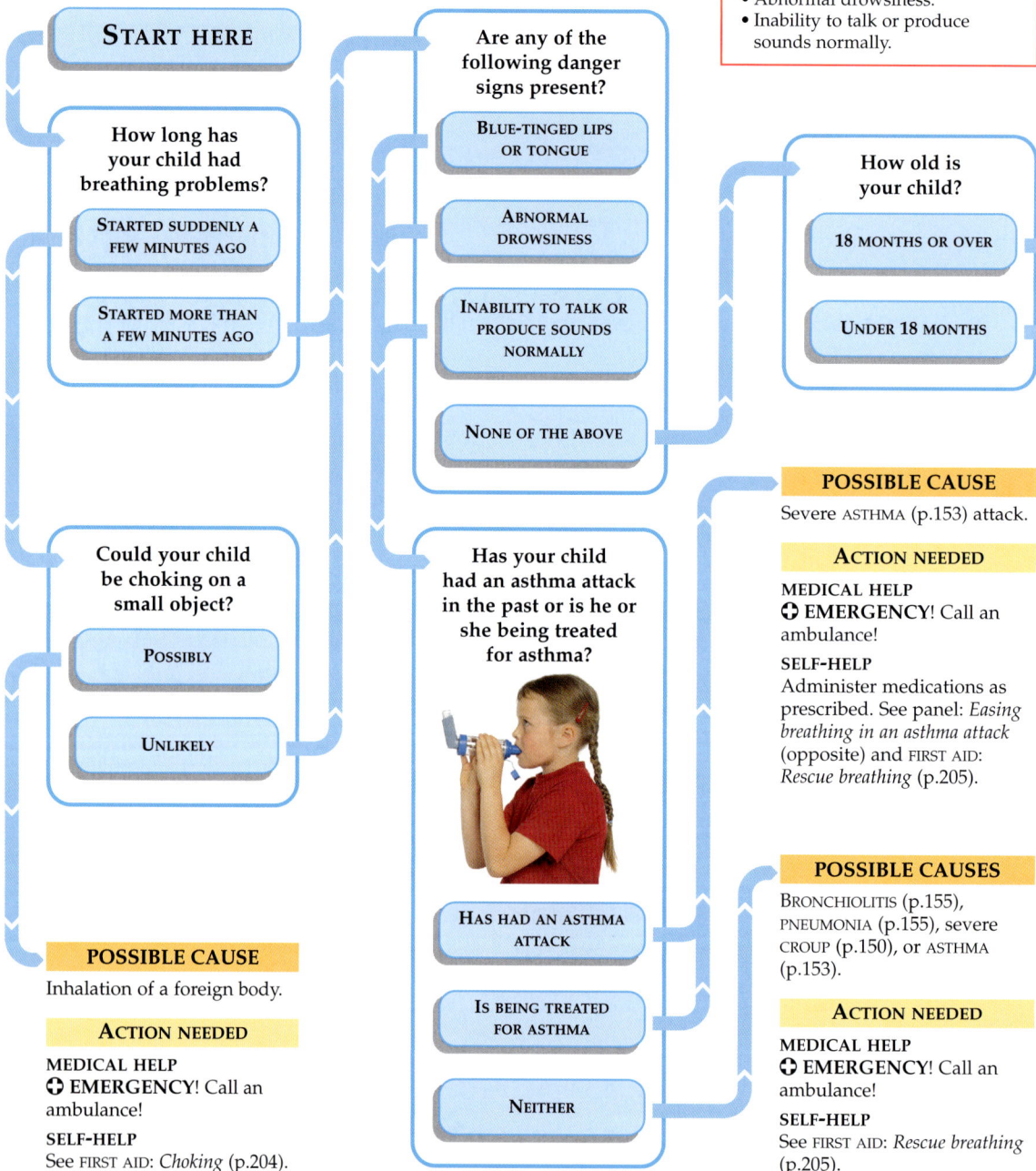

- HAS HAD AN ASTHMA ATTACK
- IS BEING TREATED FOR ASTHMA
- NEITHER

POSSIBLE CAUSE
Severe ASTHMA (p.153) attack.

ACTION NEEDED
MEDICAL HELP
✚ EMERGENCY! Call an ambulance!
SELF-HELP
Administer medications as prescribed. See panel: *Easing breathing in an asthma attack* (opposite) and FIRST AID: *Rescue breathing* (p.205).

POSSIBLE CAUSES
BRONCHIOLITIS (p.155), PNEUMONIA (p.155), severe CROUP (p.150), or ASTHMA (p.153).

ACTION NEEDED
MEDICAL HELP
✚ EMERGENCY! Call an ambulance!
SELF-HELP
See FIRST AID: *Rescue breathing* (p.205).

POSSIBLE CAUSE
Inhalation of a foreign body.

ACTION NEEDED
MEDICAL HELP
✚ EMERGENCY! Call an ambulance!
SELF-HELP
See FIRST AID: *Choking* (p.204).

Does your child suffer from repeated episodes of any of these symptoms?

WHEEZING

SHORTNESS OF BREATH

COUGHING AT NIGHT

NONE OF THE ABOVE

SELF-HELP: EASING BREATHING IN AN ASTHMA ATTACK

If your child is having difficulty in breathing, the following measures may help:
- Help your child to sit up, leaning forward against a table or the back of a chair.
- If medicine has been prescribed, make sure it is used as soon as breathing difficulties start.
- Try to keep other people away since crowds may cause further worry, making breathing harder.

Breathing position
Help your child sit up and lean against a table, using the elbows as a support.

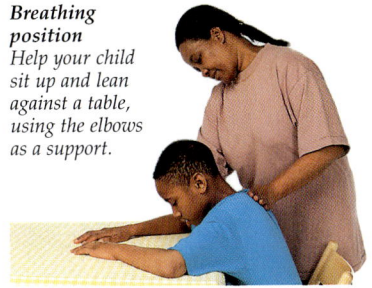

POSSIBLE CAUSE

ASTHMA (p.153).

ACTION NEEDED

MEDICAL HELP
If your child seems very sick or if breathing difficulties develop, phone your doctor immediately.

SELF-HELP
See panel: *Easing breathing in an asthma attack* (above).

POSSIBLE CAUSES

PNEUMONIA (p.155) or BRONCHIOLITIS (p.155).

ACTION NEEDED

MEDICAL HELP
✛ URGENT! Phone your doctor immediately!

SELF-HELP
See panels: *Easing breathing in an asthma attack* (above) and *Checking breathing rates* (p.90).

Has your child had noisy, crowing breathing since birth but otherwise been healthy?

NO

YES

Do either of the following apply to your child?

FAST BREATHING, FEVER, AND COUGH

HOARSE VOICE, NOISY BREATHING, AND BARKING COUGH

NEITHER

POSSIBLE CAUSE

CROUP (p.150).

ACTION NEEDED

MEDICAL HELP
✛ URGENT! Phone your doctor immediately!

Has there been a recent change in your child's breathing?

CHANGE IN BREATHING

NO CHANGE IN BREATHING

POSSIBLE CAUSE

Congenital laryngeal stridor, a harmless condition that your child will outgrow.

ACTION NEEDED

MEDICAL HELP
If there is no improvement by the age of 3 months, make an appointment to see your doctor.

POSSIBLE CAUSES

ASTHMA (p.153) or BRONCHIOLITIS (p.155).

ACTION NEEDED

MEDICAL HELP
Get medical advice within 24 hours.

SELF-HELP
See panel: *Easing breathing in an asthma attack* (above).

27 COUGHING

In very young babies, coughing is rare and may indicate a serious lung infection. In older children, however, coughing is usually caused by a minor respiratory infection, such as a cold. A sudden cough in any child who is otherwise well can be serious as it may be caused by an airway obstruction.

DANGER SIGNS
Call an ambulance at once if your child has any of the following symptoms:
- Blue-tinged lips or tongue.
- Abnormal drowsiness.
- Inability to talk or produce sounds.
Phone your doctor at once if your child has the following symptom:
- Areas between ribs appear sunken when breathing in.

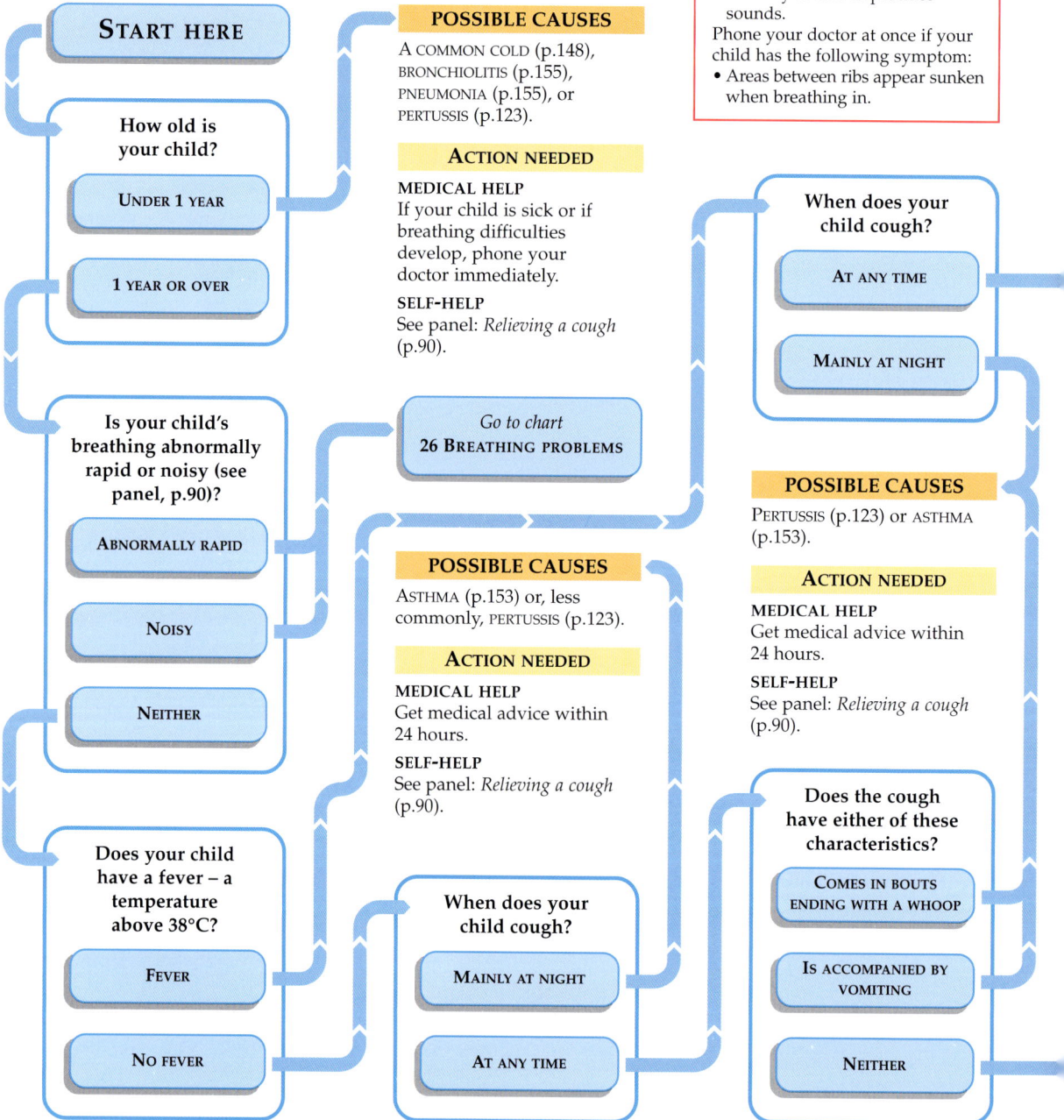

START HERE

How old is your child?
- UNDER 1 YEAR
- 1 YEAR OR OVER

POSSIBLE CAUSES
A COMMON COLD (p.148), BRONCHIOLITIS (p.155), PNEUMONIA (p.155), or PERTUSSIS (p.123).

ACTION NEEDED
MEDICAL HELP
If your child is sick or if breathing difficulties develop, phone your doctor immediately.
SELF-HELP
See panel: *Relieving a cough* (p.90).

Is your child's breathing abnormally rapid or noisy (see panel, p.90)?
- ABNORMALLY RAPID
- NOISY
- NEITHER

Go to chart
26 BREATHING PROBLEMS

POSSIBLE CAUSES
ASTHMA (p.153) or, less commonly, PERTUSSIS (p.123).

ACTION NEEDED
MEDICAL HELP
Get medical advice within 24 hours.
SELF-HELP
See panel: *Relieving a cough* (p.90).

Does your child have a fever – a temperature above 38°C?
- FEVER
- NO FEVER

When does your child cough?
- MAINLY AT NIGHT
- AT ANY TIME

When does your child cough?
- AT ANY TIME
- MAINLY AT NIGHT

POSSIBLE CAUSES
PERTUSSIS (p.123) or ASTHMA (p.153).

ACTION NEEDED
MEDICAL HELP
Get medical advice within 24 hours.
SELF-HELP
See panel: *Relieving a cough* (p.90).

Does the cough have either of these characteristics?
- COMES IN BOUTS ENDING WITH A WHOOP
- IS ACCOMPANIED BY VOMITING
- NEITHER

Do either of the following apply to your child?

- HAS A RASH
- HAS RECENTLY BEEN EXPOSED TO MEASLES
- NEITHER

Does your child have any nasal symptoms?

- STUFFY NOSE
- RUNNY NOSE
- NEITHER

POSSIBLE CAUSE

MEASLES (p.118).

ACTION NEEDED

MEDICAL HELP
Get medical advice within 24 hours.

SELF-HELP
See panel: *Bringing down a high temperature* (p.37).

POSSIBLE CAUSES

A COMMON COLD (p.148) or INFLUENZA (p.151).

ACTION NEEDED

MEDICAL HELP
If breathing difficulties develop, phone your doctor. If a rash appears, get medical advice within 24 hours.

SELF-HELP
See panels: *Relieving a cough* (p.90) and *Bringing down a high temperature* (p.37).

POSSIBLE CAUSE

A COMMON COLD (p.148).

ACTION NEEDED

MEDICAL HELP
If your child is distressed by the symptoms, consult your doctor.

SELF-HELP
See panel: *Relieving a cough* (p.90).

POSSIBLE CAUSE

Inhalation of a foreign body.

ACTION NEEDED

MEDICAL HELP
✚ URGENT! Phone your doctor immediately!

SELF-HELP
See FIRST AID: *Choking* (p.204).

POSSIBLE CAUSE

SINUSITIS (p.149).

ACTION NEEDED

MEDICAL HELP
Make an appointment to see your doctor.

SELF-HELP
If the ear infections are causing pain, see panel: *Relieving earache* (p.101).

How long has your child been coughing?

- LESS THAN 24 HOURS
- 24 HOURS OR MORE

Is your child's nose continuously runny?

- CONTINUOUSLY RUNNY
- NOT RUNNY

Does your child also have either of the following symptoms?

- FREQUENT EAR INFECTIONS
- NASAL VOICE
- NEITHER

POSSIBLE CAUSE

Overlapping colds (see COMMON COLD, p.148).

ACTION NEEDED

MEDICAL HELP
If your child seems generally sick or is upset by the cough, consult your doctor.

SELF-HELP
See panel: *Relieving a cough* (p.90).

continued on p.90, top

27 Coughing (continued)

continued from p.89, bottom

Do either of the following apply to your child?

- **HAS HAD PERTUSSIS WITHIN THE LAST FEW MONTHS**
- **HAS BEEN DIAGNOSED AS HAVING ASTHMA**
- **NEITHER**

POSSIBLE CAUSE

ASTHMA (p.153).

ACTION NEEDED

MEDICAL HELP
If there is no improvement within 24 hours, consult your doctor.

SELF-HELP
Make sure that your child is taking his or her asthma medicine as directed. See panels: *Easing breathing in an asthma attack* (p.87) and *Relieving a cough* (below).

Are there smokers in your home, or could your child have been smoking?

- **SMOKERS IN THE HOME**
- **CHILD MIGHT SMOKE**
- **NEITHER**

ASSESSMENT: CHECKING BREATHING RATES

A child whose breathing rate is unusually rapid may need medical attention. To check your child's breathing, make sure that he or she is resting, then count the number of breaths over one minute.

Normal breathing rates
As a child grows older and the breathing apparatus matures, his or her normal breathing rate (the breathing rate at rest, not when active or crying) decreases. A young baby breathes much faster than a child who is 5 years of age or over.

AGE	NORMAL RATE
Under 2 months	Less than 60 breaths per minute
2 to 11 months	Less than 50 breaths per minute
1 to 5 years	Less than 40 breaths per minute
Over 5 years	Less than 30 breaths per minute

POSSIBLE CAUSE

Cough persisting after PERTUSSIS (p.123).

ACTION NEEDED

MEDICAL HELP
If your child is upset by the cough or feels sick, or if the cough lasts for more than 3 months, make an appointment to see your doctor.

SELF-HELP
See panel: *Relieving a cough* (below).

POSSIBLE CAUSE

Irritation of the throat and lungs as a result of smoking or of being in a smoky atmosphere.

ACTION NEEDED

SELF-HELP
Make sure no one smokes around your child. If your child smokes, encourage him or her to give it up (see SUBSTANCE ABUSE, p.174).

If you cannot identify your child's problem from this chart, talk to your doctor within 48 hours.

SELF-HELP: RELIEVING A COUGH

The following measures may help to relieve your child's cough:
- Give soothing liquids, such as warm water mixed with honey (do not give honey to children under 1 because it may cause food poisoning), and plenty of other warm or cool drinks.
- Moisten the air by hanging a wet towel in front of a radiator.
- Do not overheat your child's room because this will dry out the air and increase coughing.

Relieving a coughing fit
Sit a young child on your lap, leaning slightly forward, and pat his or her back to loosen any phlegm.

28 SORE THROAT

Most sore throats in children are caused by minor viral infections that clear up quickly without treatment. However, a sore throat can indicate a more serious problem, such as streptococcal (or strep) pharyngitis. In very young children, reluctance to eat or drink may be a sign of a sore throat.

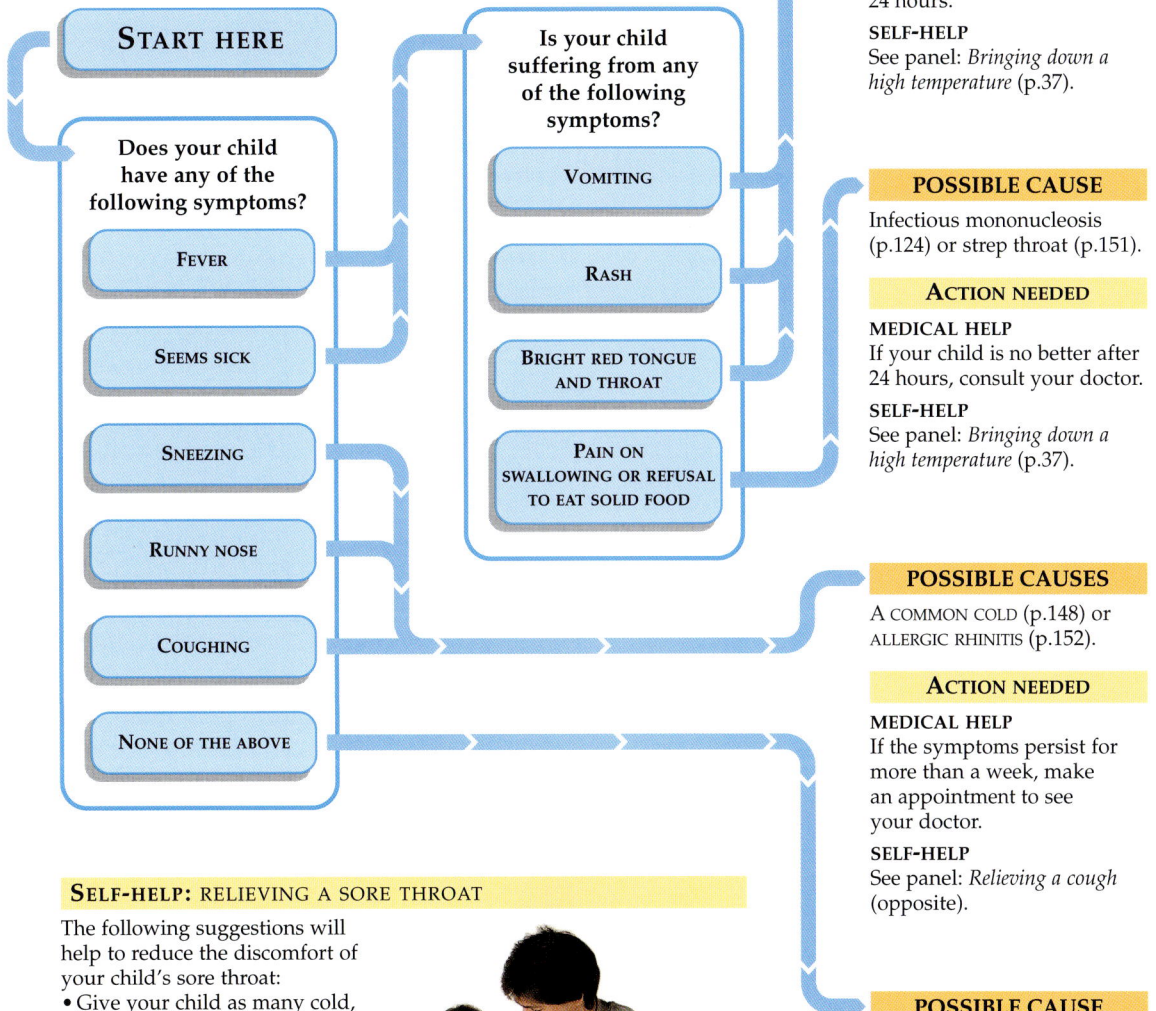

START HERE

Does your child have any of the following symptoms?

- FEVER
- SEEMS SICK
- SNEEZING
- RUNNY NOSE
- COUGHING
- NONE OF THE ABOVE

Is your child suffering from any of the following symptoms?

- VOMITING
- RASH
- BRIGHT RED TONGUE AND THROAT
- PAIN ON SWALLOWING OR REFUSAL TO EAT SOLID FOOD

POSSIBLE CAUSE

SCARLET FEVER (p.121).

ACTION NEEDED

MEDICAL HELP
Get medical advice within 24 hours.

SELF-HELP
See panel: *Bringing down a high temperature* (p.37).

POSSIBLE CAUSE

Infectious mononucleosis (p.124) or strep throat (p.151).

ACTION NEEDED

MEDICAL HELP
If your child is no better after 24 hours, consult your doctor.

SELF-HELP
See panel: *Bringing down a high temperature* (p.37).

POSSIBLE CAUSES

A COMMON COLD (p.148) or ALLERGIC RHINITIS (p.152).

ACTION NEEDED

MEDICAL HELP
If the symptoms persist for more than a week, make an appointment to see your doctor.

SELF-HELP
See panel: *Relieving a cough* (opposite).

POSSIBLE CAUSE

Inflammation of the throat caused by a minor infection or irritation.

ACTION NEEDED

MEDICAL HELP
If your child's throat is still sore after 48 hours, make an appointment to see your doctor.

SELF-HELP: RELIEVING A SORE THROAT

The following suggestions will help to reduce the discomfort of your child's sore throat:

- Give your child as many cold, nonacidic drinks, and as much ice cream and gelatin to eat, as he or she wants.
- Give regular doses (15 mgm per kg) of liquid acetaminophen.
- Offer throat lozenges if your child is old enough to suck rather than chew them.
- Let a child over 8 years old gargle with a pinch of salt in 90–120 ml of warm water.

Soothing a sore throat
Cold, nonacidic drinks, such as milk, may help to soothe your child's sore throat. A straw makes drinking easier.

29 ABNORMAL DROWSINESS OR CONFUSION

Drowsiness may simply be a result of lack of sleep or a minor illness, or it may be a symptom of a serious disease, such as meningitis. Confusion – which includes appearing dazed or agitated, or talking nonsense – is always a serious symptom that requires immediate medical attention.

DANGER SIGNS

Call an ambulance at once if your child has any of the following symptoms:
- Unconscious for 3 minutes.
- Unresponsive or difficult to rouse from sleep.
- Blood or fluid leaking from the nose or ears.
- Irregular, slow, or fast breathing.

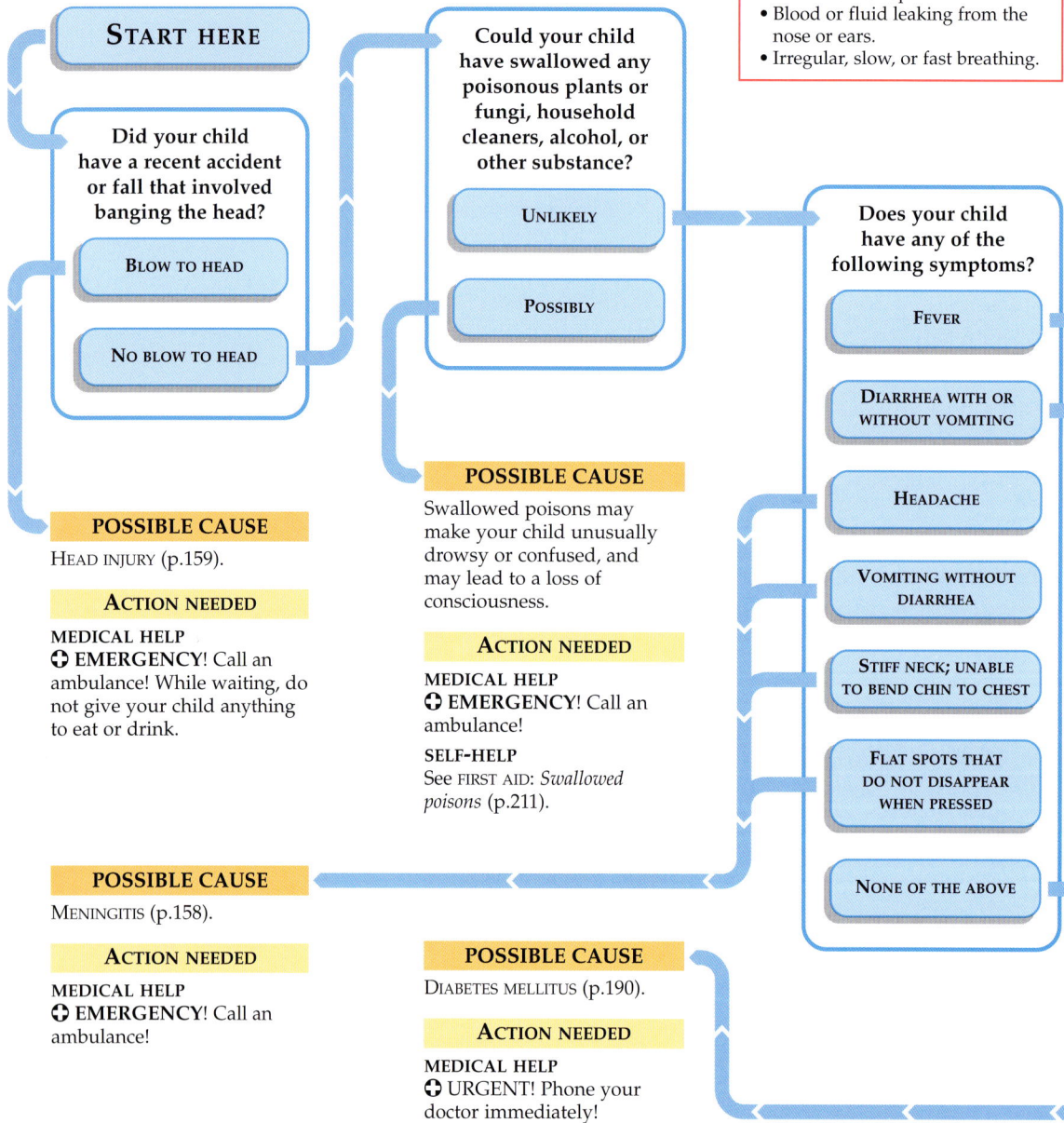

START HERE

Did your child have a recent accident or fall that involved banging the head?

- BLOW TO HEAD
- NO BLOW TO HEAD

Could your child have swallowed any poisonous plants or fungi, household cleaners, alcohol, or other substance?

- UNLIKELY
- POSSIBLY

Does your child have any of the following symptoms?

- FEVER
- DIARRHEA WITH OR WITHOUT VOMITING
- HEADACHE
- VOMITING WITHOUT DIARRHEA
- STIFF NECK; UNABLE TO BEND CHIN TO CHEST
- FLAT SPOTS THAT DO NOT DISAPPEAR WHEN PRESSED
- NONE OF THE ABOVE

POSSIBLE CAUSE
HEAD INJURY (p.159).

ACTION NEEDED
MEDICAL HELP
✚ EMERGENCY! Call an ambulance! While waiting, do not give your child anything to eat or drink.

POSSIBLE CAUSE
Swallowed poisons may make your child unusually drowsy or confused, and may lead to a loss of consciousness.

ACTION NEEDED
MEDICAL HELP
✚ EMERGENCY! Call an ambulance!
SELF-HELP
See FIRST AID: *Swallowed poisons* (p.211).

POSSIBLE CAUSE
MENINGITIS (p.158).

ACTION NEEDED
MEDICAL HELP
✚ EMERGENCY! Call an ambulance!

POSSIBLE CAUSE
DIABETES MELLITUS (p.190).

ACTION NEEDED
MEDICAL HELP
✚ URGENT! Phone your doctor immediately!

POSSIBLE CAUSES

A high fever, resulting from any infection but especially MENINGITIS (p.158) or a kidney or liver infection, may cause delirium, particularly if your child's temperature goes above 39°C.

ACTION NEEDED

MEDICAL HELP
✚ URGENT! Phone your doctor immediately!

SELF-HELP
See panel: *Bringing down a high temperature* (p.37).

POSSIBLE CAUSE

Your child may be suffering from dehydration as a result of GASTROENTERITIS (p.180).

ACTION NEEDED

MEDICAL HELP
✚ URGENT! Phone your doctor immediately!

SELF-HELP
See panel: *Preventing dehydration in babies* (p.38) or *Preventing dehydration in children* (p.53).

POSSIBLE CAUSE

DIABETES MELLITUS (p.190).

ACTION NEEDED

MEDICAL HELP
✚ URGENT! Phone your doctor immediately!

POSSIBLE CAUSE

Certain medicines, such as antihistamines given for ALLERGIES (p.152), can cause confusion or have a sedative effect on some children.

ACTION NEEDED

MEDICAL HELP
Phone your doctor to find out whether the medicine may be causing your child's symptoms and whether you should stop giving it.

POSSIBLE CAUSE

SUBSTANCE ABUSE (p.174).

ACTION NEEDED

MEDICAL HELP
Make an appointment to see your doctor.

Has your child been passing an unusually large quantity of urine?

- LARGE AMOUNT OF URINE
- NORMAL AMOUNT OF URINE

Have you noticed any of the following changes in your child's appearance or behavior?

- RED EYES
- LOSS OF APPETITE
- MOOD SWINGS
- WITHDRAWAL
- AGGRESSION
- NONE OF THE ABOVE

Is your child suffering from any of the following symptoms?

- EXCESSIVE THIRST
- LOSS OF WEIGHT
- UNCHARACTERISTIC TIREDNESS DURING THE LAST FEW WEEKS
- NONE OF THE ABOVE

Have you been giving your child any medicine?

- MEDICINE
- NO MEDICINE

If you cannot identify your child's problem from this chart, talk to your doctor at once.

30 DIZZINESS, FAINTING, AND SEIZURES

Dizziness is a spinning sensation. It may be accompanied by an attack of faintness or lightheadedness. Fainting is a brief loss of consciousness that is caused by a fall in blood pressure. A seizure may also involve a loss of consciousness, but it is a result of abnormal electrical activity in the brain.

DANGER SIGNS

Call an ambulance at once if your child has lost consciousness and any of the following occur:
- Consciousness is not regained within 3 minutes.
- Breathing becomes slower.
- Breathing is irregular or noisy.

START HERE

Does your child have any of the following symptoms?

- **FELL DOWN UNCONSCIOUS**
- **FEELS SURROUNDINGS ARE GOING AROUND AND AROUND**
- **SEEMS UNAWARE OF SURROUNDINGS FOR A FEW MOMENTS**
- **FEELS FAINT OR UNSTEADY**
- **NONE OF THE ABOVE**

During your child's loss of consciousness, did any of the following occur?

- **TWITCHING OF THE FACE OR LIMBS**
- **URINATION**
- **INJURY, SUCH AS BITING THE TONGUE**
- **NONE OF THE ABOVE**

POSSIBLE CAUSE

LABYRINTHITIS (p.164).

ACTION NEEDED

MEDICAL HELP
Make an appointment to see your doctor.

POSSIBLE CAUSE

An absence seizure (see EPILEPSY, p.157).

ACTION NEEDED

MEDICAL HELP
Make an appointment to see your doctor.

SELF-HELP
Sit your child down quietly until fully recovered.

POSSIBLE CAUSE

Low blood sugar level (hypoglycemia), caused by DIABETES MELLITUS (p.190).

ACTION NEEDED

MEDICAL HELP
If your child often feels faint, make an appointment to see your doctor.

SELF-HELP
As soon as your child feels faint, give glucose tablets or a glucose or sweet drink. See panel: *Dealing with faintness and fainting* (opposite).

Is your child being treated for diabetes mellitus?

- **YES**
- **NO**

If you cannot identify your child's problem from this chart, talk to your doctor within 48 hours.

Is your child being treated for diabetes mellitus?

YES

NO

How old is your child?

UNDER 5 YEARS

5 YEARS OR OVER

Does your child have a fever – a temperature above 38°C?

NO FEVER

FEVER

POSSIBLE CAUSE

Extremely low blood sugar level (severe hypoglycemia), caused by DIABETES MELLITUS (p.190), may cause your child to lose consciousness and, in some cases, to have a seizure.

ACTION NEEDED

MEDICAL HELP
✚ **EMERGENCY!** Call an ambulance! While waiting, give glucagon by injection.

POSSIBLE CAUSE

A seizure (see EPILEPSY, p.157).

ACTION NEEDED

MEDICAL HELP
✚ URGENT! Phone your doctor immediately!

POSSIBLE CAUSE

FEBRILE SEIZURES (p.156).

ACTION NEEDED

MEDICAL HELP
✚ URGENT! Phone your doctor immediately!

SELF-HELP
See panel: *Bringing down a high temperature* (p.37).

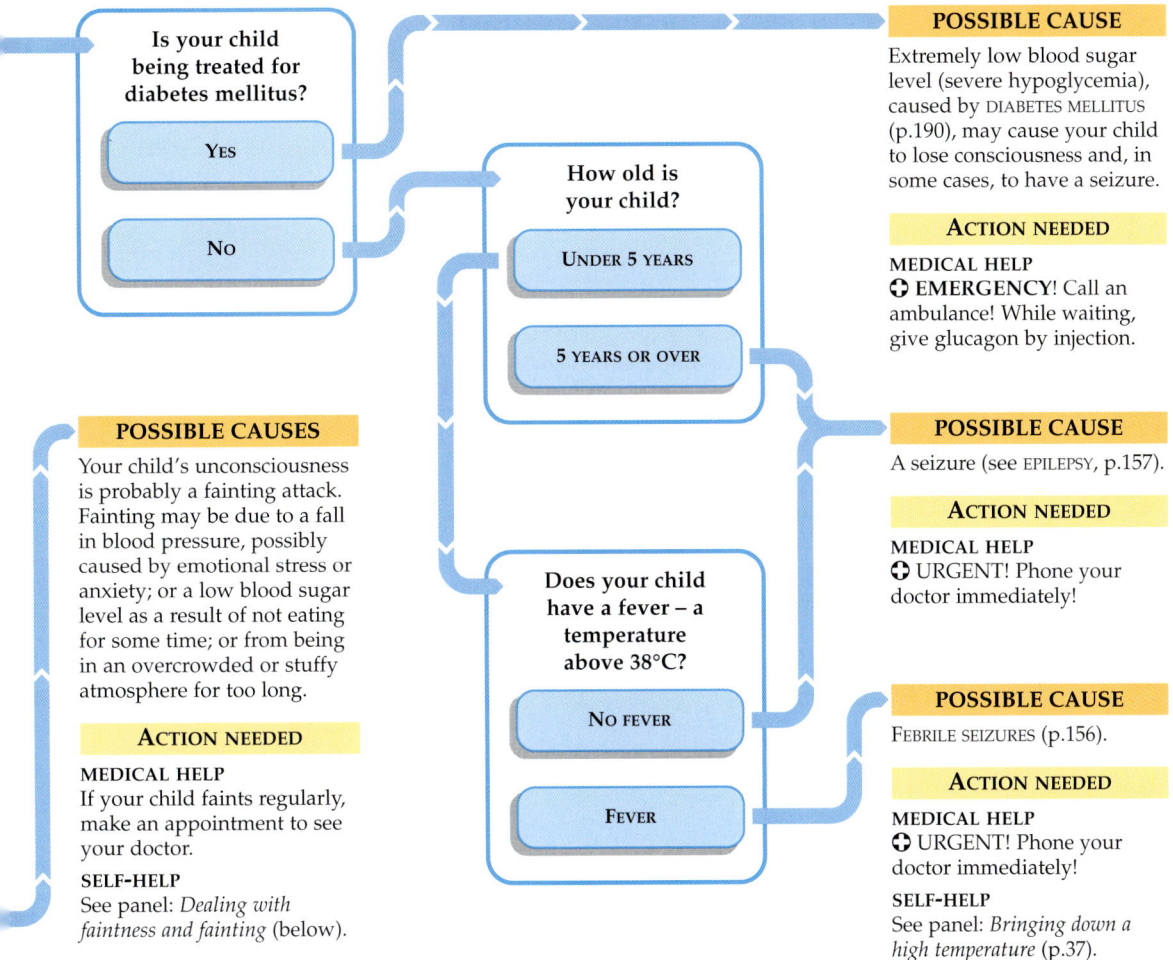

POSSIBLE CAUSES

Your child's unconsciousness is probably a fainting attack. Fainting may be due to a fall in blood pressure, possibly caused by emotional stress or anxiety; or a low blood sugar level as a result of not eating for some time; or from being in an overcrowded or stuffy atmosphere for too long.

ACTION NEEDED

MEDICAL HELP
If your child faints regularly, make an appointment to see your doctor.

SELF-HELP
See panel: *Dealing with faintness and fainting* (below).

POSSIBLE CAUSES

Hunger, a rapid heartbeat, a stuffy atmosphere, or anxiety may cause faintness. A child who is feeling faint may experience dizziness, nausea, and weakness; the child will also have a very pale face.

ACTION NEEDED

MEDICAL HELP
If your child has not shown any signs of recovery within 30 minutes, phone your doctor immediately.

SELF-HELP
See panel: *Dealing with faintness and fainting* (right).

SELF-HELP: DEALING WITH FAINTNESS AND FAINTING

A child who feels faint should be laid down with his or her legs propped up on several cushions, and the following steps should be taken:

- Loosen any tight clothing and make sure there is plenty of fresh air.
- Calm and reassure your child.
- Faintness can be caused by low blood sugar, so a sweet drink or small snack may help. Do not offer food or drink if your child is not fully conscious.
- If your child loses consciousness, monitor his or her condition using the ABCs of resuscitation (pp.202–203). Place in the recovery position (p.203) if he or she is unconscious but breathing.

First aid for fainting
Lay your child down with his or her feet raised to increase the supply of blood to the brain.

31 EYE PROBLEMS

Any child with an eye injury, or a foreign body in the eye that cannot be removed by self-help measures (opposite), should receive immediate medical attention. Most other problems, such as itching, redness, watering, and discharge, are caused by infections or irritation and are seldom serious.

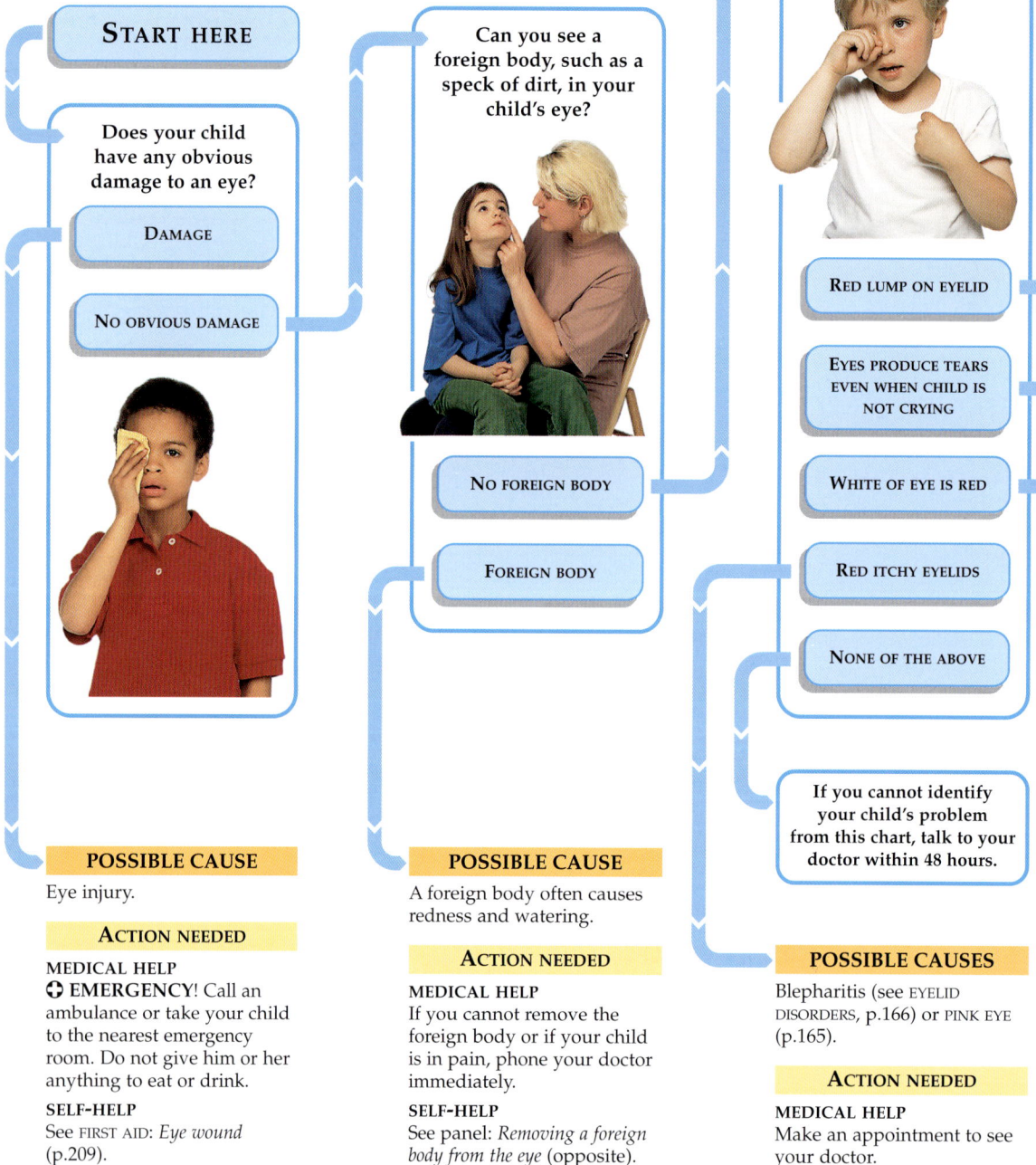

START HERE

Does your child have any obvious damage to an eye?

- DAMAGE
- NO OBVIOUS DAMAGE

Can you see a foreign body, such as a speck of dirt, in your child's eye?

- NO FOREIGN BODY
- FOREIGN BODY

Does your child have any of the following symptoms?

- RED LUMP ON EYELID
- EYES PRODUCE TEARS EVEN WHEN CHILD IS NOT CRYING
- WHITE OF EYE IS RED
- RED ITCHY EYELIDS
- NONE OF THE ABOVE

If you cannot identify your child's problem from this chart, talk to your doctor within 48 hours.

POSSIBLE CAUSE

Eye injury.

ACTION NEEDED

MEDICAL HELP
✚ EMERGENCY! Call an ambulance or take your child to the nearest emergency room. Do not give him or her anything to eat or drink.

SELF-HELP
See FIRST AID: *Eye wound* (p.209).

POSSIBLE CAUSE

A foreign body often causes redness and watering.

ACTION NEEDED

MEDICAL HELP
If you cannot remove the foreign body or if your child is in pain, phone your doctor immediately.

SELF-HELP
See panel: *Removing a foreign body from the eye* (opposite).

POSSIBLE CAUSES

Blepharitis (see EYELID DISORDERS, p.166) or PINK EYE (p.165).

ACTION NEEDED

MEDICAL HELP
Make an appointment to see your doctor.

SELF-HELP: REMOVING A FOREIGN BODY FROM THE EYE

A foreign body, such as an eyelash or a speck of dirt, can usually be removed as illustrated. If the foreign body is metal, or if it is embedded in your child's eye, do not try to remove it. See FIRST AID: *Eye wound* (p.209) and take your child to the hospital at once.

• If you can see the foreign body on your child's lower eyelid or white of the eye, use a corner of a clean, damp tissue to lift it off.

• If your child cannot dislodge the object from the upper eyelid as shown, hold the lashes, pull the eyelid outward, and fold it over a small piece of cotton ball. Remove the object with a tissue.

• If the foreign body is still not visible, seek medical assistance.

Foreign body on lower eyelid
Lift the foreign body off your child's eyelid with the corner of a clean tissue that has been moistened with water.

Foreign body on upper eyelid
Tell your child to pull the upper eyelid down over the lower one to dislodge a foreign body caught under it.

POSSIBLE CAUSE

Stye (see EYELID DISORDERS, p.166).

ACTION NEEDED

MEDICAL HELP
If the eye becomes red and painful, if the stye does not heal within 1 week, or if it recurs, make an appointment to see your doctor.

How old is your child?

> UNDER 1 YEAR

> 1 YEAR OR OVER

POSSIBLE CAUSE

BLOCKED TEAR DUCT (p.165).

ACTION NEEDED

MEDICAL HELP
Make an appointment to see your doctor.

If you cannot identify your child's problem from this chart, talk to your doctor within 48 hours.

POSSIBLE CAUSES

Eye irritation may be caused by chemicals, fumes, or viral or allergic conjunctivitis (PINK EYE, p.165). IRITIS (p.164), a more serious condition, is also a possibility.

ACTION NEEDED

MEDICAL HELP
✚ URGENT! Phone your doctor immediately if your child is in pain. If there is no pain but redness continues for more than 24 hours, make an appointment to see your doctor.

SELF-HELP
See FIRST AID: *Chemical in eye* (p.209).

Does your child's eye have a sticky discharge?

> DISCHARGE

> NO DISCHARGE

POSSIBLE CAUSE

Severe PINK EYE (p.165).

ACTION NEEDED

MEDICAL HELP
Get medical advice within 24 hours.

32 VISION PROBLEMS

Any problem with a child's vision should be investigated promptly. Usually, any defects in vision are picked up at home or at school. You or the teacher may notice that your child is having difficulty in seeing or that there are other eye problems, such as the eyes being out of alignment.

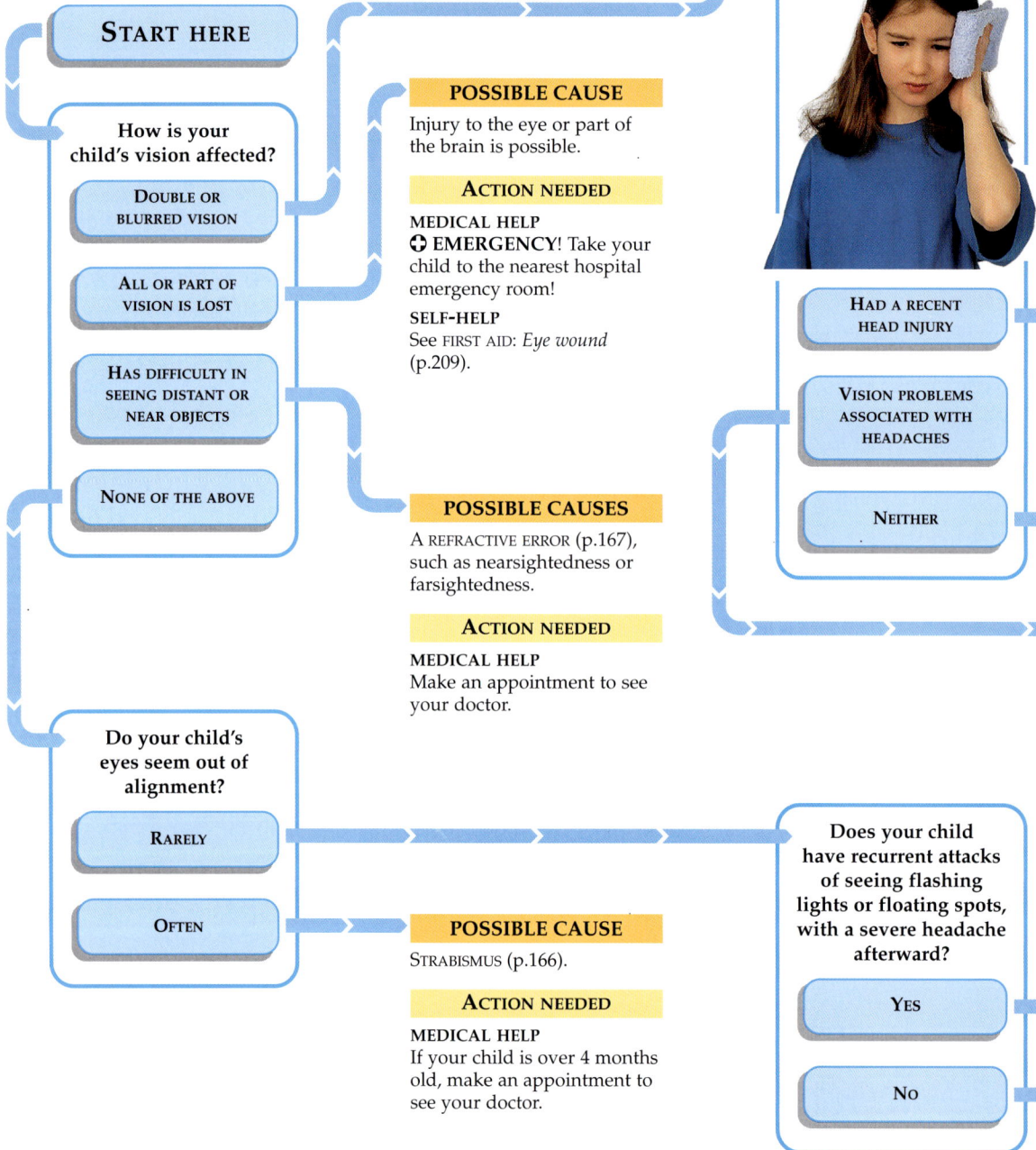

Do either of the following apply to your child?

- **HAD A RECENT HEAD INJURY**
- **VISION PROBLEMS ASSOCIATED WITH HEADACHES**
- **NEITHER**

START HERE

How is your child's vision affected?

- **DOUBLE OR BLURRED VISION**
- **ALL OR PART OF VISION IS LOST**
- **HAS DIFFICULTY IN SEEING DISTANT OR NEAR OBJECTS**
- **NONE OF THE ABOVE**

POSSIBLE CAUSE

Injury to the eye or part of the brain is possible.

ACTION NEEDED

MEDICAL HELP
✚ **EMERGENCY!** Take your child to the nearest hospital emergency room!

SELF-HELP
See FIRST AID: *Eye wound* (p.209).

POSSIBLE CAUSES

A REFRACTIVE ERROR (p.167), such as nearsightedness or farsightedness.

ACTION NEEDED

MEDICAL HELP
Make an appointment to see your doctor.

Do your child's eyes seem out of alignment?

- **RARELY**
- **OFTEN**

POSSIBLE CAUSE

STRABISMUS (p.166).

ACTION NEEDED

MEDICAL HELP
If your child is over 4 months old, make an appointment to see your doctor.

Does your child have recurrent attacks of seeing flashing lights or floating spots, with a severe headache afterward?

- **YES**
- **NO**

POSSIBLE CAUSE

Bleeding inside the skull (see HEAD INJURY, p.159).

ACTION NEEDED

MEDICAL HELP
✚ **EMERGENCY!** Call an ambulance!

Is your child taking any medicine, or could he or she have taken someone else's medicine?

- TAKING MEDICINE
- POSSIBLY TOOK SOMEONE ELSE'S MEDICINE
- NEITHER

Is one or both of your child's eyes red and painful?

- NOT RED OR PAINFUL
- RED AND PAINFUL

POSSIBLE CAUSE

Some drugs may cause blurred vision.

ACTION NEEDED

MEDICAL HELP
Phone your doctor to find out whether the medicine may be causing your child's symptoms and whether you should stop giving it.

POSSIBLE CAUSE

Accidental poisoning by drugs, particularly certain antidepressants, may cause blurred vision.

ACTION NEEDED

MEDICAL HELP
✚ URGENT! Phone your doctor immediately!

SELF-HELP
See FIRST AID: *Swallowed poisons* (p.211).

POSSIBLE CAUSES

A REFRACTIVE ERROR (p.167), such as nearsightedness or farsightedness, or STRABISMUS (p.166) is possible.

ACTION NEEDED

MEDICAL HELP
Make an appointment to see your doctor or optometrist.

POSSIBLE CAUSE

IRITIS (p.164).

ACTION NEEDED

MEDICAL HELP
✚ URGENT! Phone your doctor immediately!

POSSIBLE CAUSE

Migraine (see RECURRENT HEADACHES, p.161).

ACTION NEEDED

MEDICAL HELP
If this is your child's first attack, phone your doctor. If the attacks are frequent, make an appointment to see your doctor.

SELF-HELP
See panel: *Relieving a headache* (p.65).

> **If you cannot identify your child's problem from this chart, talk to your doctor within 48 hours.**

ASSESSMENT: CHECKING YOUR BABY'S VISION

You can use the following method to check developing vision in a baby who is at least 8 weeks old.
- Your baby should sit on another adult's lap, preferably someone with whom your baby is familiar.
- Crouch down so that your face is level with your baby's face, and at arm's length away. Your baby should fixate on your face.
- Move your head from side to side. Your baby should hold your gaze.

An alternative method
Ask another adult to sit your baby on his or her lap and hold a toy at arm's length. Note whether your baby fixates on the toy.

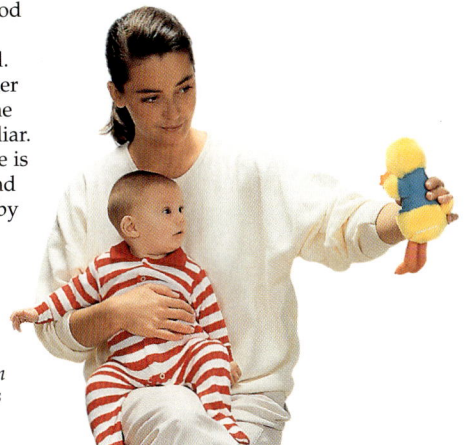

33 PAINFUL OR ITCHY EAR

Earache, in young children especially, is most often caused by upper respiratory infections. Middle ear infections are common because the tubes connecting the ears and nose are short and easily blocked. Disorders that cause symptoms such as itchiness or discharge can affect the outer ear.

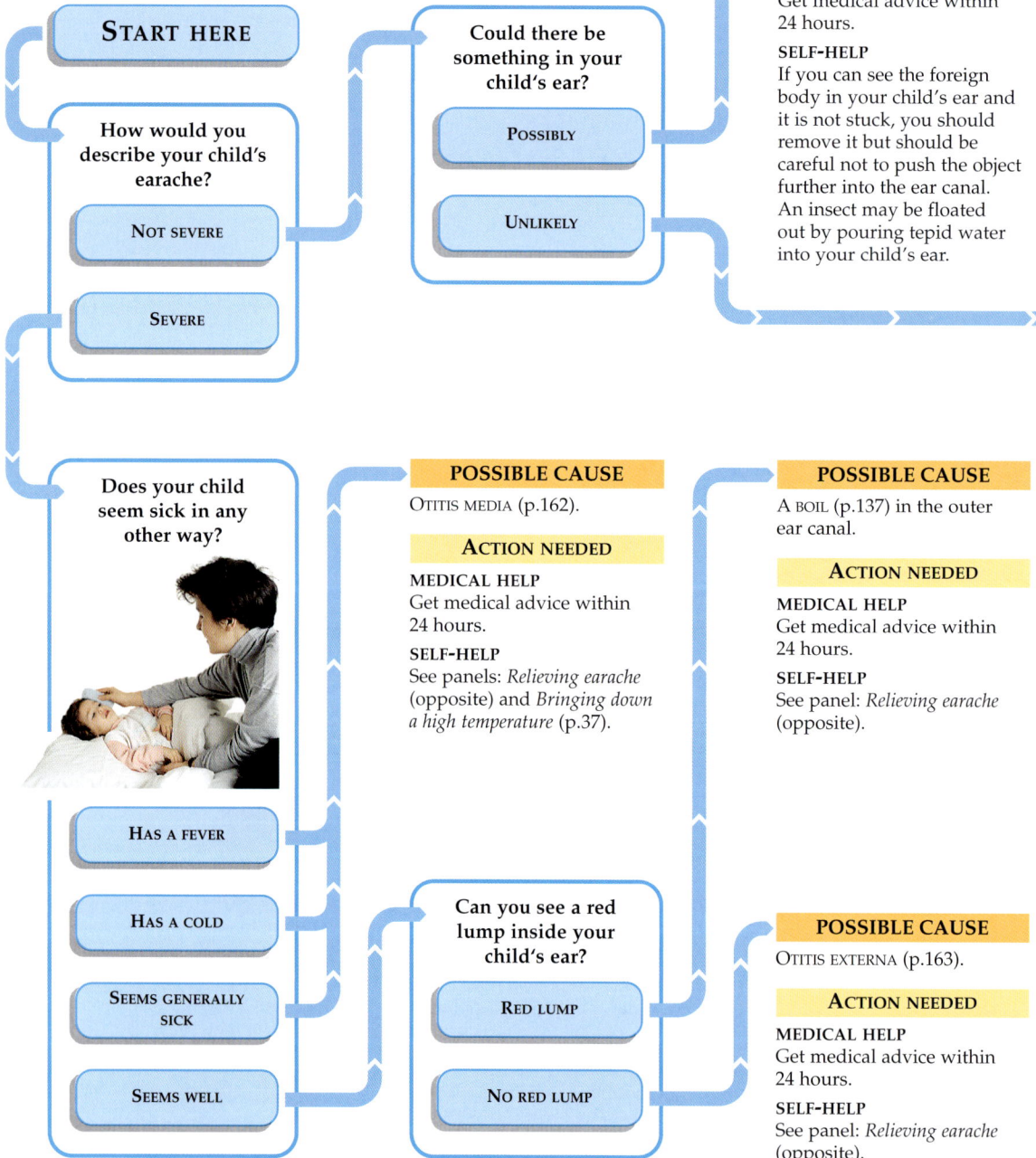

START HERE

How would you describe your child's earache?

NOT SEVERE

SEVERE

Could there be something in your child's ear?

POSSIBLY

UNLIKELY

POSSIBLE CAUSE

A foreign body, such as an insect or bead, in the ear.

ACTION NEEDED

MEDICAL HELP
Get medical advice within 24 hours.

SELF-HELP
If you can see the foreign body in your child's ear and it is not stuck, you should remove it but should be careful not to push the object further into the ear canal. An insect may be floated out by pouring tepid water into your child's ear.

Does your child seem sick in any other way?

HAS A FEVER

HAS A COLD

SEEMS GENERALLY SICK

SEEMS WELL

Can you see a red lump inside your child's ear?

RED LUMP

NO RED LUMP

POSSIBLE CAUSE

OTITIS MEDIA (p.162).

ACTION NEEDED

MEDICAL HELP
Get medical advice within 24 hours.

SELF-HELP
See panels: *Relieving earache* (opposite) and *Bringing down a high temperature* (p.37).

POSSIBLE CAUSE

A BOIL (p.137) in the outer ear canal.

ACTION NEEDED

MEDICAL HELP
Get medical advice within 24 hours.

SELF-HELP
See panel: *Relieving earache* (opposite).

POSSIBLE CAUSE

OTITIS EXTERNA (p.163).

ACTION NEEDED

MEDICAL HELP
Get medical advice within 24 hours.

SELF-HELP
See panel: *Relieving earache* (opposite).

What are your child's other symptoms?

DISCHARGE FROM EAR

ITCHY EAR

NEITHER

Did the pain start during or soon after an airplane trip?

STARTED DURING OR AFTER A FLIGHT

DID NOT START DURING OR AFTER A FLIGHT

POSSIBLE CAUSE

ALTITUDE TRAUMA (p.164).

ACTION NEEDED

MEDICAL HELP
If the earache persists or if your child seems sick, make an appointment to see your doctor.

SELF-HELP
See panel: *Relieving earache* (right).

What is the effect of gently tugging on your child's earlobe?

MAKES PAIN WORSE

NO EFFECT

POSSIBLE CAUSES

ECZEMA (p.135) or OTITIS EXTERNA (p.163).

ACTION NEEDED

MEDICAL HELP
Get medical advice within 24 hours.

SELF-HELP
See panel: *Relieving earache* (below).

POSSIBLE CAUSES

ECZEMA (p.135) or OTITIS EXTERNA (p.163).

ACTION NEEDED

MEDICAL HELP
Get medical advice within 24 hours.

SELF-HELP
See panel: *Relieving earache* (below).

POSSIBLE CAUSE

OTITIS MEDIA (p.162).

ACTION NEEDED

MEDICAL HELP
Get medical advice within 24 hours.

SELF-HELP
See panel: *Relieving earache* (below).

SELF-HELP: RELIEVING AN EARACHE

- Give liquid acetaminophen (15 mgm per kg per dose).
- Provide a hot water bottle covered with a towel to hold against the ear. For a baby, use a warmed soft cloth.
- Tell your child to sit up, with his or her head propped up with pillows.
- Do not insert either ear drops or oil into your child's ear.

Easing the pain of an earache
If lying flat makes the earache worse, prop your child up, supported by a couple of pillows or cushions.

34 HEARING PROBLEMS

Hearing defects are often first noticed by a newborn screening audiogram or by the parents. The first sign of deafness in babies is a failure to respond to sounds. In older children, the onset of hearing problems may cause school work to deteriorate. Hearing loss may be only temporary, but it should be checked.

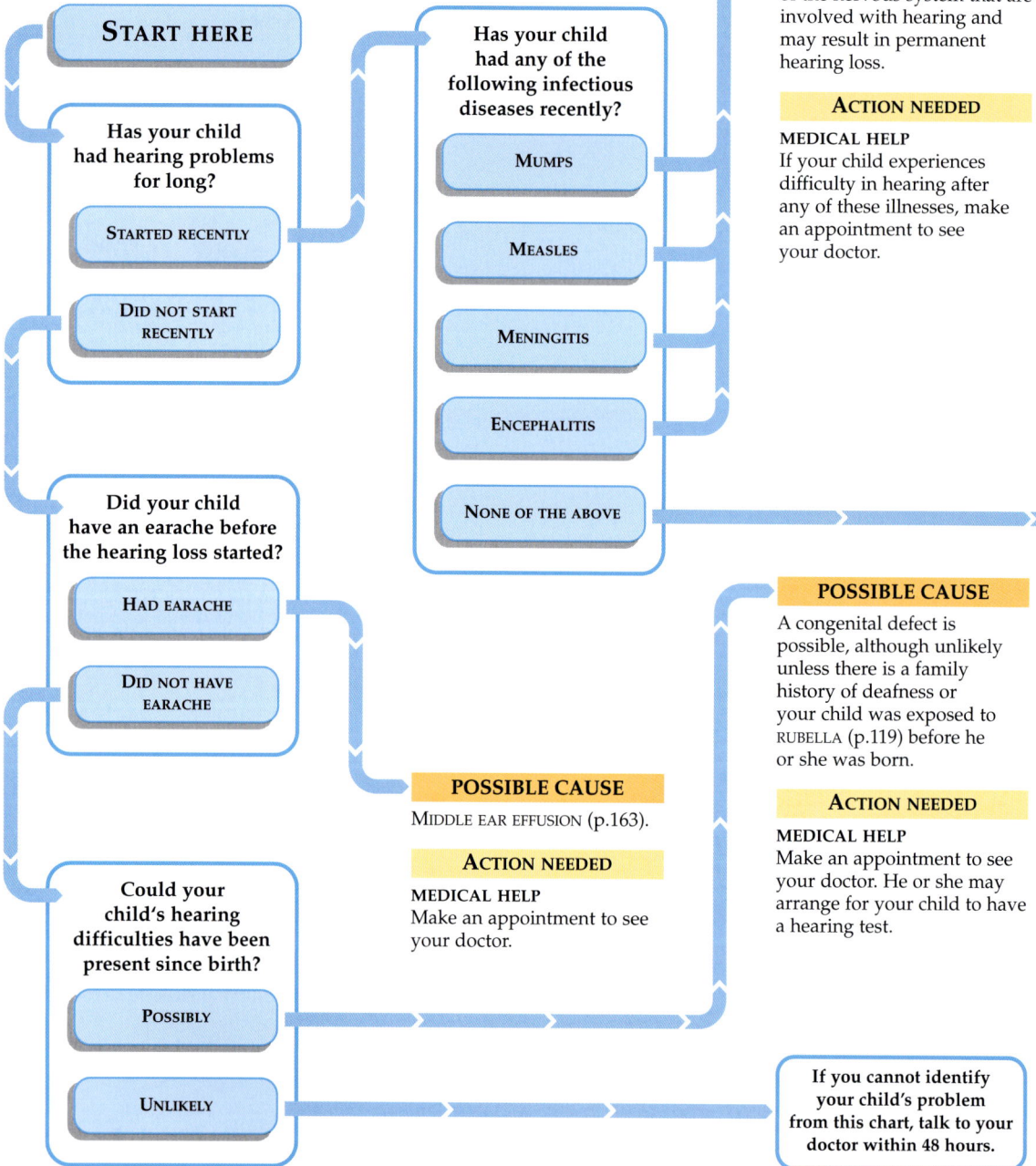

START HERE

Has your child had hearing problems for long?

- STARTED RECENTLY
- DID NOT START RECENTLY

Did your child have an earache before the hearing loss started?

- HAD EARACHE
- DID NOT HAVE EARACHE

Could your child's hearing difficulties have been present since birth?

- POSSIBLY
- UNLIKELY

Has your child had any of the following infectious diseases recently?

- MUMPS
- MEASLES
- MENINGITIS
- ENCEPHALITIS
- NONE OF THE ABOVE

POSSIBLE CAUSES

Rarely, infectious diseases, such as MUMPS (p.122), MEASLES (p.118), MENINGITIS (p.158), and ENCEPHALITIS (p.159), may damage parts of the nervous system that are involved with hearing and may result in permanent hearing loss.

ACTION NEEDED

MEDICAL HELP
If your child experiences difficulty in hearing after any of these illnesses, make an appointment to see your doctor.

POSSIBLE CAUSE

MIDDLE EAR EFFUSION (p.163).

ACTION NEEDED

MEDICAL HELP
Make an appointment to see your doctor.

POSSIBLE CAUSE

A congenital defect is possible, although unlikely unless there is a family history of deafness or your child was exposed to RUBELLA (p.119) before he or she was born.

ACTION NEEDED

MEDICAL HELP
Make an appointment to see your doctor. He or she may arrange for your child to have a hearing test.

If you cannot identify your child's problem from this chart, talk to your doctor within 48 hours.

Is your child suffering from an earache or has he or she had an earache recently?

HAS EARACHE NOW

HAD EARACHE RECENTLY

NEITHER

Did the hearing problems start during or shortly after an airplane trip?

STARTED DURING OR AFTER A FLIGHT

DID NOT START DURING OR AFTER A FLIGHT

POSSIBLE CAUSE

ALTITUDE TRAUMA (p.164).

ACTION NEEDED

MEDICAL HELP
If hearing problems persist, make an appointment to see your doctor.

SELF-HELP
See panel: *Relieving an earache* (p.101).

POSSIBLE CAUSE

OTITIS MEDIA (p.162).

ACTION NEEDED

MEDICAL HELP
Get medical advice within 24 hours.

SELF-HELP
See panel: *Relieving an earache* (p.101).

POSSIBLE CAUSES

A COMMON COLD (p.148) or ALLERGIC RHINITIS (p.152) may have caused the tubes connecting the ears and throat to become blocked.

ACTION NEEDED

MEDICAL HELP
Make an appointment to see your doctor.

Which of the following apply to your child?

HAS BEEN SNEEZING

RECENTLY HAD A COLD

NEITHER

POSSIBLE CAUSE

Earwax blockage (see OTITIS EXTERNA, p.163).

ACTION NEEDED

MEDICAL HELP
Make an appointment to see your doctor.

ASSESSMENT: CHECKING YOUR BABY'S HEARING

Although only a professional can test your child's hearing accurately, you can easily make the following observations of your baby's hearing. A negative response at any age may indicate a problem.
- Shortly after birth, your baby should respond to a sudden loud noise, such as clapped hands, by blinking or opening the eyes.
- By the age of 1 month, your baby should respond to a prolonged sound that starts suddenly, such as the noise of a vacuum cleaner.
- By the age of 4 months, your baby should react to the sound of your voice, even if you are out of sight.
- By the age of 12 months, your baby should respond to his or her own name as well as familiar words such as "mama" and "no."

Hearing development
By the age of 7 months, your baby should turn toward a soft sound made behind him or her, such as paper being crackled.

35 MOUTH PROBLEMS

Most problems of the lips, tongue, gums, and inside of the mouth are minor. Still, a sore mouth may make your child miserable, and eating and drinking painful. During the teething process, infants experience some mouth pain and they enjoy chewing on a hard or cold object at this time.

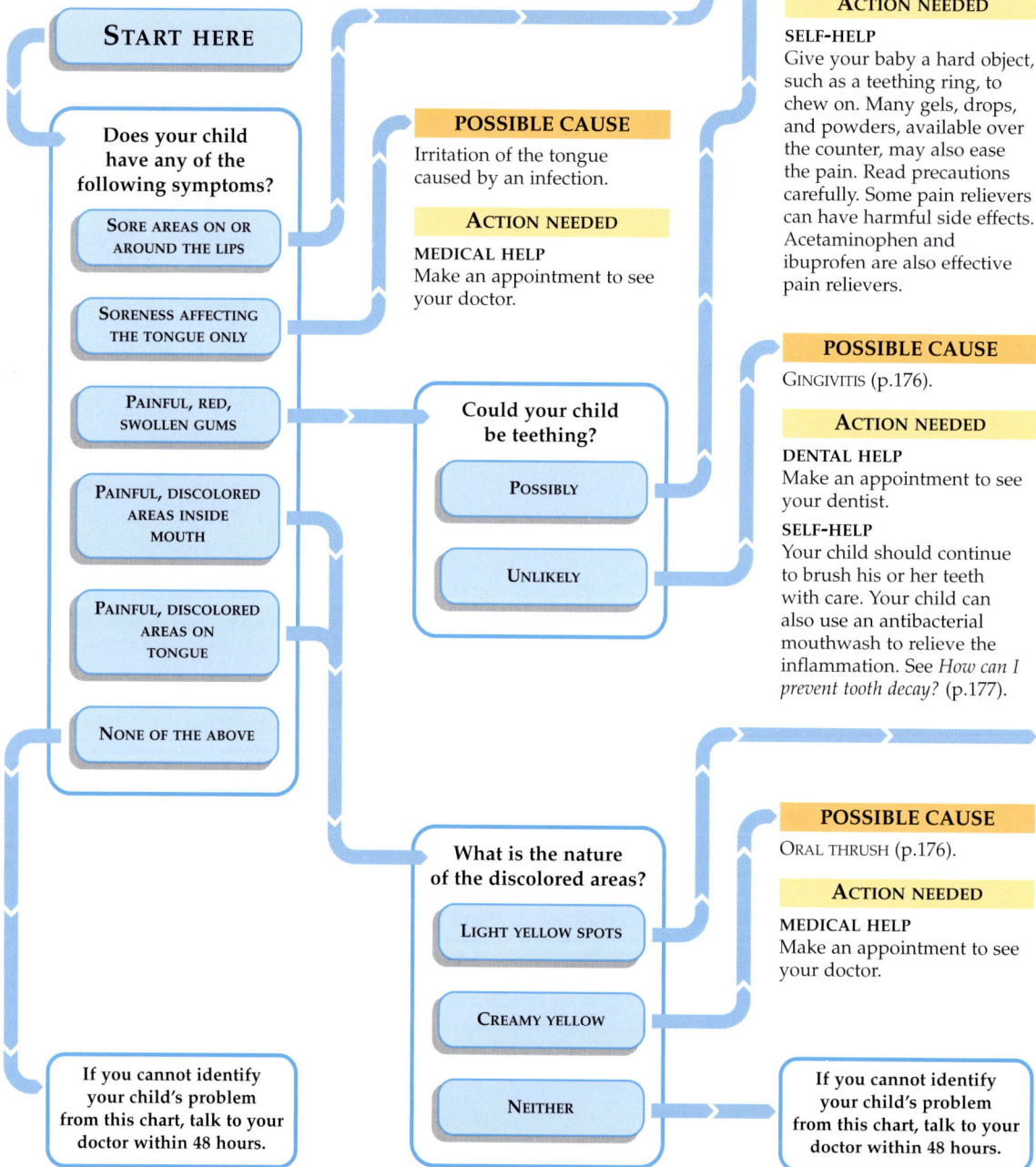

START HERE

Does your child have any of the following symptoms?

- SORE AREAS ON OR AROUND THE LIPS
- SORENESS AFFECTING THE TONGUE ONLY
- PAINFUL, RED, SWOLLEN GUMS
- PAINFUL, DISCOLORED AREAS INSIDE MOUTH
- PAINFUL, DISCOLORED AREAS ON TONGUE
- NONE OF THE ABOVE

POSSIBLE CAUSE

Irritation of the tongue caused by an infection.

ACTION NEEDED

MEDICAL HELP
Make an appointment to see your doctor.

Could your child be teething?

- POSSIBLY
- UNLIKELY

What is the nature of the discolored areas?

- LIGHT YELLOW SPOTS
- CREAMY YELLOW
- NEITHER

POSSIBLE CAUSE

TEETHING (p.33).

ACTION NEEDED

SELF-HELP
Give your baby a hard object, such as a teething ring, to chew on. Many gels, drops, and powders, available over the counter, may also ease the pain. Read precautions carefully. Some pain relievers can have harmful side effects. Acetaminophen and ibuprofen are also effective pain relievers.

POSSIBLE CAUSE

GINGIVITIS (p.176).

ACTION NEEDED

DENTAL HELP
Make an appointment to see your dentist.

SELF-HELP
Your child should continue to brush his or her teeth with care. Your child can also use an antibacterial mouthwash to relieve the inflammation. See *How can I prevent tooth decay?* (p.177).

POSSIBLE CAUSE

ORAL THRUSH (p.176).

ACTION NEEDED

MEDICAL HELP
Make an appointment to see your doctor.

If you cannot identify your child's problem from this chart, talk to your doctor within 48 hours.

If you cannot identify your child's problem from this chart, talk to your doctor within 48 hours.

What is the appearance of the affected area?

- TINY BLISTERS ON OR AROUND THE LIPS
- REDNESS AROUND MOUTH
- CRACKS AT CORNERS OF LIPS
- STRAW-COLORED CRUSTS
- NONE OF THE ABOVE

POSSIBLE CAUSE

CHAPPED LIPS (p.136).

ACTION NEEDED

SELF-HELP
Apply petroleum jelly to the affected area every few hours. Use a lip salve to moisturize and protect the lips themselves.

If you cannot identify your child's problem from this chart, talk to your doctor within 48 hours.

POSSIBLE CAUSE

COLD SORES (p.139).

ACTION NEEDED

MEDICAL HELP
If the blisters are severe, have lasted for more than 2 weeks, or are causing your child embarrassment, make an appointment to see your doctor.

SELF-HELP
Apply acyclovir cream, available by prescription only, to the sores within 36 hours of the onset of symptoms.

POSSIBLE CAUSE

IMPETIGO (p.139).

ACTION NEEDED

MEDICAL HELP
Get medical advice within 24 hours.

Does your child have any of the following symptoms?

- FEELS GENERALLY UNWELL
- HAS A FEVER
- HAS SPOTS ON THE HANDS AND FEET
- NONE OF THE ABOVE

POSSIBLE CAUSE

GINGIVOSTOMATITIS (p.176).

ACTION NEEDED

MEDICAL HELP
Make an appointment to see your doctor.

SELF-HELP
See panels: *Relieving a sore mouth* (below) and *Bringing down a high temperature* (p.37).

POSSIBLE CAUSE

HAND, FOOT, AND MOUTH DISEASE (p.120).

ACTION NEEDED

SELF-HELP
See panel: *Relieving a sore mouth* (below).

POSSIBLE CAUSE

MOUTH ULCERS (p.175).

ACTION NEEDED

MEDICAL HELP
If the mouth ulcers have failed to heal within 10 days, make an appointment to see your doctor.

SELF-HELP
See panel: *Relieving a sore mouth* (right).

SELF-HELP: RELIEVING A SORE MOUTH

The following measures may help to relieve your child's discomfort:
- A sore mouth should be rinsed out every hour with ¼ teaspoon bicarbonate of soda dissolved in 100 ml of warm water.
- If symptoms are causing pain, you can give the appropriate dose of acetaminophen (15 mgm per kg per dose).
- Your child may prefer soft foods, such as soup and ice cream.
- Avoid giving acidic drinks, such as fruit juices. Drinking through a straw may stop irritating liquids from bathing the ulcers.

Foods for a sore mouth
Give your child plenty of fluids and soft foods, including yoghurt and soup, until his or her mouth heals.

36 ABDOMINAL PAIN

Every child suffers from abdominal pain from time to time and some children have recurrent bouts of pain. Usually the cause is minor and the pain disappears within a few hours without any treatment. Rarely, however, there may be a serious underlying disorder that requires medical attention.

DANGER SIGNS

Call an ambulance at once if your child has any of the following symptoms:
- Abdominal pain for 6 hours.
- Pain or swelling in the groin or testes.
- Greenish yellow vomit.
- Blood in feces.

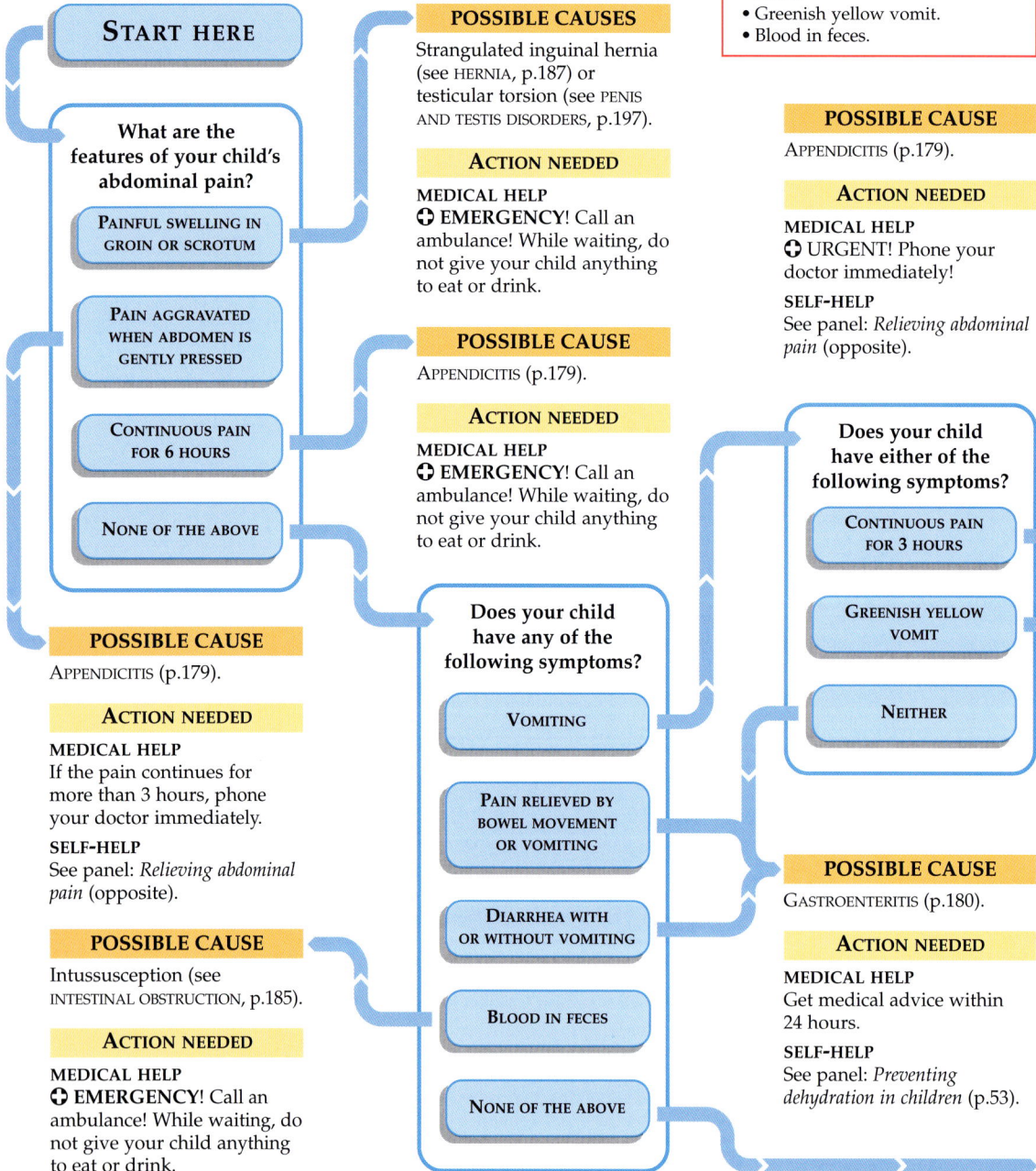

START HERE

What are the features of your child's abdominal pain?

- PAINFUL SWELLING IN GROIN OR SCROTUM
- PAIN AGGRAVATED WHEN ABDOMEN IS GENTLY PRESSED
- CONTINUOUS PAIN FOR 6 HOURS
- NONE OF THE ABOVE

POSSIBLE CAUSES

Strangulated inguinal hernia (see HERNIA, p.187) or testicular torsion (see PENIS AND TESTIS DISORDERS, p.197).

ACTION NEEDED

MEDICAL HELP
✚ EMERGENCY! Call an ambulance! While waiting, do not give your child anything to eat or drink.

POSSIBLE CAUSE

APPENDICITIS (p.179).

ACTION NEEDED

MEDICAL HELP
✚ EMERGENCY! Call an ambulance! While waiting, do not give your child anything to eat or drink.

POSSIBLE CAUSE

APPENDICITIS (p.179).

ACTION NEEDED

MEDICAL HELP
If the pain continues for more than 3 hours, phone your doctor immediately.

SELF-HELP
See panel: *Relieving abdominal pain* (opposite).

POSSIBLE CAUSE

Intussusception (see INTESTINAL OBSTRUCTION, p.185).

ACTION NEEDED

MEDICAL HELP
✚ EMERGENCY! Call an ambulance! While waiting, do not give your child anything to eat or drink.

Does your child have any of the following symptoms?

- VOMITING
- PAIN RELIEVED BY BOWEL MOVEMENT OR VOMITING
- DIARRHEA WITH OR WITHOUT VOMITING
- BLOOD IN FECES
- NONE OF THE ABOVE

POSSIBLE CAUSE

APPENDICITIS (p.179).

ACTION NEEDED

MEDICAL HELP
✚ URGENT! Phone your doctor immediately!

SELF-HELP
See panel: *Relieving abdominal pain* (opposite).

Does your child have either of the following symptoms?

- CONTINUOUS PAIN FOR 3 HOURS
- GREENISH YELLOW VOMIT
- NEITHER

POSSIBLE CAUSE

GASTROENTERITIS (p.180).

ACTION NEEDED

MEDICAL HELP
Get medical advice within 24 hours.

SELF-HELP
See panel: *Preventing dehydration in children* (p.53).

POSSIBLE CAUSE

INTESTINAL OBSTRUCTION
(p.185).

ACTION NEEDED

MEDICAL HELP
✪ **EMERGENCY**! Call an
ambulance! While waiting, do
not give your child anything
to eat or drink.

SELF-HELP: RELIEVING ABDOMINAL PAIN

The following measures may help
to relieve your child's pain:
• Give your child a hot water
bottle, filled with warm water
and wrapped in a towel, to hold
against his or her abdomen.
• Your child should not have
anything to eat, and only plain
water to drink, while in pain.
If there is any possibility of

appendicitis or another serious
disorder for which your child
might require surgery, do not
give anything to eat or drink
until you have a doctor's advice.

Easing abdominal pain
A well-wrapped hot water bottle held
against your child's abdomen, while lying
on a bed or sofa or sitting in a chair, may
soothe the pain.

POSSIBLE CAUSE

An upper respiratory tract
infection, such as a COMMON
COLD (p.148).

ACTION NEEDED

MEDICAL HELP
If your child is distressed by
his or her symptoms, consult
your doctor.

SELF-HELP
See panels: *Relieving a cough*
(p.90), *Relieving a sore throat*
(p.91), and *Relieving abdominal*
pain (above).

Does your child have any of the following symptoms?

FEVER

PAIN ON PASSING URINE

BED-WETTING (AFTER BEING DRY AT NIGHT)

- TWO OR MORE
- ONE OR NONE

POSSIBLE CAUSE

URINARY TRACT INFECTION
(p.193).

ACTION NEEDED

MEDICAL HELP
Get medical advice within
24 hours.

SELF-HELP
If your child has a fever, see
panel: *Bringing down a high*
temperature (p.37).

Does your child have any of the following symptoms?

- SORE THROAT
- COUGH
- STUFFY OR RUNNY NOSE
- NONE OF THE ABOVE

POSSIBLE CAUSES

Anxiety (see ANXIETY AND
FEARS, p.170) or food
intolerance (see REACTIONS TO
FOOD, p.182) may be the
explanation, but often there
is no obvious cause.

ACTION NEEDED

MEDICAL HELP
Make an appointment to see
your doctor.

SELF-HELP
Try to alleviate your child's
anxiety. If you think food
intolerance is the problem try
to establish and avoid the
triggers. See panel: *Relieving*
abdominal pain (above).

Does your child often have abdominal pain without seeming unwell?

- HAS RECURRENT BOUTS
- NOT USUALLY

If you cannot identify your child's problem from this chart, talk to your doctor within 48 hours.

37 CONSTIPATION

Children have bowel movements from as often as three times a day to once every 4 days; anything within this range is normal as long as the stool is not runny, hard, or painful to pass. Changes in your child's diet, minor illness, or emotional stress may temporarily affect the frequency of defecation.

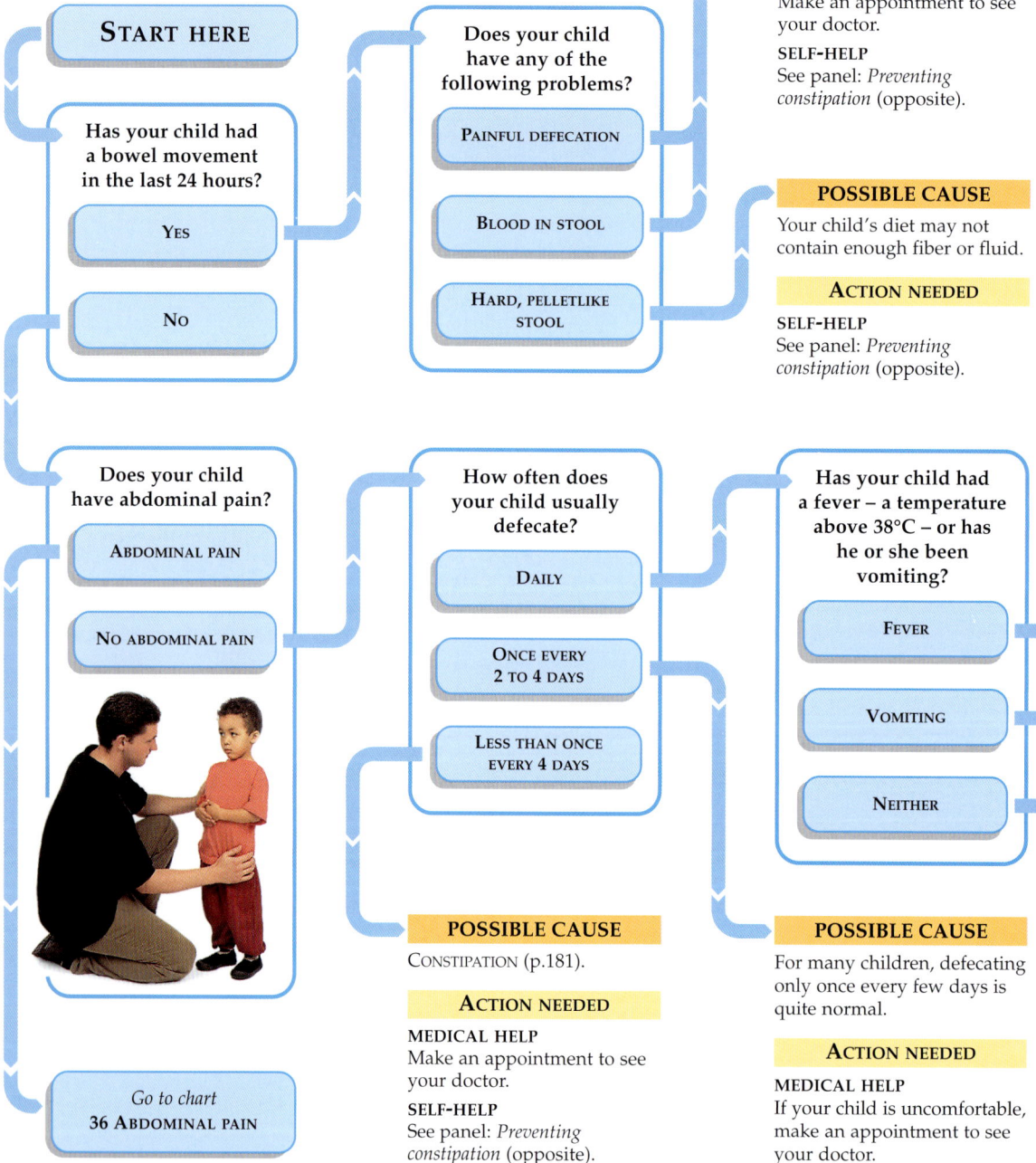

START HERE

Has your child had a bowel movement in the last 24 hours?

YES

NO

Does your child have any of the following problems?

PAINFUL DEFECATION

BLOOD IN STOOL

HARD, PELLETLIKE STOOL

Does your child have abdominal pain?

ABDOMINAL PAIN

NO ABDOMINAL PAIN

Go to chart **36 ABDOMINAL PAIN**

How often does your child usually defecate?

DAILY

ONCE EVERY 2 TO 4 DAYS

LESS THAN ONCE EVERY 4 DAYS

Has your child had a fever – a temperature above 38°C – or has he or she been vomiting?

FEVER

VOMITING

NEITHER

POSSIBLE CAUSE

Anal fissure (see CONSTIPATION, p.181).

ACTION NEEDED

MEDICAL HELP
Make an appointment to see your doctor.

SELF-HELP
See panel: *Preventing constipation* (opposite).

POSSIBLE CAUSE

Your child's diet may not contain enough fiber or fluid.

ACTION NEEDED

SELF-HELP
See panel: *Preventing constipation* (opposite).

POSSIBLE CAUSE

CONSTIPATION (p.181).

ACTION NEEDED

MEDICAL HELP
Make an appointment to see your doctor.

SELF-HELP
See panel: *Preventing constipation* (opposite).

POSSIBLE CAUSE

For many children, defecating only once every few days is quite normal.

ACTION NEEDED

MEDICAL HELP
If your child is uncomfortable, make an appointment to see your doctor.

POSSIBLE CAUSE

Loss of fluid as a result of fever or vomiting can disrupt bowel movements, which will return to normal once your child has recovered.

ACTION NEEDED

SELF-HELP
Encourage your child to drink plenty of fluids.
See also panels: *Bringing down a high temperature* (p.37), and *Preventing dehydration in babies* (p.38) or *Preventing dehydration in children* (p.53).

POSSIBLE CAUSE

Anal fissure (see CONSTIPATION, p.181).

ACTION NEEDED

MEDICAL HELP
Make an appointment to see your doctor.

SELF-HELP
See panel: *Preventing constipation* (below).

POSSIBLE CAUSE

Your child's diet may not contain enough fiber or fluid, resulting in hard stool.

ACTION NEEDED

SELF-HELP
See panel: *Preventing constipation* (below).

Have you changed your child's diet recently?

> DIET CHANGED

> DIET UNCHANGED

Has your child had either of the following symptoms in the past few days?

> PAINFUL DEFECATION

> BLOOD IN STOOL

> NEITHER

When was your child toilet-trained?

> HAS NOT STARTED YET

> A WHILE AGO

> LEARNING NOW

> RECENTLY

If you cannot identify your child's problem from this chart, talk to your doctor within 48 hours.

SELF-HELP: PREVENTING CONSTIPATION

The following steps may help relieve or prevent constipation:
- Increase the amount of fluids (except milk, which can cause constipation), fruit, vegetables, and other fiber-rich foods, such as wholegrain cereals and bread, in your child's diet.
- Encourage your child to sit on the potty or toilet at the same time every day to establish a regular bowel habit.
- Laxatives should never be used for children unless specifically recommended or prescribed by your doctor.

A fiber-rich meal
Give your child fiber-rich foods, such as wholegrain bread and salad or fruit, at all meals if possible.

POSSIBLE CAUSE

Children who are nervous about toilet-training may resist the urge to defecate.

ACTION NEEDED

MEDICAL HELP
Make an appointment to see your doctor if your child has not defecated for 4 days.

SELF-HELP
You should adopt a more relaxed attitude toward your child's toilet-training.
See also chart 14, TOILET-TRAINING PROBLEMS.

38 ABNORMAL-LOOKING STOOL

Sudden differences in color, smell, consistency, or content of stool are almost always due to changes in diet. It is very rare for any such change to last for more than a few days. However, if there are other symptoms or if the altered stool continues, you should take your child to see a doctor.

START HERE

How old is your child?

UNDER 1 YEAR

1 YEAR OR OVER

What is your child's stool like?

RED AND JELLYLIKE

GREEN; MAY BE RUNNY

NEITHER

POSSIBLE CAUSE

Intussusception (see INTESTINAL OBSTRUCTION, p.185).

ACTION NEEDED

MEDICAL HELP
✚ EMERGENCY! Call an ambulance! While waiting, do not give your child anything to eat or drink.

How is your baby fed?

BREAST- AND BOTTLE-FED

BOTTLE-FED ONLY

BREAST-FED ONLY

Is your child taking any medicines?

MEDICINE

NO MEDICINE

POSSIBLE CAUSES

If the stool is green and runny, your baby may have inflammation of the stomach and intestines (see GASTROENTERITIS (p.180).

ACTION NEEDED

MEDICAL HELP
If you think your baby may have gastroenteritis, get medical advice within 24 hours.

SELF-HELP
If you think the milk formula is responsible, you can try another brand, especially one that is lactose free. If you think your baby may have gastroenteritis, see panel: *Preventing dehydration in babies* (p.38).

POSSIBLE CAUSE

Many medicines can affect the appearance of stool.

ACTION NEEDED

MEDICAL HELP
Phone your doctor to find out whether the medicine may be causing your child's symptoms and whether you should stop giving it.

POSSIBLE CAUSE

Green runny stool is normal in breast-fed babies and is not a cause for concern.

ACTION NEEDED

MEDICAL HELP
If your baby seems sick or has other symptoms, make an appointment to see your doctor.

Has your child recently recovered from a bout of diarrhea or vomiting?

- DIARRHEA
- VOMITING
- NEITHER

POSSIBLE CAUSE

GASTROENTERITIS (p.180) may sometimes cause stool to be pale for several days.

ACTION NEEDED

MEDICAL HELP
If your child seems sick or if the stool does not return to its normal color in a few days, make an appointment to see your doctor.

SELF-HELP
See panel: *Preventing dehydration in babies* (p.38) or *Preventing dehydration in children* (p.53).

What are the characteristics of your child's stool?

- VERY PALE
- VERY PALE, FLOATING, AND FOUL-SMELLING
- BLOOD IN STOOL
- RUNNY

POSSIBLE CAUSE

MALABSORPTION (p.183), often caused by an underlying disorder, such as REACTIONS TO FOOD (p.182).

ACTION NEEDED

MEDICAL HELP
Make an appointment to see your doctor.

Does your child have any of the following symptoms?

- YELLOWISH SKIN
- YELLOWISH WHITES OF THE EYES
- DARK URINE
- NONE OF THE ABOVE

POSSIBLE CAUSES

GASTROENTERITIS (p.180), anal fissure (see CONSTIPATION, p.181), or INFLAMMATORY BOWEL DISEASE (p.184).

ACTION NEEDED

MEDICAL HELP
Get medical advice within 24 hours.

Go to chart
9 DIARRHEA IN CHILDREN

POSSIBLE CAUSE

HEPATITIS (p.188), which may cause jaundice.

ACTION NEEDED

MEDICAL HELP
Get medical advice within 24 hours.

If you cannot identify your child's problem from this chart, talk to your doctor within 48 hours.

39 URINARY PROBLEMS

For toilet-training problems, see chart 14

Urinary problems can be caused by various conditions, ranging from minor infections to serious disorders, such as diabetes mellitus. Pain on urination usually indicates a disorder, but variations in frequency of urination or in the color of urine are not necessarily symptoms of disease.

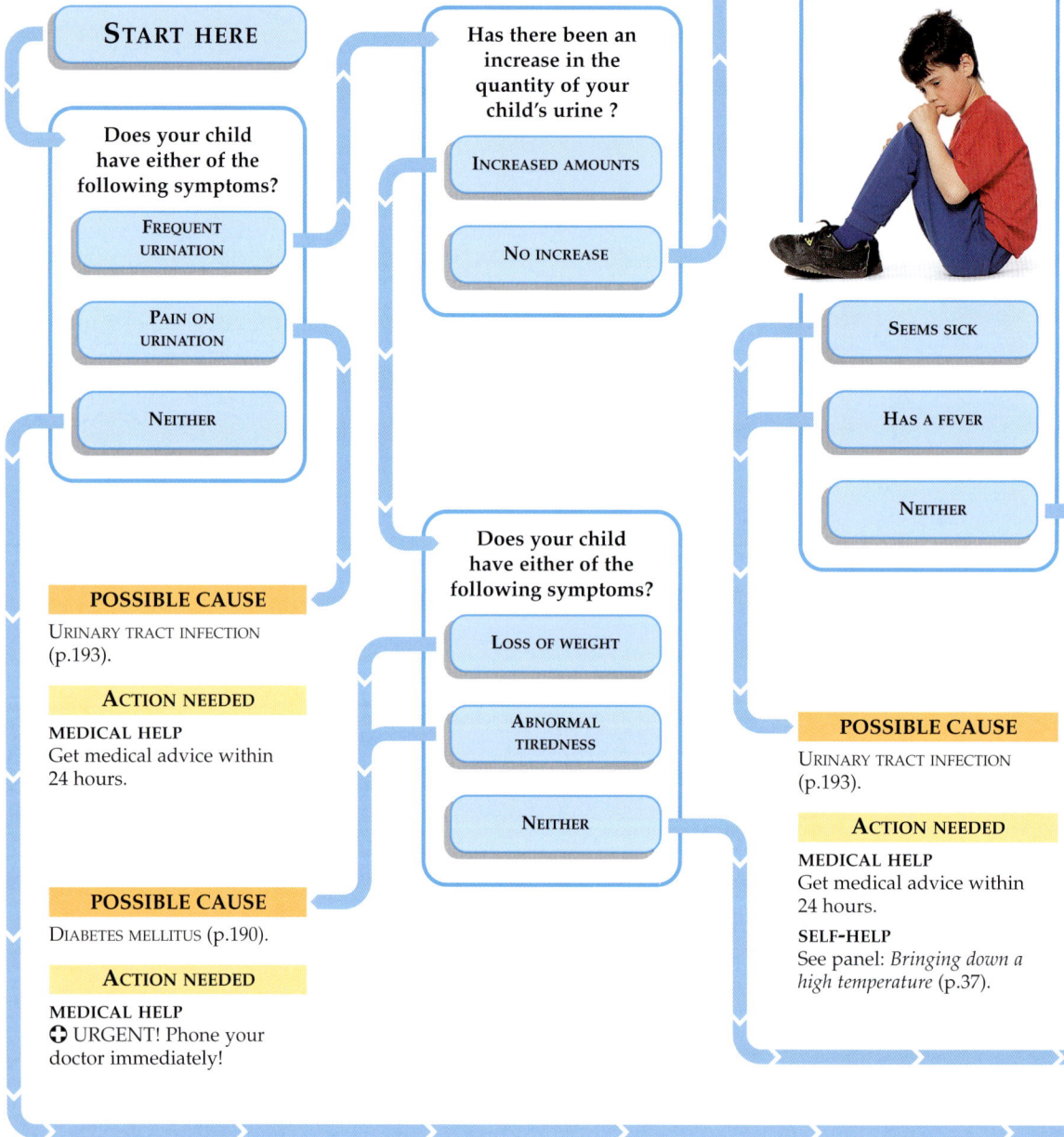

Does your child seem generally sick or does he or she have a fever – a temperature above 38°C?

START HERE

Does your child have either of the following symptoms?

FREQUENT URINATION

PAIN ON URINATION

NEITHER

Has there been an increase in the quantity of your child's urine ?

INCREASED AMOUNTS

NO INCREASE

SEEMS SICK

HAS A FEVER

NEITHER

POSSIBLE CAUSE

URINARY TRACT INFECTION (p.193).

ACTION NEEDED

MEDICAL HELP
Get medical advice within 24 hours.

Does your child have either of the following symptoms?

LOSS OF WEIGHT

ABNORMAL TIREDNESS

NEITHER

POSSIBLE CAUSE

URINARY TRACT INFECTION (p.193).

ACTION NEEDED

MEDICAL HELP
Get medical advice within 24 hours.

SELF-HELP
See panel: *Bringing down a high temperature* (p.37).

POSSIBLE CAUSE

DIABETES MELLITUS (p.190).

ACTION NEEDED

MEDICAL HELP
✚ URGENT! Phone your doctor immediately!

Has your child been taking any medicine recently?

MEDICINE

NO MEDICINE

Is there any reason why your child might be feeling insecure?

SCHOOL DIFFICULTIES

FAMILY UPHEAVAL, SUCH AS A NEW BABY

CHANGE OF ROUTINE

NONE OF THE ABOVE

POSSIBLE CAUSES

Anxiety (see ANXIETY AND FEARS, p.170) or stress may result in your child going to the bathroom more often than usual.

ACTION NEEDED

MEDICAL HELP
If the problem does not clear up within a few days, phone your doctor.

SELF-HELP
Try to establish the reason for your child's anxiety or stress, and alleviate it, if possible.

POSSIBLE CAUSE

Some drugs may cause frequent urination.

ACTION NEEDED

MEDICAL HELP
Phone your doctor to find out whether the medicine may be causing your child's symptoms and whether you should stop giving it.

POSSIBLE CAUSES

GLOMERULONEPHRITIS (p.194) or URINARY TRACT INFECTION (p.193).

ACTION NEEDED

MEDICAL HELP
✚ URGENT! Phone your doctor immediately!

If you cannot identify your child's problem from this chart, talk to your doctor within 48 hours.

POSSIBLE CAUSE

HEPATITIS (p.188).

ACTION NEEDED

MEDICAL HELP
Get medical advice within 24 hours.

What color is your child's urine?

PINK, RED, OR SMOKY

DARK BROWN AND CLEAR

DARK YELLOW OR ORANGE

GREEN OR BLUE

NONE OF THE ABOVE

What color is your child's stool?

PALE

NORMAL

POSSIBLE CAUSES

The urine has probably darkened because it has become concentrated as a result of low fluid intake, fever, vomiting, or diarrhea.

ACTION NEEDED

SELF-HELP
Make sure that your child has plenty to drink and the urine should soon return to its normal color. If your child has had been ill with a fever or diarrhea, or has been vomiting, see panel: *Preventing dehydration in babies* (p.38) or *Preventing dehydration in children* (p.53).

POSSIBLE CAUSE

Artificial coloring in food, drink, or medicine is almost always the cause of such discoloration.

ACTION NEEDED

No action is required. The artificial coloring will soon pass out of your child's system without causing any problems.

If you cannot identify your child's problem from this chart, talk to your doctor within 48 hours.

40 GENITAL PROBLEMS IN BOYS

Pain or swelling in the penis or scrotum, discharge from the penis, or pain on urination can affect boys of any age. Injuries to the genitals tend to be most common in boys of school age. Any boy who has severe or persistent genital pain needs urgent medical help.

START HERE

Does your son have any of the following symptoms?

- PAINLESS SWELLING IN GROIN OR SCROTUM
- PAINFUL SWELLING IN GROIN OR SCROTUM
- PAIN OR BURNING SENSATION ON URINATION
- SWELLING OF PENIS TIP OR DISCHARGE FROM FORESKIN
- GRAYISH YELLOW DISCHARGE FROM PENIS
- NONE OF THE ABOVE

POSSIBLE CAUSES
Inguinal hernia (see HERNIA, p.187) or hydrocele (see PENIS AND TESTIS DISORDERS, p.197).

ACTION NEEDED
MEDICAL HELP
Get medical advice within 24 hours.

POSSIBLE CAUSE
URINARY TRACT INFECTION (p.193).

ACTION NEEDED
MEDICAL HELP
Get medical advice within 24 hours.

POSSIBLE CAUSE
Balanitis (see PENIS AND TESTIS DISORDERS, p.196).

ACTION NEEDED
MEDICAL HELP
Get medical advice within 24 hours.

POSSIBLE CAUSE
A foreign body in your son's urethra.

ACTION NEEDED
MEDICAL HELP
Make an appointment to see your doctor.

If you cannot identify your son's problem from this chart, talk to your doctor within 48 hours.

POSSIBLE CAUSE
Orchitis (see PENIS AND TESTIS DISORDERS, p.197).

ACTION NEEDED
MEDICAL HELP
Get medical advice within 24 hours.

POSSIBLE CAUSE
Pain that lasts more than 2 hours after an injury may indicate damage to the testes.

ACTION NEEDED
MEDICAL HELP
✚ URGENT! Phone your doctor immediately!

Could your son have suffered an injury to his genitals?

- POSSIBLY
- UNLIKELY

Has your son had mumps in the past 2 weeks?

- YES (RARE, DUE TO IMMUNIZATION)
- NO

POSSIBLE CAUSES
Testicular torsion (see PENIS AND TESTIS DISORDERS, p.197) or strangulated inguinal hernia (see HERNIA, p.187).

ACTION NEEDED
MEDICAL HELP
✚ EMERGENCY! Call an ambulance! While waiting, do not give your son anything to eat or drink.

41 GENITAL PROBLEMS IN GIRLS

The most common genital symptoms in girls are itching and inflammation of the genital area, which may cause pain on urination or an unusual vaginal discharge. An infection or irritation by scented soaps, bubble baths, or feminine hygiene products may be the underlying cause of these symptoms.

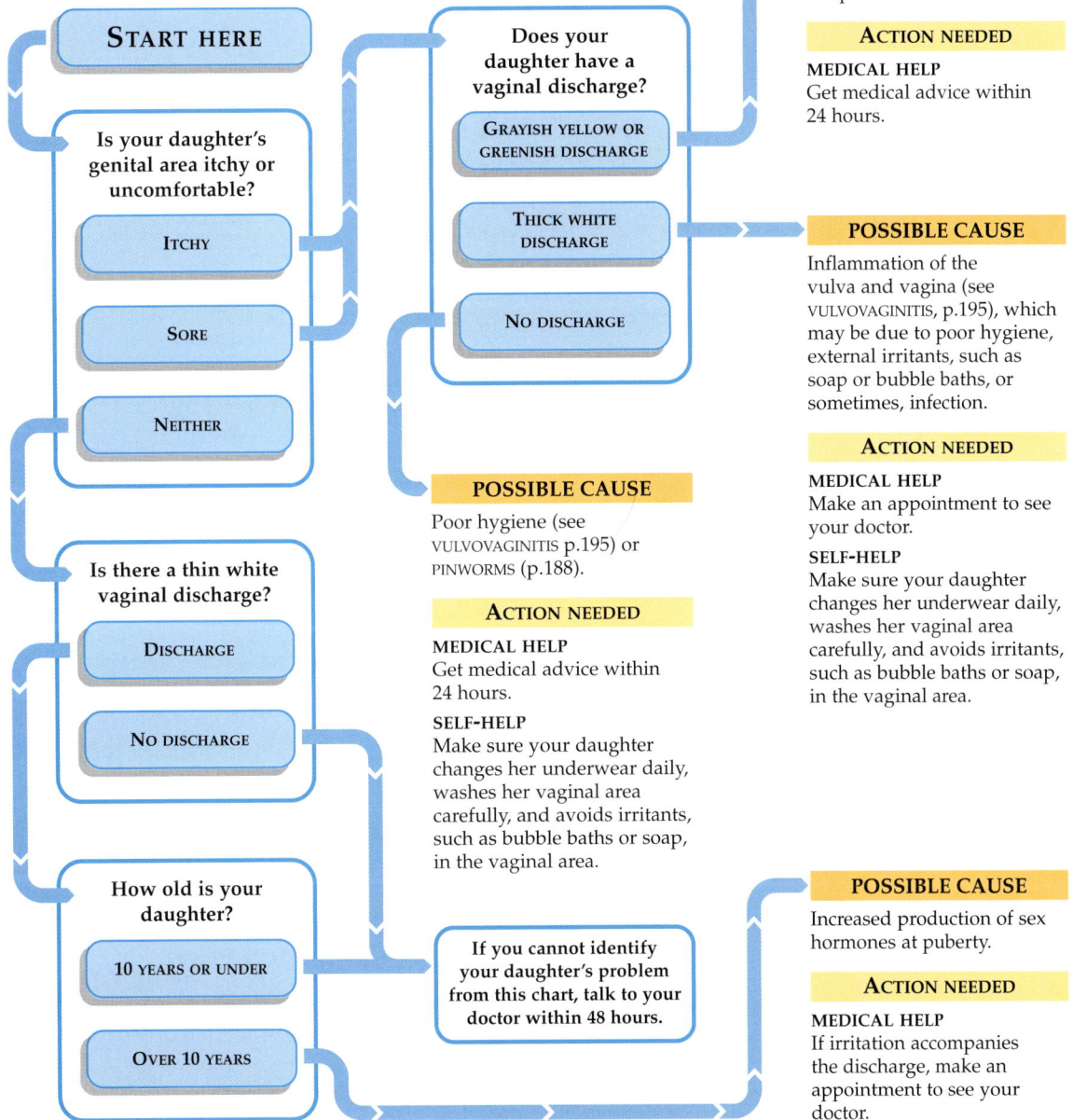

START HERE

Is your daughter's genital area itchy or uncomfortable?
- ITCHY
- SORE
- NEITHER

Is there a thin white vaginal discharge?
- DISCHARGE
- NO DISCHARGE

How old is your daughter?
- 10 YEARS OR UNDER
- OVER 10 YEARS

Does your daughter have a vaginal discharge?
- GRAYISH YELLOW OR GREENISH DISCHARGE
- THICK WHITE DISCHARGE
- NO DISCHARGE

If you cannot identify your daughter's problem from this chart, talk to your doctor within 48 hours.

POSSIBLE CAUSE

Infection of the vagina (see VULVOVAGINITIS, p.195), which, in young girls, may be caused by a foreign object or, in older girls, a forgotten tampon.

ACTION NEEDED

MEDICAL HELP
Get medical advice within 24 hours.

POSSIBLE CAUSE

Inflammation of the vulva and vagina (see VULVOVAGINITIS, p.195), which may be due to poor hygiene, external irritants, such as soap or bubble baths, or sometimes, infection.

ACTION NEEDED

MEDICAL HELP
Make an appointment to see your doctor.

SELF-HELP
Make sure your daughter changes her underwear daily, washes her vaginal area carefully, and avoids irritants, such as bubble baths or soap, in the vaginal area.

POSSIBLE CAUSE

Poor hygiene (see VULVOVAGINITIS p.195) or PINWORMS (p.188).

ACTION NEEDED

MEDICAL HELP
Get medical advice within 24 hours.

SELF-HELP
Make sure your daughter changes her underwear daily, washes her vaginal area carefully, and avoids irritants, such as bubble baths or soap, in the vaginal area.

POSSIBLE CAUSE

Increased production of sex hormones at puberty.

ACTION NEEDED

MEDICAL HELP
If irritation accompanies the discharge, make an appointment to see your doctor.

DISEASES &
DISORDERS

ELECTRON
MICROGRAPH OF
INFLUENZA VIRUS

CHILDREN TEND TO SUFFER from a variety of illnesses and problems that do not affect adults or that affect them differently. In this section all the most common childhood diseases and disorders are described, including all possible causes that are pinpointed on the symptom charts. Each article gives detailed information about a particular disease, including a list of the symptoms, causes, if and when a doctor should be consulted, medical and self-help treatment, and the outlook. Photographs and artworks show aspects of the disease or demonstrate self-help techniques that can be used at home. Turn to these pages for information that your doctor has provided but which you may have forgotten or not taken in during the consultation.

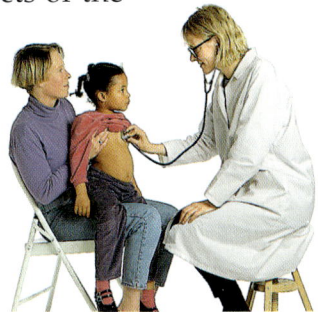

CONSULTING A DOCTOR ABOUT
YOUR CHILD'S ILLNESS

INFECTIOUS DISEASES

CHILDREN ARE MORE SUSCEPTIBLE to infectious diseases than adults because their immune systems have not yet built up resistance. Most childhood infections are not serious. A few can be dangerous. However, because of routine immunization, the main serious viral infections, such as measles, are less common. Bacterial infections can either be prevented by immunization or measurably improved by antibiotics.

MEASLES

A once common disease of childhood, measles is a viral infection that causes fever and a characteristic rash. The disease itself is not usually serious, but a child with measles typically feels very sick. There is also a slight possibility of serious complications, especially in children with chronic heart or lung disease or in those who have a depressed immune system. Measles is highly infectious, but widespread IMMUNIZATION (p.30) has now made it a rare disease in Canada and other developed countries.

Measles rash
The rash of measles appears 3 to 4 days after the first signs of illness. Initially, the rash consists of separate spots. The spots then merge to give the skin a blotchy appearance.

What are the symptoms?
The measles virus produces the initial symptoms after an incubation period of 8 to 14 days. These symptoms are:
- Fever.
- Red watering eyes.
- Runny nose.
- Dry cough.

The following characteristic features then appear:
- First, tiny white spots with a red base (Koplik's spots), which may be seen on the insides of the cheeks about two days after the first symptoms appear.
- Then, a flat, blotchy, red rash, which develops 3 to 4 days after the start of the illness. The rash appears on the face and behind the ears, and then spreads down to cover the whole body.

The rash starts to fade after 3 or 4 days. Also at this time, the child's fever subsides and he or she begins to feel better. In the majority of cases, the rash disappears within a week.

What are the complications?
Infection of the middle ear (see OTITIS MEDIA, p.162) and PNEUMONIA (p.155) are the most common complications. In about 1 in 1,000 cases of measles, a serious complication called ENCEPHALITIS (p.159) occurs; this inflammation of the brain is caused by spread of infection to the brain or by an abnormal immune response to the measles virus.

Should I consult a doctor?
Your child should be seen by a doctor within 24 hours if you suspect measles. You should phone a doctor at once if your child has any of the following symptoms: earache, abnormally rapid breathing, drowsiness, seizures, severe headache, or vomiting.

What might the doctor do?
The doctor will examine your child to confirm the diagnosis. Antibiotics may be prescribed if pneumonia or otitis media exists. If the doctor suspects encephalitis, he or she will have your child admitted to the hospital.

What can I do to help?
Let your child choose whether to stay in bed. Give him or her acetaminophen to reduce fever, and plenty of fluids.

The infectious period lasts for 2 days before the onset of the rash until 5 days after it appears. Try to keep your child away from people at risk of infection. Attempts to isolate siblings if one of them has measles may be futile. Often brothers and sisters have been infected before the disease is diagnosed.

What is the outlook?
Most children recover completely from measles within about 10 days of the onset of symptoms. A single attack of measles should give lifelong immunity.

RUBELLA

Formerly known as German measles, rubella is a mild viral infection that may cause a rash and swelling of the lymph nodes. In about a quarter of cases, there is no rash and the infection often passes unnoticed, although blood tests can show that it has occurred. If rubella is contracted early in pregnancy, it can cause serious damage to the developing baby. A once common disease, rubella has become rare because of routine IMMUNIZATION (p.30).

Rubella rash
The rubella rash consists of tiny, flat pink spots that fade when pressed. They appear on the face and spread rapidly to the trunk and limbs, eventually merging.

What are the symptoms?
After an incubation period of between 2 and 3 weeks, the rubella virus may cause the following symptoms:
• Slight fever.
• Swollen lymph nodes at the back of the neck and behind the ears. In some cases, there is enlargement of lymph nodes throughout the body, including those in the armpits and groin.
• A nonitchy rash (see illustration at right) that develops on the second or third day of illness. The rash usually disappears within about 3 days.
• In some children, joint pain.
Rare complications are inflammation of the brain (see ENCEPHALITIS, p.159) and THROMBOCYTOPENIA (p.147), a disorder in which the number of platelets (clotting agents) in the blood is abnormally low.

Should I consult a doctor?
Phone a doctor if you think your child may have rubella. Do not take the child to the doctor's office because of the risk of infecting a pregnant woman.

You should phone a doctor at once if your child develops joint pain or if a complication is signaled by any of the following symptoms: a rash of flat, dark red spots that do not fade when they are pressed, severe headache, vomiting, lack of energy, or abnormal drowsiness.

What might the doctor do?
The doctor will examine your child. To confirm the diagnosis of rubella, a sample of your child's blood may be sent to the laboratory, to be examined for antibodies to the virus. There is no specific medical treatment for rubella.

What can I do to help?
Give your child acetaminophen to reduce fever, and plenty of fluids. Try to prevent your child from having any contact with pregnant women. Rubella is infectious from 1 week before until 4 days after the rash appears.

What is the outlook?
Children usually recover completely from rubella within about 10 days of the onset of symptoms. A single attack usually gives lifelong immunity.

FIFTH DISEASE

Also known as erythema infectiosum, fifth disease is a mildly contagious viral illness. It usually occurs in small outbreaks in the spring among children over the age of 2 years. The most distinctive symptom of the disease is a red rash on both cheeks.

What are the symptoms?
After a typical incubation period of between 4 and 14 days, the following symptoms appear:
• Bright red cheeks, contrasting with a pale area around the mouth.
• Fever – usually low grade.
• A rash that usually develops 1 to 4 days after the cheeks become red. The rash appears on the arms and legs and occasionally on the trunk. It is blotchy or lacelike and may be much more pronounced after a warm bath. The rash usually lasts between 7 and 21 days.
• Rarely, joint pain.

What are the complications?
Fifth disease sometimes leads to severe illness in children who have certain uncommon blood disorders, including anemias such as SICKLE-CELL ANEMIA (p.199) or THALASSEMIA (p.200).
  If fifth disease is contracted during pregnancy, the condition can, in rare cases, lead to miscarriage.

Distinctive red cheeks
Fifth disease is sometimes referred to as "slapped cheek" disease because the first symptom is a bright red rash that suddenly appears on the cheeks. In this child, the rash has also spread to the arms.

Should I consult a doctor?
Phone a doctor if you are concerned about your child's condition, or if he or she has a blood disorder. In some cases, the doctor will arrange for a blood test to confirm the diagnosis. There is no specific treatment for the disease.

What can I do to help?
Give your child acetaminophen to reduce a fever, and plenty of fluids. Sufferers are unlikely to be infectious after the rash appears; nevertheless, for as long as the rash persists, it may be safest to keep your child away from anyone who might be pregnant.

What is the outlook?
The rash may recur over a period of several weeks or months, and it may vary in intensity in response to changes in temperature or exposure to sunlight. Once your child has been sick with fifth disease, he or she is not likely to experience a recurrence of it.

CHICKENPOX

Otherwise known as varicella, chickenpox is typically a mild viral infection that is characterized by a distinctive, itchy rash and a slight fever. Chickenpox used to be a common childhood infection, but routine immunization has greatly reduced its frequency. Cases are most numerous in late winter and spring.

What are the symptoms?

After an incubation period of usually between 2 and 3 weeks, the following symptoms of chickenpox appear:

- Mild fever or headache that develops a few hours before the rash.
- Rash, mainly on the trunk, made up of crops of spots that rapidly turn into itchy blisters. After a few days, the blisters dry up to form scabs. Spots at different stages of development are usually present at the same time.
- Sometimes, discomfort during eating caused by spots in the mouth that have developed into ulcers.
- In some cases, a severe cough.

Appearance of a chickenpox rash
A chickenpox rash initially consists of raised pimples. The pimples rapidly turn into small, fluid-filled blisters that have red bases.

What are the complications?

The most common complication is a secondary infection with streptococcal bacteria, introduced into the body by scratching. Two other possible complications are PNEUMONIA (p.155) and, rarely, inflammation of the brain (see ENCEPHALITIS, p.159). Those most at risk are children who have a depressed immune system (due to chemotherapy or taking oral corticosteroids, for example) and newborn babies, who can develop chickenpox if the mother contracted the illness late in pregnancy.

Should I consult a doctor?

Phone a doctor at once if your child is a young baby, or has reduced immunity or eczema and has been exposed to chickenpox. Also phone a doctor at once if your child develops any of the following symptoms: coughing, seizures, rapid breathing, abnormal drowsiness, persistent or recurrent fever, or unsteadiness when walking.

Have a doctor see your child if the spots ooze cloudy fluid or pus, the skin around them is red, or a high fever begins on the third day of illness.

What might the doctor do?

An oral antibiotic may be prescribed for a secondary bacterial infection. A child with eczema may be given oral acyclovir (an antiviral drug). A child at high risk of complications may receive intravenous acyclovir in the hospital or injections of varicella zoster immune globulin.

What can I do to help?

Itchiness may be relieved by applying calamine lotion to the rash; by giving oral antihistamines (available over the counter); and by bathing your child in warm water containing a handful of baking soda. Give acetaminophen to reduce a fever, and plenty of fluids.

To avoid infection, you should keep your child's fingernails short and discourage scratching.

Chickenpox is infectious from 1 day before the rash has appeared until all the blisters have formed scabs. During this period, keep your child away from anyone at high risk of complications.

What is the outlook?

Children usually recover completely from chickenpox within 7 to 10 days of the onset of symptoms. An attack of chickenpox leads to lifelong immunity from this disease, but the virus remains dormant in nerve cells in the body and may become active again in late adulthood to cause shingles.

HAND, FOOT, AND MOUTH DISEASE

This mild viral infection causes blisters to appear in the mouth, on the hands, and on the feet. The disease is common in children up to 4 years old, and occurs in epidemics during the summer and early autumn. It is usually caused by the Coxsackie virus.

What are the symptoms?

After an incubation period of usually between 3 and 5 days, hand, foot, and mouth disease causes:

- Mild fever.
- Blisters on the inside of the mouth, which sometimes develop into painful, shallow ulcers.
- Reluctance to eat.
- Blisters on the hands and feet, which typically develop 1 or 2 days after the symptoms in the mouth. The blisters are not usually itchy or painful.

Blisters on the fingers
A child with hand, foot, and mouth disease develops blisters on the hands and feet. They commonly appear on the fingers, the backs of the hands, or the top surfaces of the feet.

What is the treatment?

No specific treatment exists, apart from measures to relieve the symptoms. Give liquid acetaminophen for painful mouth ulcers. Rinsing the mouth out with salty water may also help to soothe the pain (see panel: *Relieving a sore mouth*, p.105). Give plenty of bland fluids, such as water or milk. Do not give fruit juices, which are acidic and may make the pain worse. There is no need for your child to eat solid food.

What is the outlook?

Blisters on the hands and feet usually disappear within 3 or 4 days, as does the fever. However, mouth ulcers may persist for as long as 4 weeks. A single attack provides lifelong immunity.

ROSEOLA INFANTUM

Caused by a virus, roseola infantum is a common infection of early childhood. Most children have had the illness by the time they are 2 years old. Roseola infantum characteristically causes the abrupt onset of a high fever, which lasts for about 4 days, followed by the appearance of a rash of tiny pink spots.

What are the symptoms?
Roseola occurs in two stages. After an incubation period of 5 to 15 days, the first symptoms appear:
- A raised temperature of 39–40°C, although your child may otherwise appear healthy.
- Sometimes, one or more FEBRILE SEIZURES (p.156).
Some children also have:
- Mild diarrhea.
- Cough.
- Enlargement of the lymph nodes in the neck.
- Earache.
After about 4 days, the illness enters its second stage, characterized by:
- Sudden return of the temperature to its normal level.

- Appearance of a rash, which is made up of tiny, distinct pink spots, usually distributed over the head and trunk. The rash lasts for about 4 days.

What are the complications?
A child who has a suppressed immune system may develop HEPATITIS (p.188) or PNEUMONIA (p.155). Complications are rare in otherwise healthy children.

Should I consult a doctor?
Phone a doctor at once if your child has a temperature of 39°C or above, or he or she has a febrile seizure or is drowsy or irritable. While waiting for the doctor, try to reduce the fever with acetaminophen (see panel: *Bringing down a high temperature*, p.37).

What might the doctor do?
The doctor will consider other causes of the fever and may arrange blood or urine tests to exclude bacterial infections. A lumbar puncture may be performed if MENINGITIS (p.158) is suspected. No specific treatment is needed for roseola infantum.

What is the outlook?
Recovery from roseola is usually rapid. Your child should feel completely better by the time the rash has disappeared.

Reducing a fever
For a high fever, give acetaminophen. There is no need to treat a fever that is below 39°C if your child is comfortable.

SCARLET FEVER

This illness has become rare in developed countries since the widespread introduction of antibiotics. Scarlet fever is caused by streptococcal bacteria. The most prominent feature of this illness is a rash, which gives the child a scarlet appearance.

What are the symptoms?
After an incubation period, typically lasting for 2 to 4 days, the following symptoms of scarlet fever appear:
- Vomiting.
- Fever.
- Sore throat and headache.
- Rash (see photograph right), which develops within 12 hours of the first symptoms appearing. The rash affects the neck and chest first and spreads rapidly, but does not affect the face. It is most dense on the neck and in the armpits and groin. The rash lasts for up to 6 days; the skin then peels.
- Flushed cheeks and an obvious pale area around the mouth.
- The tongue in the early stages has a thick white coating through which red spots project. The coating peels on the third or fourth day to reveal a bright red "strawberry tongue," still with the projecting spots.

Scarlet fever rash
The rash varies, but usually consists of a mass of tiny raised red spots, which temporarily disappear when pressed.

What are the complications?
Possible complications of scarlet fever are rheumatic fever, a disorder that can lead to permanent heart damage, and the kidney disorder GLOMERULONEPHRITIS (p.194). Antibiotic treatment has now made these complications rare.

Should I consult a doctor?
Consult a doctor within 24 hours of the onset of your child's symptoms. Phone a doctor at once if your child's urine becomes red, pink, or smoky (see GLOMERULONEPHRITIS, p.194) or if your child has a fever that lasts for 5 days (see KAWASAKI DISEASE, p.125).

What might the doctor do?
The diagnosis will be confirmed, based on symptoms and the positive results of a throat culture. Usual treatment is a 10-day course of an antibiotic or a single injection of penicillin.

What can I do to help?
Reduce fever and relieve pain with liquid acetaminophen. Your child must finish the course of medication, and avoid other children until this time.

What is the outlook?
Your child should feel better within a week of symptoms starting. If normal energy has not returned, you should consult the doctor because rheumatic fever is a possibility. The streptococcal infection can recur; the rash may not.

MUMPS

A mild viral infection, mumps was common among children until routine IMMUNIZATION (p.30) was introduced. Mumps causes a fever and characteristic swelling of one or both of the parotid (salivary) glands, which are situated just in front of and below the ears. This swelling (parotitis) can also be caused by a blockage or bacterial infection.

Swollen glands
The most obvious feature of mumps is the swelling of the parotid (salivary) glands. If both sides are affected, the child may have a hamsterlike appearance. The swollen glands may be painful.

What are the symptoms?
The following symptoms develop after an incubation period of 14 to 24 days:
• Fever.
• Tenderness and swelling of one or both sides of the face, which occurs 1 or 2 days after the onset of fever and typically lasts from 4 to 8 days.

What are the complications?
Occasionally, adolescent boys develop inflamed testes, a condition called orchitis (see PENIS AND TESTIS DISORDERS, p.197). It develops about a week after mumps has started. Rarely, ENCEPHALITIS (p.159) or MENINGITIS (p.158), both of which affect the brain, or pancreatitis may occur, either before or after the parotid glands have become swollen.

Should I consult a doctor?
Your child should be seen by a doctor if you think he or she has mumps. Phone a doctor immediately if your child has a severe headache (with or without vomiting) or has pain in the abdomen.

What might the doctor do?
The doctor will usually confirm the diagnosis by examining your child. A child with a severe headache will be admitted to the hospital for tests to rule out encephalitis or bacterial meningitis.

What can I do to help?
You may give your child acetaminophen to reduce fever and relieve pain. You should make sure that your child drinks plenty of fluids but do not give fruit juices: they stimulate the flow of saliva and may increase gland pain.

What is the outlook?
In most cases, a child recovers in about 10 days. Problems affecting the testes and pancreas do not usually have long-term ill effects. Contrary to popular belief, infertility following orchitis is extremely rare. However, encephalitis or meningitis can result in permanent hearing loss. A single attack of mumps usually provides lifelong immunity.

TETANUS

A serious illness affecting the central nervous system, tetanus is due to infection by bacterial spores, which enter the body through a wound. A deep wound contaminated by garden soil or animal manure is most likely to result in tetanus. The disease is now rare in developed countries because of IMMUNIZATION (p.30).

What are the symptoms?
After an incubation period of between 3 and 21 days, the following symptoms of tetanus develop:
• Inability to open the mouth (lockjaw).
• Difficulty in swallowing.
• Contraction of facial muscles, giving the appearance of a fixed smile.
• Spasms of muscles in the neck, back, abdomen, and limbs, which typically occur over a period of 10 to 14 days and may make breathing difficult.

Should I consult a doctor?
Tetanus is a medical emergency. You should consult a doctor at once if symptoms suggesting tetanus develop.

What is the treatment?
Your child will be admitted to the hospital if the doctor suspects tetanus. Mild cases may require only a light diet and sedative drugs. More severe cases of tetanus may be treated with a tracheostomy (insertion of a tube into the windpipe) to aid breathing, muscle-relaxant and sedative drugs to relieve muscle contractions, and mechanical ventilation to maintain breathing.

What is the outlook?
Tetanus is still a rare cause of death, but with prompt hospital treatment most children recover completely. The time it takes to recover depends on the severity of the illness, but it is usually within 3 weeks.

How is tetanus prevented?
Routine immunization against tetanus is usually given in early childhood (see illustration at right). If your child has a deep wound, you should take him or her immediately to the nearest emergency room, even if he or she has been immunized against tetanus.

Do not wait to see if any symptoms develop. To prevent the disease from developing, the doctor at the hospital may operate on the wound to make sure that all foreign bodies and dead tissue are removed. Your child may be given injections of tetanus vaccine.

Prevention of tetanus
Babies receive a course of three injections of vaccine. Boosters are given between 12 and 18 months, before school entry, and every 10 years thereafter.

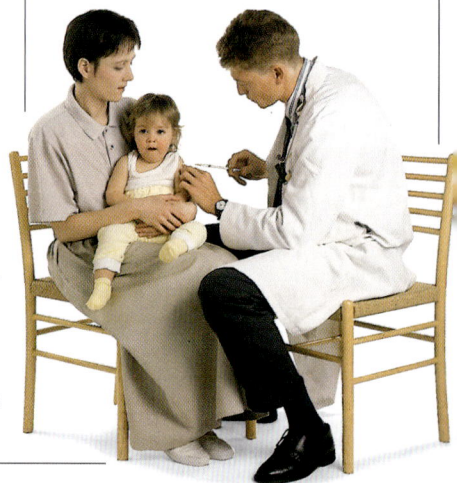

PERTUSSIS

Also known as whooping cough, pertussis is a childhood illness caused by bacterial infection. The major symptom is a cough, sometimes followed by a whoop. Infants under 6 months of age are affected most severely. Pertussis has become uncommon in developed countries because of IMMUNIZATION (p.30).

What are the symptoms?
For the first 7 to 10 days after the 7-day incubation period, the symptoms are:
• A short, dry cough usually at night.
• Runny nose.
• Slight fever.
During the next stage of the illness, which may last 8 to 12 weeks, the symptoms are easier to recognize:
• Bouts of 10 to 20 short, dry coughs that occur day and night.
• Long attacks of coughing followed by a sharp inhalation, which may produce a crowing or whooping sound. (Babies may not whoop.)
• Vomiting caused by coughing.
• Pauses in breathing (more than 10 seconds).
• Sometimes, seizures or ENCEPHALITIS (p.159).
• Appearance of stopping breathing. In rare cases, blockage of an air passage by mucus causes collapse of a segment of the lung or pneumonia.

Should I consult a doctor?
Consult a doctor within 24 hours if a child with a cough is under 6 months, if coughing causes vomiting, or if a cough does not improve after a week. Phone a doctor at once if your child's tongue or lips turn blue during a fit of coughing or if he or she has a seizure.

To confirm the diagnosis, the doctor may collect a sample from your child's throat for laboratory testing. A 10-day course of antibiotics may be prescribed for the child and any siblings. Drugs can shorten the duration of pertussis, but only if given in the early stages.

A child who has turned blue or has had a seizure may be admitted to the hospital, especially if he or she is under 6 months old. If a child continues to feel ill or if the cough has not improved after 6 weeks, your doctor may arrange for your child to have a chest X-ray.

What can I do to help?
Give your child soft, but not crumbly, food and plenty of fluids.

You may stop a coughing attack by slapping your child gently on the back. If necessary, you will be shown how to give your child simple physiotherapy to help clear lung secretions.

To avoid becoming exhausted from lack of sleep while caring for your sick child, ask other family members to take turns sleeping in his or her room.

What is the outlook?
Coughing may continue for several months. In some children, the cough recurs if they catch a viral infection in the following year. Permanent lung damage is extremely rare.

MALARIA

A serious health problem in the tropics and subtropics, malaria is increasingly occurring in other areas as a result of travel to malarial regions. It is caused by malarial parasites, which enter a human's bloodstream via a bite from an infected mosquito. The most serious form of the illness is falciparum malaria.

What are the symptoms?
Symptoms of malaria usually appear 6 to 30 days after infection. Sometimes, however, they may not appear for as long as a year if antimalarial drugs have been taken and been only partly effective. The main symptoms are:
• High fever alternating with shivering.
• Headache.
There may also be:
• Nausea and vomiting.
• Pain in the abdomen, back, and joints.
Falciparum malaria can result in very serious complications affecting the kidneys, liver, brain, and blood.

Should I consult a doctor?
Phone a doctor at once if your child has any symptoms of malaria. You should take your child to the nearest hospital emergency room if he or she develops any of the following symptoms of complications: seizures, drowsiness, yellowing of the skin, or extreme paleness of the skin.

What might the doctor do?
Your child will be admitted to the hospital, and a blood test will be performed to look for malarial parasites. Treatment is in the form of antimalarial drugs. If there are complications, your child may need treatment in an intensive care unit

How can malaria be prevented?
If you plan to visit a malarial region, you and your family will need to take antimalarial drugs. By taking measures such as wearing protective clothing and sleeping under mosquito nets, you may be able to prevent mosquito bites.

Malarial parasite   Blood cell

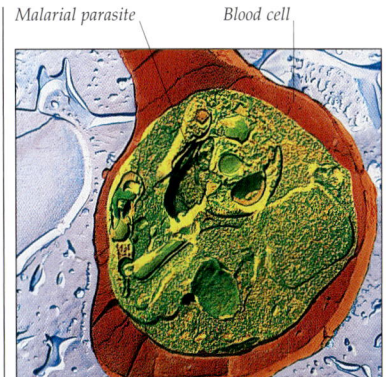

An infected red blood cell
Malarial parasites mature and multiply inside cells. The infected cells eventually burst, releasing parasites to infect more cells. Liver and red blood cells are most often affected.

What is the outlook?
With prompt treatment, recovery may take only a few days or up to 2 weeks, depending on how severe the illness is. However, falciparum malaria may be life threatening if complications affect the brain or the kidneys.

TYPHOID FEVER

Also known as enteric fever, typhoid fever is caused by bacteria called *Salmonella typhi*. The infection is usually acquired from food or water contaminated with bacteria from the feces of an infected person. Typhoid fever occurs when the bacteria pass into the bloodstream, resulting in fever and other symptoms of blood poisoning. Immunization is advisable for people traveling to developing countries, where the disease is common.

Salmonella typhi *bacteria*
After ingestion, the bacteria responsible for typhoid fever invade the wall of the small intestine and enter the bloodstream.

What are the symptoms?
After an incubation period lasting for 7 to 14 days, the following may appear:
• Fever that rises gradually to a temperature of 39–40°C and then stays at this level without daily fluctuations for up to 4 weeks.
• Headache.
• Lack of energy.
• Abdominal pain.
• Constipation or diarrhea.
• Rash, consisting of raised pink spots, on the abdomen and chest. The rash develops during the second week of illness and lasts for about a day.

Intestinal bleeding or perforation or other complications may develop in the second or third week of illness if typhoid fever is not treated.

Should I consult a doctor?
Your child should be seen by a doctor within 24 hours of the appearance of possible typhoid symptoms.

If the doctor suspects that your child might have typhoid fever, he or she will arrange for your child to be admitted to hospital. The diagnosis is confirmed by culturing a sample of stool or urine or by a blood test.

The doctor may treat your child with antibiotics, which are sometimes given intravenously if symptoms are severe.

What is the outlook?
The symptoms usually start to subside several days after the start of treatment. Most children are completely recovered within 2 or 3 weeks. Complications are unlikely to occur if treatment is prompt.

INFECTIOUS MONONUCLEOSIS

A viral infection that is commonly known as "kissing disease," infectious mononucleosis typically causes a fever, lack of energy, and swollen lymph nodes (glands). It is most often caused by the Epstein-Barr virus. The disease can occur at any age, but is most common in adolescents and young adults.

What are the symptoms?
The following symptoms occur after an incubation period of about 10 days:
• High fever (in the range of 38–40°C), which may last for a few days or for several weeks.
• Poor appetite and loss of weight.
• Lack of energy.
• Sore throat, which may be severe.
• Swollen lymph nodes in the neck and/or elsewhere in the body.
• Headache.
• Sometimes, muscle pain.
• Occasionally, a rash of raised pimples or flat spots.
• Abdominal pain.

What are the complications?
The liver condition HEPATITIS (p.188) is the most common complication. Rare complications include PNEUMONIA (p.155); rupture of the spleen; and nervous system, blood, and respiratory problems.

Should I consult a doctor?
Your child should be seen by a doctor if you suspect that he or she may have infectious mononucleosis.

A typical symptom
Children with infectious mononucleosis usually have swollen lymph nodes in the neck. The nodes can be felt just under the jaw.

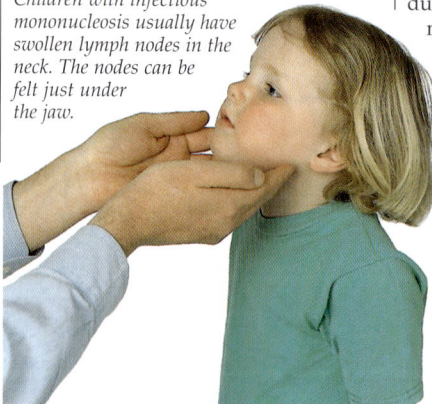

The doctor will arrange for a blood test to confirm the diagnosis and to make sure that your child does not have one of several other infections that produce similar symptoms. There is no specific medical treatment for infectious mononucleosis; antibiotic drugs do not help and may actually bring on the rash.

What can I do to help?
Give acetaminophen to reduce the fever and make sure your child drinks plenty of fluids. Your child may stay in bed during the day if he or she wishes, but may be more comfortable sitting in a chair or being up and around.

What is the outlook?
Most children feel well enough to return to school after a couple of weeks, but if your child requires extra rest for a few more weeks, attending school part-time during this period may hasten recovery. Reassure your child that the feeling of tiredness will lift in time, and help him or her to find a satisfactory balance between periods of activity and rest. Avoid contact sports as long as the spleen is enlarged.

KAWASAKI DISEASE

First observed in Japan in the 1960s, Kawasaki disease is being diagnosed increasingly in Western countries. It occurs mainly in children under the age of 5 years and is believed to be due to an infection, although no causative organism has been found. The disease causes fever, swollen lymph nodes, and symptoms that affect the skin and mucous membranes. Children who have Kawasaki disease may develop heart disease.

What are the symptoms?
Typical symptoms of the disease are:
• Fever, lasting more than 5 days.
• PINK EYE (p.165).
• Dry, cracked, swollen lips.
• Sore throat.
• Swelling of one or more lymph nodes in the neck.
• Swelling of the hands and feet.
• Blotchy, red rash over the entire body.
• Reddening of the palms and soles.
• Skin peeling from the tips of fingers and toes (in second week of illness).

What are the complications?
Possible complications of Kawasaki disease include arthritis, myocarditis (inflammation of the heart muscle), myocardial infarction (heart attack), and coronary artery disease.

Should I consult a doctor?
Your child should be seen by a doctor within 24 hours if you think he or she may have Kawasaki disease.

The doctor may admit your child to the hospital, where he or she can be monitored and treatment may be given promptly if any complications develop. Your child may be given aspirin and injections of gamma globulin to reduce the risk of heart complications.

What is the outlook?
Most children make a full recovery from the disease after about 3 weeks. Myocarditis or arthritis may last for 6 to 8 weeks. Coronary artery disease improves gradually over about a year. In perhaps 1 or 2 percent of cases, serious heart complications may occur.

HIV INFECTION AND AIDS

Most children affected by HIV (human immunodeficiency virus) got it from their mother prior to birth. Treatment of the mother during pregnancy reduces the risk of passing on the virus. HIV infection produces few symptoms, but it progressively damages the immune system, leading to AIDS (acquired immune deficiency syndrome). In AIDS, the immune system is so weak that it lets illnesses, such as PNEUMONIA (p.155), develop.

What are the symptoms?
Most infants infected before or around the time of birth will have symptoms before they are 2 years old. However, some may not develop symptoms until they are over 5 years old, and a few cases have been diagnosed as late as 12 years. Typical among the wide range of possible symptoms in children are:
• Failure to thrive.
• Recurrent diarrhea.
• Enlarged lymph nodes.
• Frequent infections.
• Attacks of pneumonia.
• Developmental delay.

Should I consult a doctor?
Children who are infected with HIV or who have developed AIDS require careful medical supervision.

What might the doctor do?
If the doctor suspects that a baby has HIV, counseling is arranged for the parents. If both parents consent, a blood test is performed. Although the mother's HIV antibodies may remain in the baby's blood for a year or more, a different test can positively confirm or exclude the infection in the first 4 months of life.

The doctor may prescribe drugs, such as zidovudine, to attack the virus and to slow the development and progress of the disease. He or she might give your child regular injections of gamma globulin and prescribe antibacterial drugs, such as cotrimoxazole, which will help to prevent or fight opportunistic infections, such as pneumonia.

What can I do to help?
If you are an HIV-positive mother, you are advised not to breast-feed because of the small risk of transmitting the virus in your milk. If you were treated while pregnant and also avoid breast-feeding, the chances of passing on the infection are less than 5 percent.

If your child has HIV infection or AIDS you will be given counseling and advice on how to manage the illness.

What is the outlook?
HIV-infected children may survive into early adulthood. However, the progressive nature of the infection is such that nearly all infected people eventually succumb to it.

An infected white blood cell
HIV particles (green spheres) are seen here on the surface a white blood cell. White blood cells play a crucial role in the body's immune system. The HIV virus destroys these cells, thus reducing the efficiency of the immune system.

MUSCLE, BONE, AND JOINT DISORDERS

CHILDREN HAVE A HIGH RISK of problems with their muscles, bones, and joints for two main reasons: they are very active, and the bones and joints are still growing and are immature. Some disorders result from genetic abnormalities or birth defects. Musculoskeletal disorders are common and orthopedics is the medical specialty that manages these problems. The outlook is generally good because children have great potential for rapid and complete recovery.

LIMPING

A child with a limp may have a minor injury that will get better on its own. However, the child may have an underlying disorder that requires prompt treatment to prevent permanent disability. Therefore, you should never ignore a limp in a child.

How is it caused?
The most common cause of a limp or a reluctance to walk is pain. Some causes of the pain are shown on the right.

Unequal leg length may also cause a limp. A bone may be short from birth or may fail to grow because of a spinal cord abnormality or CEREBRAL PALSY (p.160) involving muscular weakness of one side of the body. A limp may also be due to apparent shortening of a leg, as a result of CONGENITAL HIP DISLOCATION (p.130) that was detected late or of spinal curvature (see SCOLIOSIS, p.128).

Children who have a disorder of the muscles and/or the nervous system, such as MUSCULAR DYSTROPHY (p.133) or cerebral palsy, may have muscle weakness or incoordination, causing walking problems that resemble a limp.

Rarely, a limp develops as part of a behavioral problem in a child with emotional or psychological difficulties.

Should I consult a doctor?
A doctor should see your child if he or she has a limp, or is old enough to walk but refuses to do so, and you are

Causes of painful limp
Disorders that involve a joint, a muscle, or a bone around the hip or in the leg or foot may cause a painful limp. The site of pain can be misleading; an abnormality in the hip may cause pain in the thigh or knee.

IRRITABLE HIP (p.130), LEGG-PERTHES' DISEASE (p.131), SLIPPED FEMORAL EPIPHYSIS (p.131)

Muscle strain (see STRAINS AND SPRAINS, *opposite)*

Bone infection (see BONE AND JOINT INFECTION, p.133)

KNEE DISORDERS (p.132)

Fractured bone (see FRACTURES AND DISLOCATIONS, p.128)

JUVENILE RHEUMATOID ARTHRITIS (p.132)

unable to find an obvious cause, such as a splinter in the foot. You should phone a doctor at once if your child also has a fever, rash, or hot, swollen joints; these symptoms could indicate bone or joint infection, conditions that require immediate medical treatment.

What might the doctor do?
Your child will be examined and blood tests, X-rays, and/or scanning may be carried out in order to help diagnose the cause of the problem. The child may be referred to a pediatrician or orthopedic surgeon and admission to the hospital may be required for tests or observation. The treatment will depend on the underlying cause.

What is the outlook?
A limp due to a minor injury should disappear in a few days. A limp due to most other causes should disappear once the underlying problem has been treated. In a few cases, the underlying cause, such as unequal leg length or muscular weakness, cannot be cured, and walking problems may be lifelong.

Joint infection (see BONE AND JOINT INFECTION, p.133).

A plantar wart (see WARTS, p.141) *or a sharp object in the sole of the foot*

STRAINS AND SPRAINS

A strain, which is also known as a pulled muscle, occurs when a muscle is overstretched and some of the muscle fibers are damaged. A joint is sprained when one or more of its ligaments (the fibrous bands that connect bones at joints) are overstretched or torn. Strains and sprains often result from falls or strenuous physical activity. Treatment for the injuries can usually be given at home; medical attention is needed only if they are severe.

Tibia

Fibula

Strained ligament

Sprained ankle
The ankle is the most commonly sprained joint. The injury may occur during a fall when the foot is twisted onto its outside edge.

What are the symptoms?
The severity of symptoms depends on how badly the muscle or ligaments are damaged. The symptoms may include:
• Pain and tenderness, which increase with movement of the affected area.
• Swelling at the site of injury.
• Muscle spasm (tightness of a muscle produced by involuntary contractions).
• A limp, if a leg is affected.
• Bruising, which may appear a few days after the injury.

What can I do to help?
For about the first 48 hours after injury, a strain or a sprain is best treated by means of RICE – rest, ice, compression, and elevation (see panel: *Treating strains and sprains*, p.73). You should not apply heat to the injury for the first 48 hours. You may give your child acetaminophen in order to help relieve the pain.

After 1 or 2 days of rest, the pain and swelling should begin to subside, and your child may begin gently to exercise the sprained or strained limb.

Should I consult a doctor?
Your child should be seen by a doctor if pain and swelling are severe just after the injury (for example, if a child cannot walk on an injured ankle) or if milder symptoms have not shown any improvement within a few days.

What might the doctor do?
After an examination the injured area may be X-rayed to check for a fracture. Growing children may be X-rayed 7 to 10 days later as well; some fractures are not visible at first. The injured part may be wrapped in a compression bandage or strapped. Your child may need to use crutches or a sling for a while.

If the strain or sprain is very severe, nonsteroidal anti-inflammatory drugs (NSAIDs), such as ibuprofen, may be prescribed to reduce pain and swelling and speed healing. Your child may have to wear a splint or plaster cast for a severe sprain.

Once the pain has disappeared, the doctor may suggest exercises that will strengthen the affected part or may refer your child to a physiotherapist.

How can I prevent strains and sprains?
Always encourage your child to warm up before doing any strenuous physical activity. Movements that warm up the muscles and mobilize the joints, followed by gentle stretches, are ideal.

What is the outlook?
A strain or a sprain should heal within 2 weeks. If the affected ligament or muscle is allowed to heal properly and is exercised, it will regain full mobility and will not be permanently weakened.

CRAMPS

The onset of a cramp, a strong, painful contraction (spasm) of a muscle, is usually sudden and severe. However, cramps usually last only a few minutes. As well as being painful, the muscle feels hard and tight, and a lump or distortion may be visible in the affected area. Cramps frequently affect the calf muscle.

How is it caused?
A cramp may be triggered by strenuous exercise, by repetitive movement, or by lying or sitting awkwardly. Exercise-related cramps may be partly caused by loss of salt from sweating. Rarely, a recurrent or prolonged cramp may be caused by lack of calcium in the blood.

What can I do to help?
Your child's cramps can be relieved by gently massaging and stretching the affected muscle. You can teach your child to stretch the calf muscle by using the method shown in the illustration (at right). The exercise may be repeated until the pain starts to subside. If there is still some pain, apply a hot water bottle wrapped in a towel to the affected area or have your child take a hot bath or shower. Acetaminophen or ibuprofen may also be given. Cramps can be frightening; reassure your child that cramps are common and temporary.

To help prevent cramps, have your child drink plenty of fluids during exercise, particularly in hot weather.

If the cramps continue and there is no obvious cause, you should consult a doctor to exclude the possibility of an underlying disorder.

Relieving cramps
First, gently pull the toes of the affected leg toward you. Then push the foot back so that the toes point upward. Each position should be held for a few minutes.

FRACTURES AND DISLOCATIONS

Bones commonly fractured (broken) in children are those of the leg and arm, and the clavicle (collarbone). A dislocation occurs when the ligaments that hold the bones of a joint are stretched or torn, so that the bones are displaced. The elbow is the joint most often dislocated in children. When a joint is dislocated, bones may also be fractured. Fractures and dislocations usually result from falls, sports activities, or traffic accidents.

Dislocated elbow joint
This X ray shows severe displacement of the ball-like end of the humerus from its normal position in the socket of the ulna.

What are the symptoms?
A minor fracture may cause only mild symptoms and may be mistaken for a STRAIN OR SPRAIN (p.127). More severe fractures and dislocations may cause:
• Severe pain; the child will not want to move the injured part.
• Extreme tenderness if pressure is put on the area directly over the site of the injury.
• Swelling and skin discoloration at the site of the injury.
• Visible deformity (in the case of a dislocated joint and some serious fractures).
A fracture or a dislocation may damage surrounding tissues, nerves, and blood vessels. If a fractured bone breaks the skin, infection is a risk.

Should I consult a doctor?
Do not move your child if his or her neck or back might be injured; call an ambulance. If you suspect a fracture or dislocation of another part of the body, take your child to an emergency room immediately or

call an ambulance. While waiting for an ambulance, you can immobilize an affected arm or leg (see BROKEN ARM, p.211; BROKEN COLLARBONE, p.210; BROKEN LEG, p.210).

What might the doctor do?
An X ray will be taken of the injured area to confirm whether a bone is fractured and/or dislocated, and to pinpoint the site of the injury and its severity. The doctor may give your child a local or a general anesthetic and manipulate any displaced bones back into position. Repositioning bones and repairing damage to surrounding tissues may require surgery. The affected limb may be immobilized so that the bones heal properly. Fiberglass or plaster casts or splints are used to immobilize some fractures; traction

Greenstick fracture
Because children's bones are supple, the long bones of the arms and legs tend to bend and to crack on only one side.

may also be used. Metal screws, rods, pins, or plates may be inserted to hold bones in position.

Fractures in children heal much more quickly than they do in adults. A small bone that does not bear weight, such as a finger bone, may take only a week or two to heal; large, weight-bearing bones such as the femur (thighbone) may take several months. Dislocations usually heal within a week or two.

As soon as it is safe for your child to use the affected part, physical therapy will be given to prevent muscles and joints from becoming stiff and weak.

What is the outlook?
As long as bones have been properly repositioned and immobilized, your child should recover completely from a fracture or dislocation; stiffness may take several weeks or months to disappear. Joint fractures slightly increase the risk of arthritis in later life.

SCOLIOSIS

Abnormal sideways curvature of the spine is called scoliosis. Usually, scoliosis has no known cause. Rarely, it is due to a structural abnormality of one or more vertebrae or to a local muscle weakness. Scoliosis most often affects girls, starting around the time of the adolescent growth spurt.

What are the symptoms?
The main symptoms are:
• Sideways curve of the spine.
• Shoulders are not level.
• Chest is more prominent on one side than the other.

Appearance of scoliosis
In scoliosis, the spine curves to one side, usually the right, and one shoulder is higher than the other.

The curve of the spine will probably be accentuated when your child bends forward to touch his or her toes with the knees kept straight.

What is the treatment?
A doctor should be consulted if you think your child has scoliosis. After examining your child, the doctor will refer him or her to an orthopedic surgeon, who will monitor your child

to see whether the curvature is getting worse. A mild curvature that is not progressive does not usually need any treatment. In progressive cases, a child may be fitted with a plastic body cast or brace to prevent the curvature of the spine from becoming worse.

What is the outlook?
As long as scoliosis is treated promptly, it should not become any worse and your child is unlikely to have any long-term ill effects. If progressive scoliosis is not treated, it may, in some children, eventually cause severe deformity of the spine and rib cage. The deformity may lead to breathing difficulties and recurrent chest infections.

MINOR SKELETAL PROBLEMS

When a child first starts to stand and walk, parents often worry that the position of his or her legs or feet may be abnormal. The most common sources of concern are in-toeing or out-toeing (walking pigeon-toed or splay-footed), bowlegs, knock-knees, and flat feet. In most cases, these conditions result from the position of the baby in the uterus or are a normal variation. In a very few cases, they may indicate an underlying disorder.

Bowlegs
Outward-curved legs prevent the knees from touching; the shinbone is rotated inward.

Knock-knees
The legs are curved inward so that the knees touch and the feet lie apart.

IN-TOEING; OUT-TOEING

Both conditions are common. Inward rotation of the whole leg from the hip, or the tibia from the knee, are frequent causes of in-toeing. Other causes are curving of the front of the foot (below) and bowlegs (right). Out-toeing is caused by outward rotation of the leg at the hip, or the tibia at the knee.

In-toeing
Inward curving of the front part of the foot (known as hooked forefoot) is a common cause of in-toeing. The web space between the big toe and the second toe is also often increased.

Should I consult a doctor?
Consult a doctor if you are worried about the position of your child's legs or feet. Inward-curving feet usually get better on their own by the age of 3 or 4 years. If severe, they can be treated by gentle manipulation of the feet and immobilization in casts. On occasion,

surgery is needed. Hip rotation usually corrects itself by the age of 8 years. An operation is rarely required for a persistent problem.

Out-toeing almost always corrects itself within a year of the child's starting to walk. Even if out-toeing does persist, it does not cause problems.

BOWLEGS; KNOCK-KNEES

Slight outward curving of the leg bones is normal in toddlers; in bowlegs, the outward curve is exaggerated and the tibia (shinbone) is rotated inward. In knock-knees, the legs curve inward. Bowlegs usually correct themselves by the age of 3 or 4 years; knock-knees are usually outgrown by the age of 11 years.

Should I consult a doctor?
If you are worried, you should consult a doctor, who will probably reassure you that nothing is wrong with your child. Very rarely, an operation is required to correct a severe or persistent deformity, which can be the result of a disorder of bone growth, such as rickets.

FLAT FEET

It is normal for children to have flat feet (meaning that the soles of the feet rest on the ground) up to the age of about 2 or 3 years. In some children, they last but are not associated with any problems. Orthotics (shoe inserts) may help sore legs caused by flat feet. Rarely, flat feet are due to an underlying abnormality of the bones or joints that makes the feet painful, stiff, and weak.

Should I consult a doctor?
Consult a doctor if you are worried about your child's feet. The doctor will check the appearance, mobility, and strength of the feet. If all these features are normal, no treatment is needed.

If there is an underlying disorder, treatment may include immobilizing the feet in casts and, rarely, surgery.

CLUBFOOT

In this congenital deformity, the foot is twisted out of shape or position. Clubfoot affects three times more male babies than female babies, and in half of all cases, both feet are affected. Clubfoot is detected during the routine examination at birth.

Features of clubfoot
The heel of the foot is turned inward, and the rest of the foot is bent downward and inward. In some cases, the tibia (shinbone) is turned inward and the leg muscles are underdeveloped.

How is it caused?
Clubfoot may be due to the position of the baby's foot in the uterus (postural clubfoot) or to an abnormality of the bones in the foot (structural clubfoot).

What might the doctor do?
The doctor will check the mobility of the foot. If it is normal, your child has postural clubfoot, and no treatment is required. Restricted mobility indicates structural clubfoot. Treatment consists

of manipulation of the foot followed by adhesive strapping and splinting to hold the foot in position. If the foot has not straightened by the age of 6 months to 3 years, an operation to straighten it may be performed. The foot is then put in a cast for at least 3 months.

What is the outlook?
Postural clubfoot corrects itself within a few weeks of birth. In about half of all cases of structural clubfoot, the baby's

foot is corrected after 2 to 3 months of manipulation and strapping but it may never be completely normal. If unsuccessful, a cast or exercise may be tried. In most of the remaining cases, an operation corrects the deformity. In a few cases, a series of operations over a 5-year period may improve but not completely correct structural clubfoot.

CONGENITAL HIP DISLOCATION

One newborn baby in about 250 has congenital hip dislocation. In this condition, the head of the femur (thighbone) lies outside the socket of the pelvis or is unstable and likely to slip out of position. Babies are screened for congenital hip dislocation soon after birth, and tests for the condition are included in routine checkups during the first year of life. Congenital hip dislocation runs in families and is more common in girls than in boys.

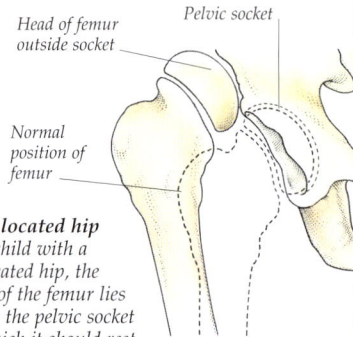

A dislocated hip
In a child with a dislocated hip, the head of the femur lies above the pelvic socket in which it should rest.

How is it caused?
Although the underlying cause is not known, one or both of a baby's hips may be dislocated or unstable because the fibrous capsule surrounding the hip joint is weak or because the pelvic socket is abnormally shallow.

What are the symptoms?
Congenital hip dislocation is usually detected soon after birth. The technique shown below or, in some hospitals, ultrasound may be used to diagnose the condition. The problem may be found later, during one of the routine checkups in the first year of life. Occasionally, the disorder may not be discovered until your child begins to walk, when you may notice:
• A limp.
• The back of the affected leg has more skin folds below the buttock than the unaffected leg.
Your child should be seen by a doctor if you suspect that he or she may have congenital hip dislocation.

What is the treatment?
An unstable hip often corrects itself soon after birth. If this has not happened by the time of the baby's 2-week checkup, an imaging study may be done and a splint applied to move the head of the femur into the socket and keep it there. The splint is usually worn for 2 to 4 months. You will be advised about how to care for your baby while the splint is on. When it is removed, the hip joint should be normal. However, if your baby's congenital hip dislocation is not discovered until his or her next routine examination (which is carried out at 6 weeks or more) the head of the femur may have to be moved into the socket and held in place by traction for several weeks. After traction, your child will probably have to wear a splint or cast for several months.

If your child begins to walk before the condition is discovered, a series of operations will probably be necessary to correct the disorder.

What is the outlook?
The earlier that treatment is given, the better the outlook. If a child is treated in early infancy, he or she should be able to walk normally and is not likely to suffer from any ill effects later in life. However, if treatment is delayed or if no treatment is given, there may be a risk of a permanent limp and the early onset of arthritis in the affected hip.

Examining a baby's hips
The doctor manipulates a newborn baby's thighs and hips to check for congenital hip dislocation. A dislocated hip may cause a jolt or jerk as the head of the femur moves in and out of the partially formed socket.

HIP PAIN

This condition, called toxic synovitis, occurs when the lining of the hip joint becomes inflamed and fluid accumulates inside the joint. The cause is unknown, but hip pain often develops within 2 weeks of a mild upper respiratory tract infection, such as a cold. Children 2 to 12 years of age are most susceptible to hip pain.

What are the symptoms?
The symptoms of hip pain start suddenly and may include:
• A limp.
• Pain in the hip, groin, thigh, or knee.
• Sometimes, mild fever.
Your child should be seen by a doctor within 24 hours if he or she has pain in the hip, groin, thigh, or knee, and/or a limp without an obvious cause.

What is the treatment?
The doctor will probably advise you to give painkillers, such as acetaminophen, and to make sure that your child rests until the pain improves, which usually takes 1 to 7 days.

If the pain is severe, a child may be hospitalized and blood tests may be carried out to exclude an infection. X rays and ultrasounds of the hip may be taken to rule out conditions such as LEGG-PERTHES' DISEASE (opposite) or joint infection (see BONE AND JOINT INFECTION, p.133). Traction may be applied to the hip to relieve muscle spasm and pain.

What is the outlook?
Once the pain has subsided, a child can usually return to normal activities. If a child becomes active too early, symptoms may return and nonsteroidal anti-inflammatory drugs (NSAIDs), such as ibuprofen, may be required. If pain recurs in the hip despite treatment, the problem may be due to Legg-Perthes' disease or JUVENILE RHEUMATOID ARTHRITIS (p.132).

SLIPPED FEMORAL EPIPHYSIS

The growth of a long bone occurs near the ends at growth plates, which separate regions called the epiphyses from the main shaft. A slipped femoral epiphysis occurs when the upper epiphysis of the femur (thighbone), which forms part of the hip joint, slips into an abnormal position. This rare disorder affects adolescents during the growth spurt (about 10 to 14 years of age in girls and 12 to 16 years of age in boys). Children who are overweight or growing very rapidly are most susceptible to the condition.

NORMAL POSITION   SLIPPED EPIPHYSIS

Slipped femoral epiphysis
In this condition, the growth plate shears and the upper epiphysis (end) of the femur slips and comes to lie below and behind its normal position, causing the leg to rotate outward.

How is it caused?
In growing children, the femur grows mainly at the upper end. The growth plate, where new bone is formed, is made of cartilage and so is an area of relative weakness in the bone; the upper epiphysis is therefore vulnerable to displacement (see illustration at right). A femoral epiphysis may slip suddenly out of position as a result of an injury that shears the growth plate, or it may slip gradually, for unknown reasons.

What are the symptoms?
The symptoms may include:
- Pain in the hip, knee, or thigh.
- Inability to bear weight on affected leg.
- A limp or a splay-footed walk because the leg is rotated outward.
- Restricted movement of the hip.

If your child has a painful hip, thigh, or knee and/or a limp, he or she should be seen by a doctor within 24 hours, immediately if there is hip pain accompanied by a high fever.

What is the treatment?
The doctor will examine your child and have the hip X-rayed. If the X ray shows a slipped femoral epiphysis, an operation will be performed. A mildly slipped epiphysis may be left where it is and fixed with screws to halt slipping. In the same operation, the epiphysis of the other hip joint may be strengthened similarly. For a more severe slip, a wedge of bone may be removed from below the upper epiphysis so that the epiphysis is returned to its normal position within the pelvic socket.

What is the outlook?
Provided that the hip is treated promptly, the long-term outlook is good, and after recovering from the operation, your child will probably be able to lead a normal, active life. A subsequent slipped femoral epiphysis is unlikely to occur, especially once the growth spurt is over. In a few cases, however, the affected hip may become stiff and painful, and there may be vulnerability to arthritis in later life.

LEGG-PERTHES' DISEASE

Progressive softening, followed by re-forming and hardening, of the head of the femur (thighbone) is known as Legg-Perthes' disease. It is caused by poor blood supply to the head of the femur. The condition affects children, particularly boys, aged 4 to 8 years. Although Legg-Perthes' disease gets better by itself in 2 to 4 years, treatment should be carried out as early as possible in order to prevent the hip joint from becoming deformed.

What are the symptoms?
The main symptoms of the disease are:
- A limp.
- Pain in the hip or knee.
- Restricted movement at the hip.

If your child has pain in the hip or knee and/or a limp, he or she should be seen by a doctor within 24 hours.

What is the treatment?
The doctor will examine your child and may send him or her to the hospital for an X ray of the hip joint to establish the cause of the symptoms. The type of

Flattened head of femur   Pelvic socket

Femur

Femoral deformity
If the hip joint continues to bear a child's weight while he or she has Legg-Perthes' disease, the head and neck of the femur may become deformed.

Shortened neck of femur

treatment depends on the severity of the disease. In less severe cases, bed rest for 1 to 2 weeks until the joint pain subsides, with regular monitoring by X ray, may be all that is required. If the joint is at risk of becoming deformed, your child may have to wear calipers, splints, or a plaster cast. In very severe cases, an operation may be performed to fix the head of the femur more firmly within the pelvic socket, which reduces the risk of hip joint deformity.

What is the outlook?
The younger a child is when Legg-Perthes' disease is discovered and treatment is given, and the less severe the disease, the better the outcome is likely to be. Usually, deformity of the hip joint can be prevented and the joint will function normally. In some very severe cases, joint deformity cannot be prevented, even with treatment, and arthritis of the hip is a risk later in life.

KNEE DISORDERS

The most common knee disorders that affect children are chondromalacia patellae and Osgood-Schlatter disease. They occur mainly in adolescents. Both conditions may be brought on by overuse of the joint, usually as a result of strenuous physical activity. One or both knees may be affected.

Tendon from quadriceps muscle
Patella
Tibia
Point of attachment

Osgood-Schlatter disease
The large tendon from the quadriceps muscle of the thigh extends to the patella and then to the tibia, where it is attached. Exercise can cause inflammation of the tendon at its point of attachment.

CHONDROMALACIA PATELLAE

In this condition, the cartilage at the back of the patella (kneecap) becomes soft, swollen, and roughened. Girls 15 to 18 years of age are the group most susceptible to chondromalacia patellae.

The main symptom is aching pain behind the patella. The pain is made worse by exercise (especially climbing stairs) and gets better with rest.

What is the treatment?

The treatment is rest. Your child should avoid any activities that make the pain worse or that involve repetitive knee-bending, such as cycling. You may give acetaminophen to relieve the pain. If pain is severe or is no better after 24 hours, have a doctor see your child to exclude a more serious disorder.

What is the outlook?

Bouts of pain behind the patella may recur throughout life. Most children are symptom-free within a year of growth ceasing. In a few cases, early arthritis may develop.

OSGOOD-SCHLATTER DISEASE

In this disorder, there is inflammation of the tibia (shinbone) just below the knee at the point where a large tendon is attached (see illustration above right). Osgood-Schlatter disease mainly affects boys 10 to 14 years of age.

The main symptoms are tenderness, pain, and swelling just below the knee, which usually worsens with exercise. Your child should be seen by a doctor, but referral to an orthopedic surgeon is not necessary.

What is the treatment?

The doctor may ask your child to avoid strenuous physical activities, such as football, for several months. If the pain is severe or persists for more than a few months despite avoiding strenuous activities, the knee, in rare cases, may be immobilized in a cast for 6 to 8 weeks. This almost always cures the problem.

As long as the child exercises only moderately until after about 14 years of age, the problem is unlikely to recur.

JUVENILE RHEUMATOID ARTHRITIS

Three types of rheumatoid arthritis (inflammation of the joints) affect children. Pauciarticular arthritis affects four or fewer large joints (such as the knee). The polyarticular type affects small joints, such as those of the hands. Systemic juvenile arthritis also affects small joints and produces symptoms of general illness.

How is it caused?

The cause is unknown, but the disorder may be inherited. Joint inflammation may result from a viral infection or, in the case of Lyme disease, from a tick bite (see INSECT BITES AND STINGS, p.138).

What are the symptoms?

The main symptoms are:
• Pain, redness, swelling, and stiffness of affected joints.
• A limp, if the feet or legs are affected.
• In polyarticular arthritis, a mild fever.
In systemic arthritis, the following symptoms may appear several weeks or months before the joints are affected:
• A temperature above 39°C.
• Swollen glands throughout the body.
• A blotchy, nonitchy rash.
A known complication is IRITIS (p.164).

Arthritis affecting the hands
The joints of the fingers are red and swollen because of arthritis. Other small joints that may be affected are those of the neck and jaw.

Should I consult a doctor?

Your child should be seen by a doctor within 24 hours of the onset of joint pain or stiffness, a limp, or a rash with a fever. The doctor will examine your child and arrange for blood tests in order to exclude other disorders.

What is the treatment?

An important part of treatment consists of physical therapy to maintain muscle strength and joint mobility. Splints may need to be worn at night to prevent joint deformity and sometimes during the day in order to rest the joints.

The doctor may prescribe aspirin and nonsteroidal anti-inflammatory drugs (NSAIDs), such as ibuprofen, to relieve pain and swelling. If these drugs are ineffective, more powerful drugs, such as corticosteroids, may be prescribed. In very severe cases, an operation may be performed to replace joints that are damaged and painful or to lengthen muscles that are causing deformity.

Until your child has recovered from arthritis, his or her eyes will probably be examined regularly for signs of iritis.

What is the outlook?

One third of children recover from juvenile arthritis completely; another third continues to have symptoms for many years. In the remaining cases, the condition worsens.

BONE AND JOINT INFECTION

Infection of a bone or joint most commonly occurs when bacteria are carried through the bloodstream from an infected site, such as a wound or a BOIL (p.137), elsewhere in the body. In some cases, infection spreads directly from nearby infected tissue.

BONE INFECTION

Children 3 to 14 years of age, especially boys, are susceptible to bone infection. The long bones of the arms and legs are most often affected. Without prompt treatment, bone infection may become chronic and difficult to eradicate.

What are the symptoms?
The symptoms may include:
- Severe pain in the affected arm or leg, which the child is reluctant to move or allow to be touched.
- Fever.
- If treatment is delayed, swelling and inflammation of the skin overlying the infected bone.

Phone a doctor at once if you think that your child might have a bone infection.

What might the doctor do?
The doctor will examine your child and admit him or her to the hospital for tests, including a blood culture and a bone scan. Treatment is with antibiotics. In a few cases, an operation may be carried out to remove infected bone. Your child should make a complete recovery if he or she is treated promptly.

JOINT INFECTION

Infection of a joint is most common in children up to the age of 2 years and in adolescents. The joint becomes inflamed and fluid collects within it. If treatment is delayed, the cartilage that covers bones inside the joint may be damaged, causing stiffness and deformity of the joint.

What are the symptoms?
The symptoms are similar to those of bone infection, but the joint is usually also swollen and hot. Phone a doctor at once if you think that your child might have a joint infection.

What might the doctor do?
The doctor will examine your child and may send him or her to the hospital for an ultrasound of the joint. To confirm the diagnosis, fluid is taken from the joint for analysis (see illustration below). Blood tests may also be carried out. Treatment is with antibiotic drugs. An operation may be performed to drain the infected fluid from the infected joint. Once the infection has cleared up, your child may receive physical therapy, which will keep the joint flexible. As long as the infected joint is treated promptly, your child should make a complete recovery.

Femur

Patella

Fluid

Diagnosing joint infection
In order to diagnose bacterial joint infection, fluid may be removed from the joint for microscopic analysis. Here, a needle is inserted into the knee, and the fluid flows into a syringe.

Tibia *Syringe*

MUSCULAR DYSTROPHY

The main features of this disorder are progressive weakness and wasting of muscle. There are several types of muscular dystrophy. The most common and most serious type is Duchenne muscular dystrophy; it affects only boys and appears before 5 years of age.

How is it caused?
Duchenne muscular dystrophy is due to an abnormal gene. A boy born to a woman who is a carrier has a 50 percent chance of having the disorder; his sisters have a 50 percent chance of being carriers.

What are the symptoms?
The first symptom is weakness in the leg muscles, which may cause your child to:
- Walk late (at over the age of 18 months) and waddle.
- Climb stairs with difficulty.
- Fall easily and roll onto his front, and climb or "hand walk" up his own legs.

Other symptoms may include:
- Enlarged calf muscles.
- Inward curvature of the lower spine.

Your child should be seen by a doctor if you think that muscular dystrophy might be a possibility.

What might the doctor do?
The doctor will examine your child and may send him to a neurologist. Hospital tests may be arranged in order to confirm the diagnosis. At present, there is no cure for

Weak leg muscles
A child with weak leg muscles gets up from the floor by pushing against his ankles, knees, and thighs.

Duchenne muscular dystrophy. Instead, physical therapy is given to maintain mobility, and you will be shown how to help your child exercise.

How can Duchenne muscular dystrophy be prevented?
A woman who has a family history of Duchenne dystrophy and who plans to have a baby may be tested to see if she is a carrier. If she is a carrier, she will be offered genetic counseling to explain the risks of a baby's being affected. Tests can also be done during pregnancy to see if the fetus of a woman is affected; if it is, termination can be considered.

What is the outlook?
The child's muscle weakness increases and gradually spreads to affect more and more muscles until the child needs a wheelchair, usually by 8 to 11 years of age. The boy becomes increasingly vulnerable to chest infections and may not survive past his early 20s.

SKIN DISORDERS

YOUNG SKIN IS SENSITIVE, and skin reactions are common in childhood. A rash or other change in the skin may be caused by irritation (for example, by chemicals in detergents), infection, or allergy. Skin reactions may also be part of a generalized illness, such as roseola. Disorders confined to the skin are often minor and usually get better rapidly. The first step in dealing with a skin disorder is to identify its cause, and a doctor is the best person to do this.

SEBORRHEIC DERMATITIS

This common inflammation of the skin has no known cause. It may affect the body and face and/or the scalp. Seborrheic dermatitis may appear initially in the first few months of a baby's life. The symptoms vary in severity over a number of months, but generally clear up by the age of about 2 years. However, seborrheic dermatitis may reappear after puberty and then recur periodically throughout life.

What are the symptoms?
The main symptoms of the infant form of seborrheic dermatitis are:
- A scaly, blotchy rash, most commonly in the skin creases of the diaper area but also sometimes in other areas of the body (see illustration below).
- Occasionally, slight itchiness.
- Thick yellowish scales on the scalp (cradle cap). Scaly areas on the forehead, behind the ears, and in the eyebrows may accompany cradle cap.

Scalp

Sites of seborrheic dermatitis in infants
Babies may be affected by seborrheic dermatitis at one or more of the sites shown here.

— *Face*
— *Neck*
— *Armpits*
— *Chest (occasionally)*
— *Diaper area*

The main symptoms of the adolescent form of seborrheic dermatitis are:
- A scaly, blotchy rash, which may appear on the face, behind the ears, on the neck, chest, and back, and in the armpits and groin.
- Occasionally, itchiness.
- Dandruff, if the scalp is affected. White flakes of dead skin can be seen in the hair, usually near the scalp.

Scratching the affected area sometimes leads to a bacterial infection, such as IMPETIGO (p.139), causing the rash to become raw and weepy.

What can I do to help?
Affected areas of skin should be kept clean with emulsifying ointment, rather than soap, which may irritate the rash. After cleaning the affected areas of skin, apply a corticosteroid cream. This treatment is most effective if started as soon as symptoms appear.

Cradle cap often disappears on its own within a few weeks or months. However, you can remove unsightly cradle cap scales by gently massaging baby oil or olive oil into your baby's scalp and leaving it overnight. The next day, comb your baby's hair in order to dislodge the softened scales, and then wash them away. Over-the-counter shampoos containing salicylic acid are also available for treating cradle cap.

Regular use of a special shampoo or combing your baby's hair daily may stop the scaly patches from forming.

Dandruff can be controlled very easily by using an over-the-counter antidandruff shampoo.

Should I consult a doctor?
Your child should be seen by a doctor if the rash is extensive or looks infected, the scalp is inflamed, other symptoms develop, or the condition does not improve within a few weeks. The doctor may prescribe a corticosteroid cream or ointment, which may contain an antibiotic or an antiseptic. With treatment, the rash should clear up within a few weeks.

Cradle cap
Scaly yellowish patches of skin on the scalp are the main feature of cradle cap. Although the patches are unsightly, cradle cap is harmless.

ECZEMA

About 1 child in 20 develops the itchy rash of eczema. The rash usually first appears before a child is 18 months old, and may vary in severity over a number of years. The cause of eczema is unknown. Most affected children have a close relative with eczema or an allergic disorder, such as ASTHMA (p.153) or hay fever (see ALLERGIC RHINITIS, p.152). Rarely, intolerance to certain foods may be responsible (see REACTIONS TO FOOD, p.182).

What are the symptoms?
The symptoms of eczema vary, depending on the age of the child. In children less than 4 years old:
- The rash consists of itchy, inflamed skin, which may be mildly weepy.
- The scalp, cheeks, forearms, fronts of the legs, and trunk are most often affected, although the rash may appear anywhere on the body.
The rash often disappears before a child reaches the age of 4 years and, in some individuals, never returns. The rash may reappear (or appear for the

Appearance of eczema
The insides of the elbows are often affected by eczema. The rash seen here has the typical appearance of eczema in children aged 4 years or over: it is scaly, red, and dry, with a rough surface.

first time) in some children between the ages of 4 and 10 years. At this age:
- The rash consists of itchy, dry, scaly patches, and the skin may be cracked.
- The face, neck, insides of the elbows, wrists, backs of the knees, and ankles are most commonly affected (see illustration above right).
- Skin in affected areas may become thickened over time.
Regardless of your child's age, the first sign of an impending flare-up of eczema is generally a small, slightly inflamed area on the skin.

What are the complications?
If your child scratches the rash, the skin may become infected with bacteria, resulting in weeping blisters. A much rarer, but more serious, complication is an illness called eczema herpeticum, which can occur if a child with eczema is infected by the herpes simplex virus (which causes COLD SORES, p.139). This disorder causes a widespread rash

Sites of eczema
In children aged 4 years and over, the areas shown here are those most often affected by eczema. The rash tends to affect sites at joints where there are folds of skin.

Face

Neck

Insides of the elbows

Wrists

Backs of the knees

Ankles

consisting of blisters and open sores, which is often accompanied by a high fever of 40–41°C. The lymph nodes may also be enlarged.

Should I consult a doctor?
Your child should be seen by a doctor within 24 hours if he or she has not had the rash before. If your child has already been diagnosed as having eczema and the rash does not respond to treatment or gets worse, he or she should be seen by a doctor because the rash may be infected.

What might the doctor do?
A corticosteroid or immunomodulator ointment may be prescribed by the doctor to reduce inflammation and itchiness during flare-ups of eczema. Continue to apply the cream to affected areas of skin, according to the doctor's instructions, until the normal texture of

the skin has returned. (Limit use of corticosteroid cream or ointment on the face). When slight inflammation indicates that a flare-up of eczema is imminent, apply the prescribed cream to affected areas to prevent the rash developing. If the itchiness is keeping your child awake at night, an antihistamine may be prescribed. The doctor may suggest you exclude certain foods from your child's diet if the eczema is severe or widespread.

For a bacterial infection, the doctor may prescribe a cream or ointment containing a corticosteroid and an antibiotic. He or she may also prescribe an oral antibiotic.

Your child may be sent to the hospital if eczema herpeticum develops. In the hospital, the antiviral drug, acyclovir may be given intravenously.

What can I do to help?
Apart from applying any creams or ointments as directed by the doctor, you may be able to prevent some symptoms by keeping the skin from becoming too dry. Bathe your child daily in tepid water, and use a mild cleanser such as a baby soap or a water-based cream. You may make the bath water less irritating by adding a bath oil that is formulated for eczema, but avoid using bubble bath.

Keep your child's skin soft and well moisturized by regularly applying an emollient, such as a water-based cream or emulsifying ointment. The emollient should be used several times a day on the affected areas. It may be especially effective if it is applied to the skin when it is still warm and wet after your child's daily bath.

In some children, eczema is worse in cold weather, while in others hot weather prompts a flare-up. Make sure that your child always wears cotton clothing next to the skin as this will help reduce irritation.

Your child should avoid close contact with anyone who has cold sores.

What is the outlook?
As your child grows older, the rash will probably become less extensive, and by adolescence most children no longer have eczema. However, up to 50 percent of children who are affected by eczema develop other allergic conditions, such as asthma or hay fever.

DIAPER RASH

A baby's skin may become irritated if a wet or soiled diaper is worn for too long. Diaper rash affects most babies at some time, but illness and diarrhea may increase a child's susceptibility. Some children seem to be more prone to diaper rash than others.

Preventing diaper rash
Protecting your baby's diaper area with a barrier ointment or cream helps prevent diaper rash.

What are the symptoms?
The main symptoms of diaper rash are:
• A sore diaper area.
• Red raw spots in the diaper area.
An infection by bacteria (see IMPETIGO, p.139) or by the yeast *Candida albicans* (see ORAL THRUSH, p.176) may cause the area to become blistery and weepy.

What is the treatment?
Leave the diaper off and expose your baby's bottom to warm, dry air as much as you can. You should make an appointment to see a doctor if the rash does not improve after a few days. The doctor may prescribe a corticosteroid cream to reduce inflammation. If the rash is infected, a corticosteroid cream combined with an anti-infective drug may be prescribed. With treatment, an infected rash should take between a few days and a week to clear up.

How can diaper rash be prevented?
To help prevent a rash, change your baby's diaper as soon as possible after he or she has urinated or defecated. After washing and drying the diaper area, protect your baby's skin by applying water-repellent zinc cream or petroleum jelly.

CONTACT DERMATITIS

Dermatitis (inflammation of the skin) resulting from contact with irritating substances may occur in infants and children. Common irritants include nickel (in jewelry), rubber, fabric dyes, adhesive bandages, plants such as poison ivy, bubble bath, detergents, medicinal creams, and cosmetics.

Contact dermatitis
This red, dry, scaly rash on a child's wrist was probably caused by a reaction to the nickel in a metal watchband or bracelet.

What are the symptoms?
The rash may be confined to one area if due to jewelry, for example; or it may be widespread if due to products such as bubble bath or scented soaps. The main symptoms are:
• An inflamed, scaly rash.
• Intense itchiness.
• Sometimes, blistering and weeping (often caused by contact with plants).

The symptoms may take several days to appear after contact; the length of time they last depends on the irritant.

What is the treatment?
If you know what the cause of the dermatitis is, remove it or encourage your child to avoid contact with it. You may apply calamine lotion or a corticosteroid cream to the rash to help relieve the symptoms.

If you cannot discover the cause, consult a doctor, whose questions about your child's activities usually help to identify the irritant. Rarely, suspected irritants are applied to small areas of skin and the reaction noted.

CHAPPED LIPS

A child with chapped lips has a rash around his or her mouth. The rash, called perioral dermatitis, is caused by saliva irritating the lips and surrounding skin as a result of excessive lip-licking or thumb-sucking. It will clear up when the habit disappears.

What are the symptoms?
The symptoms of chapped lips are:
• Inflamed, scaly skin around the lips.
• Sore, dry lips.

What can I do to help?
Apply a corticosteroid cream (available over the counter) to the skin around the lips for a few days to reduce the inflammation, then use petroleum jelly often to protect the skin from saliva. Applying lip balm to the lips will help to moisturize and protect them.

Children often grow out of lip-licking or thumb-sucking before they reach school age. The habit may be given up more quickly if, whenever it occurs, you gently draw your child's attention to something more interesting. Nagging your child may make the habit worse.

Protecting dry lips
Lip balm helps to protect your child's lips from irritating saliva and also relieves discomfort.

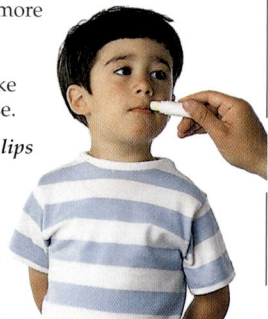

Psoriasis

In this chronic skin condition, red, scaly, thickened patches develop on the limbs, trunk, or scalp. Children over the age of 10 years are most likely to be affected. The rash does not usually itch, but psoriasis can be uncomfortable and your child may be distressed by its appearance. Psoriasis tends to fluctuate in severity; it often becomes worse during periods of illness or emotional stress, such as impending school examinations.

How is it caused?

The cause of psoriasis is unknown, but it tends to run in families and may be inherited. The psoriasis rash sometimes first appears after an acute infection such as tonsillitis (see SORE THROAT, p.150) or an infection of the middle ear (see OTITIS MEDIA, p.162).

Psoriasis rash
This rash is characteristic of psoriasis. The affected area is a sharply defined, raised red patch covered by silvery white scales of dead skin. A large patch such as this may appear on the elbows or knees.

A psoriasis rash forms when new skin cells are produced at a faster rate than old skin cells are shed. The excess new cells build up to produce the thickened areas, which may be covered with dead, flaking skin.

What are the symptoms?

The psoriasis rash tends to vary in appearance. However, the most common symptoms are:
- Patches of thickened red skin that are covered with silvery scales. The patches are most often located on the elbows, knees, or scalp.
- Numerous small, red, slightly scaly patches, which tend to be scattered over the trunk and face.
- Pitted and thickened nails.
- Pain or discomfort if cracks appear in the affected skin.

What can I do to help?

If your child's psoriasis is mild, you may be able to prevent flare-ups by keeping the skin well moisturized with an emollient cream. Exposing affected areas to the sun sometimes helps clear up the rash, but take care not to let your child get sunburned.

Should I consult a doctor?

Your child should be seen by a doctor if the rash is severe, widespread, or distressing. The doctor will probably refer your child to a dermatologist. For psoriasis limited to a few small areas, such as the scalp, knees, or elbows, the dermatologist may prescribe a cream or ointment containing coal tar, salicylic acid, or a corticosteroid. If the psoriasis is widespread, an ointment containing dithranol may be prescribed. Other treatments, such as bathing in water containing a coal tar preparation and moderate exposure to ultraviolet light, may also be recommended.

What is the outlook?

Psoriasis cannot be cured and is likely to recur throughout life. However, individual attacks can be controlled if they are treated promptly.

Boil

A boil is a painful, pus-filled swelling in the skin. It can occur when a hair follicle becomes infected by bacteria. The source of the infection is not usually known, although the bacteria are carried in the nose. Boils most commonly occur in damp areas, such as the armpit and groin, and at the back of the neck.

What are the symptoms?

A boil usually starts as a small red lump that becomes larger as it fills with pus. The main symptoms are:
- Pain and tenderness around the boil.
- A white or yellow "head" of pus at the center of the boil.

Most boils burst, releasing their pus, although occasionally pus drains away into surrounding tissues. In most cases, healing occurs within 2 weeks.

What can I do to help?

If a boil is coming to a head, you should apply hot compresses to it or soak it in warm water. This treatment may make it burst more quickly and

Appearance of a boil
The lump covered by white flakes of dead skin is a boil. Pus has escaped from the boil to form a greenish scab at its center. The surrounding skin is red because the infection has spread.

hasten healing. When the boil bursts, carefully wipe away the pus with a cotton ball, apply an antibiotic cream to the affected skin, and cover with a bandage. You should avoid poking or squeezing the boil to make it burst, because by doing so you may cause the infection to spread.

Your child should be seen by a doctor if a boil lasts longer than 2 weeks or is very large or painful, or if your child suffers from recurrent boils.

What might the doctor do?

The doctor may prescribe some oral antibiotics to clear up the infection. In some cases, he or she may make a small cut in the boil in order to release pus. If boils keep recurring, the doctor may prescribe an antibiotic cream to apply inside your child's nose. He or she may suggest that your child use an antiseptic soap both for washing and when taking a bath.

INSECT BITES AND STINGS

Most children experience only localized itchiness or pain when they are stung or bitten by an insect. However, some children, particularly those with allergies, may have a severe, possibly life-threatening, reaction to insect stings, especially those of bees and wasps. This reaction is called ANAPHYLACTIC SHOCK (p.154). The most common insect bites are those of mosquitoes. The risk of a child being stung or bitten increases with warm weather.

INSECT BITES

The reaction to an insect bite causes:
• A small red pimple.
• Local itchiness.
• In some cases, a weal (a smooth, raised red area) or a firm swelling.
• Rash (tick bite).
The symptoms may last from a few hours to several days. In some children, most commonly those 2 to 7 years of age, bites result in groups of itchy, raised spots that last for 2 to 10 days. The tick bite rash starts as a small, round red area that quickly gets larger.

What can I do to help?
Scratching may cause infection. Cool compresses or calamine lotion relieve itching. When insects are active, have your child use an insect repellent (containing 10 percent DEET) on exposed skin, wear long pants and socks, and avoid infested areas.

INSECT STINGS

The reaction to an insect sting most commonly results in:
• Local irritation or pain.
• Redness and swelling.
The symptoms of an insect sting usually disappear within 48 hours.

Children who are allergic to the venom of bees, wasps, and yellow jackets develop HIVES (below) and/or anaphylactic shock, a severe generalized allergic reaction.

Should I consult a doctor?
Call an ambulance or take your child to the nearest emergency room at once if he or she develops ANAPHYLACTIC SHOCK (p.154). If your child has had a severe reaction to a sting, your doctor may give you a kit with an adrenaline-filled syringe you can use to prevent anaphylactic shock if your child is stung by an insect again.

TICK BITES

A bite from an infected tick that has been embedded in the skin for at least 36 hours can cause Lyme disease. Ticks, usually found on deer and mice, are common in Canada, but instances of Lyme disease remain rare.

What are the symptoms?
Symptoms of Lyme disease include:
• Fever and headache.
• Weakness and fatigue.
• A mild stiff neck and body aches.
The classic "bull's-eye" rash may also occur in the groin, armpit, or thigh.

What can I do to help?
If you find a tick, grab it close to the skin with tweezers; pull it up slowly without squeezing. Wash your hands and the bite area. Save the tick.

Call a doctor if your child has played in tick-infested areas or has symptoms. If the classic rash is present, a blood test may be done, and antibiotics may be given for 2 to 4 weeks. Tests done early on may give false-positive results; they are more accurate several weeks later.

What is the outlook?
Most people recover. If Lyme disease is untreated, JUVENILE CHRONIC ARTHRITIS (p.132) or MENINGITIS (p.158) can occur.

HIVES

An intensely itchy, raised rash characterizes hives. In many cases, the cause is not known. The most common known cause is an allergic reaction to a specific food, such as fish (see REACTIONS TO FOOD, p.182), a drug (such as penicillin), an insect sting (above), or a plant. Viral and bacterial infections can also cause this rash.

What are the symptoms?
There are two forms of hives. Acute hives last between 30 minutes and several days; chronic hives may persist for up to several months. Both types may recur. The symptoms of chronic and acute hives are:
• Smooth, raised white or yellow lumps surrounded by an inflamed area of skin.
• Extreme itchiness.
The rash may affect a small area or it may be widespread. Very rarely, hives are part of ANAPHYLACTIC SHOCK (p.154), a severe, generalized allergic reaction. The symptoms of anaphylactic shock include swelling of the face or mouth, noisy or difficult breathing, difficulty in

Hives rash
The patches of affected skin in hives vary in size and shape. The patches are raised, pale, and have red edges, which distinguish them from the surrounding normal skin.

swallowing, and abnormal drowsiness. You should call an ambulance or take your child to the nearest hospital emergency room at once if he or she has any of these symptoms.

What is the treatment?
If your child has recurrent attacks of hives, try to identify the cause so that your child can avoid it, if possible. During attacks, an over-the-counter oral antihistamine may relieve the symptoms. It should be continued for several weeks after the rash disappears.

If antihistamines do not help severe hives, your child should be seen by a doctor. An oral corticosteroid may be prescribed and/or your child may be sent to a dermatologist for tests to establish the cause of the problem. As your child gets older, attacks of hives will probably diminish.

COLD SORES

Caused by a strain of the herpes simplex virus, cold sores are small blisters that develop on and around the lips. The initial infection by herpes simplex often goes unnoticed but may cause GINGIVOSTOMATITIS (p.176). After this first infection, the virus lies dormant in nerve cells but may be reactivated later to cause cold sores. Cold sores may be triggered by an acute infection, anxiety or emotional stress, or exposure to the sun or cold winds.

What are the symptoms?
Cold sores may appear singly or in clusters. The main symptoms are:
- A tingling sensation around the mouth, which occurs 4 to 12 hours before any blisters appear.
- Small blisters, which may be itchy or sore, surrounded by a slightly inflamed area. The blisters burst within a few days to form a crust and heal on their own within 2 weeks.

What can I do to help?
For most children, cold sores are a minor inconvenience for which no treatment is necessary.

However, if the sores are causing any discomfort, a cold drink or an ice pop may relieve the soreness. If the blisters recur frequently or are severe, a cream containing the antiviral drug acyclovir may be used. The cream, which is only available by prescription, reduces the severity and duration of an attack. It is most effective if it is applied as soon as there is a tingling sensation around the mouth, before any blisters appear.

If you are able to identify a particular trigger factor for your child, you can take appropriate preventive action. For example, if cold sores tend to develop after exposure to the sun, you may be able to prevent them by applying a sunscreen or sunblock to your child's lips before he or she goes outside.

To reduce the chance of spreading the virus to other people and to other parts of your child's body, try to prevent your child from touching the blisters or sucking his or her fingers; encourage frequent handwashing. Make sure your child understands the importance of using his or her own towels only.

What is the outlook?
There is no cure for cold sores, and they will probably recur throughout your child's life. However, outbreaks usually become less frequent with time.

Cold sore cluster
Often appearing in clusters, cold sore blisters are clear at first; they become cloudy and then form crusts. Cold sores are smaller and more regular in shape than impetigo sores (below).

IMPETIGO

This common, highly contagious bacterial skin infection occurs mainly in young children, especially babies. Impetigo most often affects the mouth and nose area in children, and the diaper area in babies, although it may appear anywhere on the body. The bacteria that cause impetigo are able to enter and infect the skin when it is broken by a cut, an insect bite, or a skin condition such as ECZEMA (p.135) or SCABIES (p.143).

Appearance of impetigo
Impetigo starts as small blisters. Here, the blisters have burst to form large, irregular sores covered in straw-colored crusts.

What are the symptoms?
The symptoms of impetigo change as the infection develops:
- Initially, the skin reddens and crops of small blisters appear.
- The blisters burst, leaving raw, moist sores that gradually enlarge.
- Straw-colored crusts form as the surface of the sores dries.

Impetigo sores do not hurt, although they may be slightly itchy. Without treatment, the condition may last for weeks or even months.

Should I consult a doctor?
Your child should be seen by a doctor within 24 hours if you think he or she has impetigo. The doctor may prescribe an antibiotic ointment, which should be applied to the sores several times a day. If the infection is widespread, an oral antibiotic may be prescribed instead.

What can I do to help?
Bathe your child with an antibacterial soap. Before applying the ointment, remove the crusts by gently dabbing them with gauze soaked in salt solution and then dry the area. To prevent the infection from spreading, your child should not touch the sores. Keep your child's bedding, washcloth, and towels separate. Your child should stay away from other children until the infection has cleared up. With treatment, impetigo usually gets better within about 5 days.

How can I prevent impetigo?
Your child should shower or bathe daily. Keeping your baby's diaper area clean and protected from moisture helps to prevent DIAPER RASH (p.136), and reduces the chance of impetigo. Making sure that your child's nails are kept short and clean makes infection less likely to be introduced through scratching. When your child has a cold or a runny nose, applying a little petroleum jelly to the nose and upper lip should help to protect the skin from being broken by constant wiping.

ACNE

The most common skin disorder in adolescents, acne consists of inflamed spots on the face and other parts of the body. Acne tends to appear at the onset of puberty, usually between the ages of 12 and 14 years. It may be at its worst in the late teens, after which it begins to subside. The condition often runs in families and is usually more common and severe in boys than in girls. Although acne cannot be prevented, it can be controlled.

Acne affecting the face
The spots on this boy's face are typical of acne. The slightly indented purplish marks are the result of spots that have healed.

How is it caused?
At puberty, there is an increase in the production of sebum (an oily substance produced by sebaceous glands in hair follicles), which is probably triggered by increased levels of sex hormones. Acne spots occur when excess sebum and, sometimes, dead skin cells form a plug that blocks a hair follicle; trapped bacteria multiply, causing the skin surrounding the follicle to become inflamed.

Oily substances on the skin, such as cosmetics or hair oil, may make the problem worse. However, diet has no effect.

What are the symptoms?
Acne principally affects the face (see illustration at left), neck, shoulders, chest, upper arms, and back. The main symptoms are:
• Pimples (small, raised red spots).
• Blackheads (tiny black spots).
• Whiteheads (tender, inflamed lumps with a white center).
• Cysts (fluid-filled swellings).
• Purplish marks left by healed spots, which gradually fade.
If it is very severe, acne may leave scars and pits in the skin. The condition may also make your child feel extremely embarrassed by his or her appearance, because it coincides with the increased self-consciousness of adolescence.

What is the treatment?
Your child should wash his or her face twice daily with ordinary soap and water. An over-the-counter acne cream or lotion may then be applied to the affected areas. These preparations promote skin peeling, which helps to unblock the pores, and also control bacteria. They are available in different strengths; your child should try the mildest first. Exposure to sunlight may help to clear up acne spots. Your child should avoid picking, squeezing, or scrubbing the spots, all of which may cause the bacteria to spread.

If the acne has not improved after your child has been using an acne preparation for 2 to 3 months, consult a doctor. Treatment with several courses of oral antibiotics may be suggested. Each course the doctor prescribes will last for between 3 and 6 months.

If antibiotics do not help, the doctor may prescribe a retinoid drug, which reduces sebum production. Retinoid drugs are usually effective but may cause side effects, such as dryness of the lips, eyes, and nose.

What is the outlook?
Acne cannot be cured. However, its severity can be reduced and scarring prevented with treatment. Because of the availability of effective remedies, few children should have severe acne. The condition gradually improves and often disappears in the early 20s.

PITYRIASIS ROSEA

A rash of flat, scaly spots, pityriasis rosea most frequently affects the trunk, arms, and legs. It is believed to be caused by a viral infection, although no specific virus has been isolated. Pityriasis rosea most frequently affects adolescents.

What are the symptoms?
The main symptoms are:
• An initial spot, called the herald patch, which is oval or round, flat, scaly, and 1–2 cm in diameter.
• Flat, oval, copper-colored or dark pink spots, which appear 3 to 10 days after the herald patch. After a week, each spot develops a scaly margin.
• Occasionally, itchiness.
The rash appears initially on the trunk, running along the lines of the ribs. It may then spread up toward the neck and down along the arms and legs, fading below the elbows and knees. The rash seldom appears on the face.

Should I consult a doctor?
Although pityriasis rosea is not serious and gets better without treatment, your child should be seen by a doctor within a few days. The doctor will examine your child to make sure he or she does not have a more serious skin disease.

What is the treatment?
The doctor treats the symptoms rather than the condition itself. He or she may prescribe a mild corticosteroid cream to alleviate the itchiness. If the itchiness is severe, the doctor may prescribe an oral antihistamine. Keeping the skin cool, for example by avoiding exertion in hot weather, and moisturizing the affected areas may also relieve the symptoms. Exposure to sunlight may help the rash to clear up more rapidly.

What is the outlook?
Pityriasis rosea usually takes between 3 and 8 weeks to clear up. Once your child has had the condition, he or she is very unlikely to have it again.

WARTS

Caused by a virus, warts are harmless growths on the surface of the skin. They most commonly appear on the hands and feet. Warts are contagious, but some people are more susceptible to them than others. Most warts disappear naturally within a few months, but some last for years if they are not treated.

What are the symptoms?
There are several different types of warts, any of which may occur singly or in clusters. The ones that most often affect children are:
• Common warts. These are firm, raised growths, usually with a hard, rough surface. They usually occur on the hands, feet, knees, and face.
• Flat warts. These smooth growths are level with the skin or slightly raised. They occur on the hands or face and may cause slight itchiness.
• Plantar warts (verrucas). These hard, horny warts occur on the sole of the foot. They appear flat and are often painful because the child's weight has pushed them into the skin.

What can I do to help?
Warts often disappear if left untreated. However, if your child would like to have a wart removed, home treatment is safe for warts on the hands and feet. Never attempt to remove a wart on your child's mouth or face.

Plantar wart
This wart on the sole of the foot has a hard, rough, calloused surface and is dotted with tiny blood clots (black spots).

The simplest technique for treating common and flat warts is to cover the wart with salicylic acid tape, which should be changed daily. If the wart does not respond to this treatment in about 3 weeks, you could try using wart medication. The directions must be followed carefully. To protect normal skin surrounding the wart, cover it with a little petroleum jelly before you apply the medication.

If your child has a plantar wart, rub the wart's surface with a pumice stone to remove as much of the overlying skin as possible. Apply a piece of salicylic acid tape the exact size of the wart. Replace the tape every day until the wart disappears, which may take up to 3 months.

Tell your child not to touch the warts because picking or scratching them may lead to a secondary infection.

Should I consult a doctor?
Consult a doctor if home treatment has not been successful or if a wart on the face or mouth is causing your child discomfort or embarrassment.

The doctor may send your child to a dermatologist. Most warts are removed by freezing (cryotherapy). A plantar wart may be scraped off (curettage).

What is the outlook?
Most warts eventually disappear, even without treatment. However, warts sometimes recur, even if treated, and may require several treatments before they finally disappear for good.

MOLLUSCUM CONTAGIOSUM

This mild viral infection causes small, shiny pimples to appear on the skin. Molluscum contagiosum is common in children between 2 and 5 years of age. It is easily spread, either by direct contact or indirectly – for example, in a public swimming pool or by touching infected clothing or towels.

Molluscum contagiosum pimples
The pimples, which are between 2 and 5 mm in diameter, usually appear in groups although they sometimes occur singly.

What are the symptoms?
The pimples appear 2 to 7 weeks after infection. They occur mainly on the trunk, face, hands, and (rarely) on the palms or soles. The pimples are:
• Dome shaped with a central dimple.
• Pearly white or flesh colored.

Should I consult a doctor?
The presence of this infection is not an emergency. If the condition is untreated, it will probably disappear within a few weeks to a few months. However, molluscum contagiosum should be treated by a doctor. If it is left alone, the condition may spread to other parts of the body and may become unsightly. It can also spread to other children, although not very easily. An open pimple is usually the source of a transmitted infection.

What might the doctor do?
If molluscum contagiosum affects only a small area of your child's body, the doctor may decide to treat the condition by piercing the pimples with an instrument dipped in podophyllin paint. This treatment releases the white cheesy substance in the pimples and destroys them. If your child has a large number of pimples, the doctor may send him or her to a dermatologist. The dermatologist will treat molluscum contagiosum by scraping away the pimples (curettage) or by freezing them (cryotherapy).

FUNGAL INFECTIONS

The skin, hair, and nails may all be affected by fungal infections. Of these infections, the most familiar are ringworm and athlete's foot. Ringworm appears in schoolchildren and may affect the scalp or the skin of the body or face. Adolescents are susceptible to athlete's foot, which usually affects the skin between the toes.

RINGWORM

Children can catch ringworm directly from another person, from an animal, or from soil; or indirectly from hats, combs, clothing, or household items, such as carpets or chairs.

What are the symptoms?
Ringworm of the body or face causes:
- Oval or circular, flaky patches with raised, mildly inflamed borders.
- Itchiness.

Ringworm affecting the scalp causes:
- Flakes resembling severe dandruff.
- Hair loss, with hair tending to break just above the scalp.
- Occasionally, the development of an inflamed, pus-filled area (a kerion).
- Usually, itchiness.

Your child should be seen by a doctor if you think he or she has ringworm.

What is the treatment?
For infections on the body or face, the doctor may recommend that you use an antifungal lotion or cream. If the infection on your child's body or face is very widespread, or if his or her scalp is affected, antifungal medicine, including oral drugs, may be prescribed.

To help prevent ringworm, keep your child away from infected people or animals, and discourage the sharing of personal items, such as combs.

ATHLETE'S FOOT

This condition is particularly common during the summer months, especially among adolescents who wear sneakers. Athlete's foot is commonly caught from the floors of locker rooms and showers at communal places, such as swimming pools and gyms.

What are the symptoms?
The main symptoms are:
- Cracked, sore skin between the toes, often the fourth and fifth toes.
- Usually, itchiness.
- Occasionally, thick, discolored, and easily broken toenails.

What is the treatment?
Various powders, creams, and sprays are available over the counter to treat athlete's foot (see illustration at right). With treatment, the condition usually begins to clear up after 1 to 2 weeks. If athlete's foot lasts for longer than 2 weeks, or the toenails are infected,

make an appointment for your child to see a doctor. He or she will determine whether athlete's foot is present and may prescribe antifungal tablets.

Athlete's foot is less likely to occur if your child thoroughly dries his or her feet after washing and puts on clean cotton socks every day. Wearing open-toed sandals and going barefoot when practical may also help.

Athlete's foot powder

Treating athlete's foot
Your child should wash and dry his or her feet thoroughly and sprinkle athlete's foot powder (or apply a cream or spray) between the toes twice a day. Socks and shoes should be dusted with athlete's foot powder.

TINEA VERSICOLOR

This common skin condition results in discolored patches of skin. It is caused by overgrowth of a yeast normally present on the skin, possibly triggered by exposure to sunlight or a hot, humid environment. The condition usually occurs after puberty.

Appearance of tinea versicolor
Areas of dark or tanned skin that are affected by tinea versicolor appear as round, flat, pale patches with clearly defined borders.

What are the symptoms?
Discolored patches of skin are the main symptom. The patches typically have the following characteristics:
- On pale skin, they are usually darker than surrounding skin; on dark skin, they are usually lighter.
- Slight flakiness.
- Well-defined borders.
- Sometimes, mild itchiness.

Your child should be seen by a doctor if he or she has symptoms of tinea

versicolor. Although it is not harmful or contagious, the condition may last indefinitely if it is not treated.

What is the treatment?
The doctor will prescribe an antifungal cream or lotion. You should apply the preparation once a day to the affected areas. This treatment reduces the yeast to its normal levels in about a week. However, the antifungal preparation should be used for 3 weeks in order to reduce the chance that the condition will recur. Exposing the affected areas to the air as much as possible also helps to discourage regrowth. The skin may take weeks or months to regain its normal appearance.

SCABIES

This extremely itchy, contagious condition is due to infestation of the skin by parasitic mites. The female mites burrow into the skin to lay their eggs, causing intense itching. Scabies is passed from person to person by close bodily contact. Anyone can catch scabies; it has nothing to do with lack of personal hygiene.

What are the symptoms?
After infestation, the symptoms of scabies might take up to 6 weeks to appear. They could include:
• Intense itchiness, especially at night.
• Thin gray lines (the mites' burrows) between the fingers, on the wrists, in the armpits, between the buttocks, or around the genitals. In infants, the palms and soles may be affected.
• Sores, blisters, and scabs, resulting from scratching.
• Inflamed lumps on the body.

Scabies mite burrow
Thin gray lines on the skin are the burrows made by female mites. Burrows may be obscured by sores and scabs caused by scratching.

Your child should be seen by a doctor if he or she is scratching intensely or has any other signs of scabies. Scabies will not clear up without treatment, and scratching can result in IMPETIGO (p.139).

What is the treatment?
The doctor will prescribe a lotion that kills scabies mites. It should be applied to all areas of your child's body except for the head and neck, and should be washed off after 24 hours. You need to treat all members of your household at the same time, even if they to do not have any obvious signs of scabies. After treatment, you should wash and iron all clothing and bed linen.

The mites usually die within 3 days of treatment. However, itchiness may persist for up to 2 weeks afterward. The doctor may prescribe an ointment to relieve the itchiness.

People with whom you and your child have had contact should be told about the scabies so that they can be examined and treated if necessary.

HEAD LICE

Head lice are very small, flat, wingless insects that live on the scalp and suck blood. Schoolchildren can catch these insects easily through direct contact or by sharing hats or combs. If your child has head lice, you need not worry that he or she is not washing properly: the insects actually prefer clean hair and skin.

What are the symptoms?
The main symptoms of head lice are:
• Intense itchiness of the scalp.
• Tiny red spots (bites) on the scalp.
Adult head lice are very small, almost transparent, and therefore hard to see. The eggs (nits) are more easily seen, particularly after the insects have hatched. The empty nit shells can be seen as small white bumps near the bases of the hairs.

What can I do to help?
If you suspect that your child has lice, examine his or her hair for nits. You can also see if lice are present by wetting your child's hair and combing it with a fine-tooth comb over a white piece of paper. Any lice will be visible as they crawl on the paper.

If your child is infested, check all other members of the family for head lice and tell your child's school so that other parents can be alerted.

Head lice and eggs
The tiny white ovals are louse eggs. They are firmly attached to the hair shafts. Several head lice are also visible clinging to hairs.

Should I consult a doctor?
You can treat head lice at home without consulting a doctor first. However, if your child is less than 2 years old or has allergies or asthma, you should talk to a doctor before starting treatment.

What is the treatment?
Special lotions and shampoos are available over the counter for the treatment of head lice. Some preparations can be applied just once; others must be applied repeatedly over a number of days. All family members and contacts should be treated at the same time (even if they have no symptoms) to eradicate the head lice completely and to prevent the possibility of your child's becoming reinfested. You should wash all combs and brushes in boiling water in order to kill any lice or eggs that might be attached to them.

As long as all close contacts are treated simultaneously, one course of treatment is usually all that is necessary to rid your child of head lice.

How can head lice be avoided?
To reduce your child's chances of catching lice, discourage him or her from sharing hats, combs, and brushes with family members or with school friends. If there is an outbreak of lice at school, be sure to check your child's hair each evening (without alarming him or her), and begin treatment if necessary. Reassure your child that this condition is completely curable.

Eradicating head lice
Head lice can be eradicated by washing the hair with a special shampoo or lotion. Follow the directions on the package, and comb your child's hair carefully afterward with a fine-tooth comb to remove the dead lice and nits.

Fine-tooth comb

BLOOD AND CIRCULATORY DISORDERS

CONGENITAL HEART DEFECTS are the most common serious birth defects, but, in most cases, their causes remain unknown. Fortunately, many are now curable. High cure rates are also now usual for most of the serious blood disorders, such as leukemia, that formerly were fatal. However, the early recognition of the symptoms of these blood disorders is still important to maximize the chance of a cure.

CONGENITAL HEART DISEASE

A child with congenital heart disease is born with one or more malformations of the heart. The risk of a woman having a child with a heart defect is increased if she has poorly controlled diabetes, takes certain drugs during pregnancy, has had another child with a heart defect, or, rarely, has had RUBELLA (p.119) in early pregnancy. About 1 child in 140 is born with a heart defect. Some get better without treatment, but others need surgery.

Oxygenated blood to body
Deoxygenated blood to lungs
Aorta
Right atrium
Left atrium
Oxygenated blood from lungs
Right ventricle
Left ventricle
Septum

NORMAL

Deoxygenated and oxygenated blood are mixed
Pulmonary artery
Pulmonary valve
Aortic valve
Ventricular septal defect

ABNORMAL

What are the types of heart defect?
The most common type of congenital heart abnormality is a ventricular septal defect (see illustrations above). Another relatively common defect is patent ductus arteriosus, in which the ductus arteriosus (a blood vessel that acts as a bypass in a baby's circulation before birth) fails to close after birth.

Other common heart abnormalities are atrial septal defect, a hole between the atria (upper heart chambers); aortic stenosis, narrowing of the aortic valve; and pulmonary stenosis, in which the pulmonary valve is narrowed.

Ventricular septal defect
A hole in the septum allows blood to flow from the left to right ventricle. Oxygenated blood that should flow into the aorta and out to body tissues instead returns to the lungs.

Other rarer defects, which may be more serious, include: transposition of the great arteries, in which the position of the aorta and pulmonary artery are reversed; coarctation of the aorta, which is narrowing of the aorta; and tetralogy of Fallot, a combination of four defects, including a ventricular septal defect, pulmonary stenosis, a displaced aorta, and a thickened right ventricle.

What are the symptoms?
Symptoms of congenital heart disease depend on the nature and severity of the defect or defects that a child has. In some cases, symptoms are detected when a doctor carries out his or her routine examination of the newborn baby. In other cases, symptoms of heart disease are not apparent until later in childhood or even until adult life.

Among the various possible features of congenital heart disease are:
- A heart murmur (abnormal heart sounds). A doctor will be able to hear the heart murmur when he or she listens to the child's heart through a stethoscope. Most murmurs do not indicate congenital heart disease, but in some cases the murmur is due to a narrowed pulmonary or aortic valve or some other form of heart defect.
- Feeding problems and loss of weight. In some babies with congenital heart disease, heart failure (inability of the heart to pump efficiently) causes slow feeding and inability to finish feedings. An affected baby may breathe rapidly and sweat, especially after feeding.
- Bluish discoloration of the tongue and lips (cyanosis). Several heart defects prevent effective circulation of the blood through the lungs. This means that the blood supplied to the body by the heart carries less oxygen than it should, which causes some tissues to appear blue.
- Breathlessness on exertion.
Children with congenital heart disease may grow at a slower rate than children who have healthy hearts.

What are the complications?

Children with congenital heart disease, even if it is mild, may be susceptible to bacterial endocarditis. In this condition, the heart valves become inflamed due to infection by bacteria that have entered the bloodstream, usually during dental treatment or a surgical operation.

Should I consult a doctor?

Your child should be seen by a doctor if you suspect that he or she might have a congenital heart abnormality.

If you are aware that your child has congenital heart disease, consult a doctor without delay if he or she has a fever, lacks energy, and has a poor appetite; these symptoms indicate that your child might have bacterial endocarditis.

What might the doctor do?

The doctor will examine your child. If he or she suspects that your child might have congenital heart disease, your child will be referred to a pediatrician or pediatric cardiologist. The specialist will arrange for a chest X ray, an electrocardiogram (a recording of heart rate and rhythm), and also an ultrasound of the heart to be carried out in the hospital. These investigations will reveal the nature and the severity of any congenital heart abnormality.

In many cases of congenital heart disease, the defects get better on their own without the need for surgery.

In some cases, however, emergency surgery needs to be performed to save a child's life. In other cases, surgery to correct a defect can be delayed until later in childhood. Sometimes, more than one operation may be necessary.

Your child will be monitored by a pediatrician or cardiologist and will also have periodic hospital assessments. Your family doctor can provide you with any immediate advice you require. To minimize the risk of your child's contracting bacterial endocarditis, preventive antibiotics will be prescribed whenever dental treatment is required or if your child needs surgery.

Listening to a child's heart
The doctor will use a stethoscope to listen to your child's heart. Abnormal sounds may indicate the presence of a defect.

What can I do to help?

Unless the doctor tells you otherwise, you should encourage your child to lead a completely normal life, with a normal amount of exercise. In a very few cases, particularly if your child has a heart abnormality that causes bluish discoloration of the tongue and lips, the doctor may tell you to restrict the amount of exercise your child performs.

Make sure that your child takes the full course of any antibiotics that have been prescribed to prevent bacterial endocarditis. Also make sure that your child always carries a card (obtained from the doctor) stating that he or she has congenital heart disease.

What is the outlook?

The outlook depends on the type of heart defect and on its severity. In most cases, ventricular septal defects close on their own before the child is 5 years old. Those that do not close and many other heart abnormalities, such as atrial septal defect, patent ductus arteriosus, or narrowing of a pulmonary or aortic valve, are treatable by surgery or other intervention. As a result of surgical advances over the last 20 years, children with heart disease, even those with very severe defects, usually grow up to lead normal lives.

ANEMIA

The term anemia refers to a deficient amount of hemoglobin in the blood. Hemoglobin is the pigment in red blood cells that carries oxygen from the lungs to body tissues. If hemoglobin is deficient, the tissues receive an insufficient oxygen supply.

How is it caused?

Red blood cells are manufactured in the bone marrow, then released into the bloodstream. They normally circulate for about 120 days before they become defective and are destroyed. Anemia can result from inadequate production or excessive destruction of red cells.

Inadequate red cell production usually results from deficiency of a substance that is essential for healthy red blood cell formation. The most common type is IRON-DEFICIENCY ANEMIA (p.146).

Excessive destruction of red blood cells is often due to a genetic fault. The fault causes the production of abnormal red cells that are destroyed at a high rate. Examples are SICKLE-CELL ANEMIA (p.199) and THALASSEMIA (p.200).

What are the symptoms?

A child may have no symptoms if the anemia is mild. In more severe cases, the following symptoms are typical:
• Pale skin.
• Lack of energy.
• Breathlessness after exertion.
Other symptoms may occur, depending on which type of anemia the child has.

Should I consult a doctor?

Your child should be seen by a doctor if you think that he or she might have anemia. The doctor will ask about your family history and your child's general health and diet. If the doctor suspects that your child has anemia, he or she will arrange for blood tests to confirm the presence of the condition and its severity. Your child's blood will be analyzed to determine the number, shape, size, and color of the blood cells. The analysis reveals which type of anemia is present. Subsequent tests, such as iron measurements, might be required to make a precise diagnosis. The treatment will depend on the cause of your child's anemia. If the anemia is due to a genetic fault, your child will require lifelong treatment.

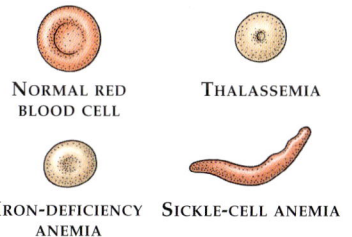

NORMAL RED BLOOD CELL

THALASSEMIA

IRON-DEFICIENCY ANEMIA

SICKLE-CELL ANEMIA

Red blood cells
In many types of anemia, red blood cells are small and pale. In sickle-cell anemia, however, the shape of the red blood cells is distorted.

145

IRON-DEFICIENCY ANEMIA

This type of ANEMIA (p.145) is the result of a deficiency of iron, which is one of the essential components of hemoglobin, the oxygen-carrying pigment in red blood cells. Iron-deficiency anemia is the most common form of anemia affecting children.

What are the symptoms?

Mild iron-deficiency anemia may not produce any symptoms. In more severe cases, symptoms may include:
• Pale skin.
• Lack of energy.
• Breathlessness after exertion.
Long-term iron-deficiency anemia in children is serious. It has been known to cause impaired mental development and function.

Should I consult a doctor?

You should consult a doctor if you think that your child might be anemic. The doctor can arrange for blood tests to find out whether your child has anemia and to assess its severity. The type of anemia may be identified by examination of red blood cells: when iron-deficiency anemia is present, they are smaller and paler than normal.

What is the treatment?

The doctor will probably ask about your child's diet and may give you advice on food to offer your child.

Your child may be prescribed iron in medicine form, typically for about 3 months, in order to build up his or her iron stores.

If your child is under the age of 6 months and was born prematurely, he or she will probably already have been prescribed supplements of iron. If not, the doctor may prescribe them at this time. Typically, premature babies are not born with sufficient iron stores to compensate for the low iron content of a milk-only diet during the first 6 months of life, before they start on solids.

What can I do to help?

Try to ensure that there is enough iron in your child's diet. Iron from green vegetables is best absorbed by the body when the meal contains protein (meat, eggs, cheese). If your baby is not eating solids by the age of 6 months, there is a risk that he or she will develop iron-deficiency anemia despite receiving milk formula enriched with iron. This may become apparent between the ages of 12 and 18 months. If your child refuses to eat iron-rich foods, talk to the doctor about giving him or her an iron supplement.

What is the outlook?

Children are less likely to develop iron-deficiency anemia as they grow and eat a varied diet.

An iron-rich diet
Give your child foods that are rich in iron, including meat and green vegetables. A child who does not eat meat should eat plenty of green vegetables.

LEUKEMIA

In leukemia, a form of cancer, the bone marrow produces many abnormal (leukemic) white blood cells, and a reduced number of normal white cells, red cells, and platelets. The leukemic cells infiltrate the liver, spleen, and lymph glands. The most common form of leukemia in childhood is acute lymphoblastic leukemia.

NORMAL	LEUKEMIA

Acute lymphoblastic leukemia
Seen under a microscope, blood taken from a person with leukemia shows a large number of abnormal white blood cells (dark purple).

What are the symptoms?

Acute lymphoblastic leukemia may produce the following symptoms:
• Pale skin.
• Pink or purple flat spots on the skin.
• Easily bruised skin.
• Lack of energy.
• Swollen lymph nodes in the neck, armpits, and groin.
• Fever.
• Pain in limb bones and joints.
• Bleeding gums.
Consult a doctor at once if you suspect that your child might have leukemia.

What might the doctor do?

The doctor will examine your child and may arrange for blood tests. If the tests cannot exclude leukemia, your child will be admitted to the hospital for a bone marrow biopsy. This procedure, which involves removing cells from the bone marrow for analysis, can show whether your child has leukemia.

Treatment for acute lymphoblastic leukemia is divided into two phases.

During the first phase, which generally lasts for several weeks, drugs are given to destroy the leukemic cells. This phase continues until a bone marrow biopsy indicates that no abnormal cells are present. At this point, your child is described as being in remission.

The second phase of treatment lasts for another 2 years. During this time, your child will undergo periods of intensive drug treatment that are aimed at destroying any leukemic cells that might still be present in the body.

What can I do to help?

Your child should lead as normal a life as possible. Because drug treatment increases susceptibility to infection, he or she should, however, be kept away from anyone who has a viral infection, such as chickenpox or measles.

What is the outlook?

Treatments currently available lead to full recovery (at least 10 years) in about 80 percent of children diagnosed as having acute lymphoblastic leukemia.

HENOCH-SCHÖNLEIN PURPURA

In Henoch-Schönlein purpura, small blood vessels become fragile and allow blood to leak from them. Bleeding into the skin results in an easily identifiable rash, while leakage of blood into joints, the kidneys, or the digestive tract causes various other symptoms. The disease is fairly common in children between the ages of 2 and 10 years, and is not usually serious. The cause is unknown but may involve an allergic reaction or bacterial infection.

What are the symptoms?
Henoch-Schönlein purpura may cause the following symptoms:
- Rash (present in all cases), made up of pink, red, or purplish blood-filled spots that do not fade when pressed. The rash appears first on the buttocks and the backs of the arms and legs, especially around the ankles and elbows, then spreads to the fronts of the limbs (see illustration at right).
- Joint pain and swelling.
- Abdominal pain, in many cases with vomiting and diarrhea.
- Blood in the stool.

Inflammation of the kidneys (see GLOMERULONEPHRITIS, p.194) is a possible complication. It does not usually cause symptoms.

Should I consult a doctor?
You should consult a doctor within 24 hours of the onset of symptoms that might indicate your child has Henoch-Schönlein purpura.

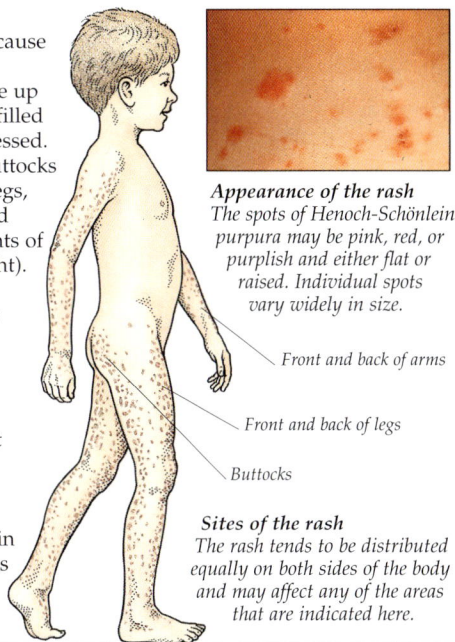

Appearance of the rash
The spots of Henoch-Schönlein purpura may be pink, red, or purplish and either flat or raised. Individual spots vary widely in size.

Front and back of arms

Front and back of legs

Buttocks

Sites of the rash
The rash tends to be distributed equally on both sides of the body and may affect any of the areas that are indicated here.

What might the doctor do?
The doctor will examine your child. If a diagnosis cannot definitely be made from your child's symptoms, he or she will arrange for blood tests to rule out other possibilities. A sample of your child's urine will be sent for laboratory examination. The presence of red blood cells and protein in the urine indicates that the kidneys are inflamed.

If symptoms are mild, no treatment is required. Corticosteroids may be given for severe abdominal pain and may bring about rapid improvement. If the kidneys are affected, repeat urine and blood tests may be performed to make sure that the condition is improving.

What can I do to help?
If your child's symptoms cause intense pain or discomfort, you may give him or her acetaminophen. Your child may stay in bed if he or she wishes to.

What is the outlook?
Henoch-Schönlein purpura may last from only a few days to up to a month, during which time the symptoms may come and go. Most children who have the illness make a complete recovery, and there are no long-term ill effects. In most cases, any inflammation of the kidneys disappears in a few days, but in some children the kidneys remain inflamed for years.

THROMBOCYTOPENIA

In this condition, the number of platelets in the blood is abnormally low. In children, thrombocytopenia most frequently occurs as part of a disorder called idiopathic thrombocytopenic purpura (ITP). The cause of this disorder is unknown, but it usually develops within 2 weeks after a viral infection.

What are the symptoms?
The symptoms of ITP are caused by abnormal bleeding due to the reduced number of platelets (which are essential for blood clotting). They may include:
- A widespread, flat purple rash caused by bleeding into the skin; the rash does not fade when pressed.
- Bruising from only minor pressure.
- Nosebleeds.
- Bleeding in the mouth.
- Blood in the urine as a result of bleeding in the kidneys.

Brain hemorrhage (bleeding around or within the brain) is a rare, but serious, possible complication of the condition.

Should I consult a doctor?
You should consult a doctor at once if your child has symptoms that might be caused by ITP. If the doctor has any doubts about the diagnosis, admission to the hospital may be arranged so that tests can be performed to confirm that your child has ITP and not another illness that produces similar symptoms.

What is the treatment?
Most children do not require treatment. However, strenuous activities should be avoided until symptoms clear up, which is usually within a few weeks.

If your child has bleeding from the nose or mouth or a very low blood platelet count, he or she will be treated in the hospital. Your child may be given a short course of corticosteroid drugs or, in some cases, intravenous gamma globulin to speed recovery and reduce the risk of severe bleeding.

What is the outlook?
Most children are free from symptoms within about 2 weeks. However, in a few children, blood platelet levels may take up to 6 months, or occasionally longer, to return completely to normal.

RESPIRATORY SYSTEM DISORDERS

INFECTION BY BACTERIA or viruses is the most common cause of respiratory tract disorders in children. Young children are particularly prone to infection because they have not had time to build up an immunity. Allergic disorders, such as asthma and allergic rhinitis (hay fever), are the other main respiratory problems affecting children. Asthma is becoming increasingly common.

COMMON COLD

A viral infection of the nose and throat, the common cold is a minor contagious illness that occurs frequently in children. Most children have at least six colds a year, with the frequency usually increasing when they begin daycare or nursery school. Some children, who are otherwise healthy, have up to ten colds a year.

What are the symptoms?
Symptoms typically begin 1 to 3 days after infection, usually starting with a tickly or scratchy feeling in the throat. Symptoms that follow may include:
- A runny nose.
- Sneezing.

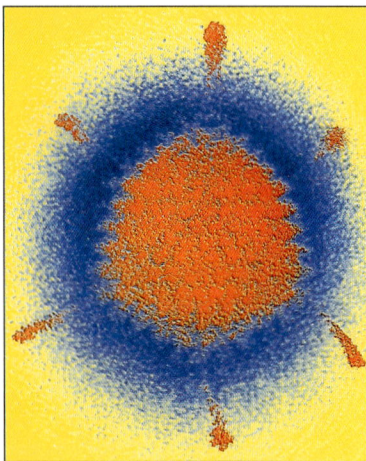

Cold virus
The adenovirus shown in this micrograph is one of more than 200 strains of virus that are known to cause the common cold.

- A blocked nose, which may make feeding difficult for a baby.
- A cough and sore throat.
- Watering eyes.
- Muscular aches.
- Sometimes, a fever.

What are the complications?
Cold viruses may spread to the lungs, causing BRONCHIOLITIS (p.156) or PNEUMONIA (p.156), which may be complicated by secondary bacterial infection. Bacterial infection may also affect the ears, causing OTITIS MEDIA (p.162), or the sinuses, causing SINUSITIS (opposite). In children who suffer from ASTHMA (p.153), a cold may trigger an asthmatic attack.

How is it caused?
Many different viruses can cause the common cold. Immunity gained from infection with one strain does not give protection against another, so infections can occur repeatedly. Children attending nursery school or elementary school are particularly susceptible to colds because they are exposed to a wide variety of viruses to which they have not yet become immune. Cold viruses are spread in droplets that are sneezed or coughed out and inhaled by others. The viruses may also spread through contact with infected people or objects.

What can I do to help?
Most colds clear up within a week without any treatment. Meanwhile, the following suggestions should help relieve the symptoms.

Keep your child's room warm (but not too hot) and increase the moisture in the atmosphere (see illustration: *Humidifying the air,* p.150).

Have your child drink plenty of fluids. Feed a baby with a cold in small amounts, and more often than usual. You may need to clear the baby's nose before feeding and relieve a sore throat and aches with liquid acetaminophen.

Should I consult a doctor?
Call a doctor within 24 hours if your child refuses food and liquids, has a fever over 39°C, or if he or she appears ill. A baby less than 3 months old with a fever should be seen as soon as possible. Consult the doctor if a cough has not improved after 5 days, other symptoms have lasted beyond 10 days, or new symptoms develop.

How can colds be prevented?
To reduce the risk of infection, keep babies away from infected people and crowded places, such as supermarkets. Hand washing is very helpful.

ENLARGED ADENOIDS

The adenoids are pads of tissue at the back of the nose that form part of the body's defenses against infection. In some children, the adenoids become enlarged after repeated infections. As a result, they may block the passage of air or obstruct normal drainage of the middle ears through the eustachian tubes.

What are the symptoms?
The symptoms may include:
- Snoring.
- Frequent waking at night due to breathing problems, leading to excessive tiredness the next day.
- Breathing through the mouth.
- Nasal voice.
- Sleep apnea.

If the eustachian tubes are blocked by the enlarged adenoids, recurrent ear infections (see OTITIS MEDIA, p.162) may result, and may lead to MIDDLE EAR EFFUSION (p.163) and hearing loss.

Should I consult a doctor?
If your child's symptoms are mild, no treatment is usually required because the adenoids shrink naturally with age.

If your child suffers from severe snoring or speech problems, or has frequent ear infections, you should make an appointment to see a doctor. The doctor may refer your child to an ear, nose, and throat specialist, who will assess the size of the adenoids from an X-ray picture taken of the area. Surgical removal of the adenoids may be recommended. The operation, called an adenoidectomy, is performed in the hospital under general anesthesia.

What can I do to help?
To relieve a dry mouth caused by constant mouth breathing, keep the air in your child's room moist (see *Humidifying the air*, p.150). Encourage your child to sleep on his or her side or front to reduce snoring.

What is the outlook?
In children whose adenoids have not been removed, symptoms usually start to diminish around the age of 7 years, when the adenoids begin to shrink and the airway becomes larger with growth. They will probably disappear by the time your child reaches adolescence.

A child whose adenoids have been removed will breathe more easily through his or her nose and will stop snoring at night.

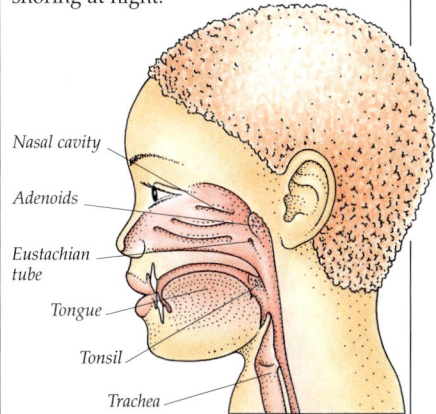

Nasal cavity
Adenoids
Eustachian tube
Tongue
Tonsil
Trachea

Location of the adenoids
Made up of lymphatic tissue, the adenoids are located at the back of the nasal cavity above the tonsils. Lymphatic tissue is rich in white blood cells, which fight infection.

SINUSITIS

Most often affecting adolescents, sinusitis is an inflammation of the lining of the sinuses (air-filled cavities in bones around the nose and in the forehead). It is usually caused by a secondary bacterial infection associated with a COMMON COLD (opposite).

What are the symptoms?
The first indication may be symptoms of a common cold, such as a runny nose and coughing, that last 10 days or more. The specific symptoms of sinusitis may then develop:
- Persistent nasal drainage.
- Swelling of the face over the sinuses.
- Headache that worsens with bending forward.
- Cough.
- Frequent ear infections.
- A persistent fever in some children.

How is it caused?
Mucus produced in the sinuses traps bacteria. Cilia (hairlike structures) that project from the lining of the sinuses move the yellowish green or clear mucus along until it drains through narrow passages into the nose and throat. If a viral infection, such as a cold, causes inflammation of tissues, these passages may be blocked. As a result, mucus collects in the sinuses, enabling the bacteria in it to multiply.

Should I consult a doctor?
Have your child see a doctor within 24 hours. If sinusitis is likely, antibiotics and nose drops will be prescribed, and the infection clears up in 7 to 10 days. Be alert to a fever above 39.4°C and a headache in the forehead area.

What can I do to help?
Give your child acetaminophen to relieve the pain; you should also provide him or her with plenty of fluids to drink. A steam inhalation can relieve a stuffy nose (see illustration below) and keeping the air moist may also help (see illustration: *Humidifying the air*, p.150).

Steam inhalation
Towel keeps vapor in
Bowl placed on a table, not your child's knees

Relieving congestion
Have your child inhale steam rising from a bowl of boiling water. To avoid the risk of scalding, do not place the bowl on your child's knees. Treatment may be repeated three times a day.

CROUP

Usually caused by a viral infection, croup is inflammation and narrowing of the main airway to the lungs. It most commonly affects children between the ages of 6 months and 3 years. Croup is usually a mild illness; occasionally, however, it causes severe breathing difficulties and requires emergency treatment.

What are the symptoms?
Croup starts with the symptoms of a COMMON COLD (p.148), including a runny nose and sneezing. After 1 or 2 days, the following symptoms develop:
• Noisy breathing.
• Persistent, barking cough.
• Hoarse voice.
In severe cases, a child may have:
• Difficulty in breathing.
• Abnormally fast breathing.
Episodes of croup tend to occur in the early morning and last for a few hours.

If your child has an attack of croup, call a doctor at once. If symptoms worsen or severe symptoms develop, call an ambulance or take your child to a hospital emergency room.

What might the doctor do?
After assessing the severity of the croup and excluding other conditions such as EPIGLOTTITIS (below), the doctor may treat mild croup with oral or injected steroids. Self-help measures (right) may be recommended to relieve symptoms.

Children with severe croup are usually hospitalized. To ease breathing, oxygen and medicated inhalations are given. Rarely, the airways are severely obstructed, and a tube may be inserted through the nose into the windpipe to bypass the blockage. Recovery from severe croup usually takes a few days.

What can I do to help?
Give liquid acetaminophen and frequent warm drinks, and keep the air in your child's room moist (see illustration). To ease the symptoms of an acute attack, take your child into the bathroom and turn on the hot water to humidify the air rapidly. Going outside into cool air also helps.

What is the outlook?
Some children have recurrent attacks of croup. In particular, those with ASTHMA (p.153) may be prone to further attacks. For these children, drugs for treating asthma may be recommended. Some doctors may also prescribe inhalations of corticosteroids to be taken at the first signs of a serious attack of croup. Your child should be better within 5 days.

Humidifying the air
Keeping the air in your child's room moist should help him or her to breathe more easily. Place wet towels on a chair near a radiator or use a vaporizer to moisten the air.

EPIGLOTTITIS

A potentially fatal infection usually caused by the bacterium *Haemophilus influenzae*, epiglottitis mainly affects children 2 to 6 years old. The epiglottis, a flap of cartilage at the entrance to the larynx, becomes inflamed and swells, obstructing the passage of air. Immunization has decreased the incidence of this disease.

What are the symptoms?
Epiglottitis comes on suddenly. The main symptoms are:
• Severe difficulty in swallowing.
• Pain on swallowing.
• Drooling because the child cannot swallow his or her saliva.
• Noisy breathing that becomes quieter as the illness worsens.
• Increasing difficulty in breathing. The child will probably want to sit upright in order to ease breathing.
• Fever.
• Bluish tongue and, sometimes, skin.
If your child develops difficulty in swallowing and breathing, call an ambulance or take him or her to a hospital emergency room: there is a risk of complete airway obstruction.

You should not attempt to look down your child's throat because he or she may start to cry. Crying increases the production of secretions, which may totally block the narrowed airway.

What is the treatment?
After an initial examination and X ray, your child will be examined in an operating room while sedated with an inhaled agent. If epiglottitis is present, a breathing tube is inserted until the infection is under control, usually in a few days.

Prompt treatment assures a complete recovery, usually within a week. A child who has had this infection becomes immune.

How can I prevent epiglottitis?
Infection with *Haemophilus influenzae* can be prevented by IMMUNIZATION (p.30). Children are routinely offered immunization with HIB vaccine against the bacterium.

SORE THROAT

The sore throat most commonly results from pharyngitis, the inflammation of the throat that often recurs as part of a COMMON COLD (p.148). Pharyngitis often occurs with tonsillitis (inflammation of the tonsils) in children up to 8 years of age. Both conditions may be caused by viruses or streptococcal bacteria.

Tonsil   Uvula   Pharynx (throat)

Swollen tonsils
In tonsillitis, the tonsils are swollen and fiery red (as seen here) and are sometimes flecked with yellow or white pus. Rarely, the tonsils become so enlarged that they block the airway.

What are the symptoms?
Both pharyngitis and tonsillitis have similar symptoms, although those of tonsillitis are usually more severe. The main symptoms are:
• Sore, inflamed throat.
• Fever.
• Discomfort during swallowing (young children may refuse to eat).
• Enlarged, tender glands in the neck.
• Earache, occasionally.
• In tonsillitis, red swollen tonsils.
In the majority of cases, the symptoms disappear within 3 days. Rarely, an abscess may form around a tonsil. It causes a high fever and increasing difficulty in swallowing.

Should I consult a doctor?
If the symptoms persist for more than 24 hours or get worse, phone a doctor at once. The doctor will examine your child and, if a bacterial infection is likely, will swab the throat to confirm the diagnosis. Antibiotics will be given for a strep positive swab. An abscess may need surgical drainage in hospital.

What can I do to help?
Give your child liquid acetaminophen (see also panel: *Relieving a sore throat*, p.91) and plenty of fluids. Your child is infectious for about 3 days after a sore throat starts and should be kept away from other children during this time.

What is the outlook?
Most children become immune to the common viruses. Occasionally, removal of the tonsils is recommended for children who have recurrent bouts of tonsillitis that are due to confirmed streptococcal infections (six per year or ten in two years) or cause sleep apnea.

INFLUENZA

Commonly known as flu, influenza is a viral infection of the upper respiratory tract that may affect children of all ages. The influenza virus is spread by coughing and sneezing, and by direct contact. There are outbreaks of influenza every year.

What are the symptoms?
The symptoms develop 1 to 3 days after infection and usually come on rapidly. They may include:
• Fever, usually above 39°C.
• Dry cough.
• Muscular aches.
• Stuffy nose.
• Tiredness and weakness.
• Headache.
• Usually, a sore throat.
The symptoms are usually most severe during the first 2 to 5 days of the illness. In most cases, influenza clears up completely within about 10 days.

What are the complications?
The influenza virus may spread to the lungs, causing PNEUMONIA (p.155), or BRONCHIOLITIS (p.155) in infants, often complicated by secondary bacterial infection. Bacterial infection may also affect the sinuses (see SINUSITIS, p.149) or ears (see OTITIS MEDIA, p.162). Children at high risk of such complications include those with chronic heart, lung, or kidney disease, DIABETES MELLITUS (p.190), CYSTIC FIBROSIS (p.201), or a depressed immune system. Babies may have FEBRILE SEIZURES (p.156).

Influenza virus
The influenza virus can change its structure, producing new strains to which a child has not developed an immunity. For this reason, repeated attacks of influenza can occur.

Should I consult a doctor?
If symptoms persist for more than 24 hours or get worse, phone a doctor. If a bacterial infection is likely, antibiotics may be prescribed and a throat swab sent for analysis. If your child has a streptococcal infection, the course of antibiotics must be finished.

What is the treatment?
Mostly, treatment is supportive. The flu does not respond to antibiotics, and cold remedies have limited value. If a bacterial infection is present, the doctor may prescribe antibiotics. A child who has severe symptoms or is at risk for complications may be hospitalized.
   If the child remains at home, he or she should stay in bed in a warm, well-ventilated, and humidified room (see *Humidifying the air*, p.150) until the fever is gone. Offer drinks frequently. You may give your child liquid acetaminophen for aches and fever.

How can I prevent influenza?
Annual vaccination against influenza is recommended for children with a chronic disorder or any defect of the immune system, and for infants aged between 6 months and 2 years.

ALLERGIES

An allergy is a condition in which the immune system responds to a substance inappropriately. The result is an allergic reaction that may produce a wide range of symptoms, such as HIVES (p.138), coughing, or vomiting. A child is more likely to suffer from an allergy if there is a family history of allergic disorders.

How is an allergic reaction caused?
The body's immune system responds to foreign material (such as bacteria or viruses) by producing antibodies and sensitized white blood cells that can recognize and then destroy the foreign substance. An allergic reaction is similar except that it is misdirected at normally harmless substances (called allergens), such as dust or a food.

The initial exposure to an allergen sensitizes the immune system to the substance. On subsequent exposures, the immune response to the allergen is fast and strong, producing an allergic reaction. This reaction may occur when a chemical comes into contact with the skin (see CONTACT DERMATITIS, p.136); a particular food is swallowed (see REACTIONS TO FOOD, p.182); or airborne particles, such as pollen, are inhaled (see ALLERGIC RHINITIS, below; ASTHMA, opposite). Insect venom (see INSECT BITES AND STINGS, p.138) and certain drugs (for example, penicillin or penicillin-based drugs) may also cause a reaction. In a small number of cases, a very severe, life-threatening reaction may occur (see ANAPHYLACTIC SHOCK, p.154).

What are the symptoms?
The symptoms of allergies range from mild to severe, and may affect one area or part of the body (such as the skin, the eyes, or the lining of the nose or airways), or may be more widespread. Symptoms may include:
- Rash.
- Sore, itchy, runny red eyes.
- Blocked, runny nose.
- Coughing.
- Faintness.
- Abdominal pain.
- Nausea, vomiting, or diarrhea.

What is the treatment?
Call an ambulance if there are symptoms of anaphylactic shock, such as difficulty breathing, a tightness in the throat, or a feeling of doom.

It is helpful to identify and remove or avoid the allergens, for instance, by keeping your house as dust-free as possible or by not eating certain foods.

Antihistamines and corticosteroids may be used for allergic symptoms. Some allergies lessen or disappear altogether with time.

ALLERGIC RHINITIS

Inflammation of the lining of the nose due to an allergic reaction (see ALLERGIES, above) is called allergic rhinitis. Allergic rhinitis takes two forms. The seasonal variety, commonly known as hay fever, causes symptoms in the spring, summer, or fall months, while the perennial variety affects people throughout the year. Allergic rhinitis often runs in families and is most common among children with other allergies.

How is it caused?
Allergic rhinitis occurs when a person inhales an allergen (a substance that causes an allergic reaction). Allergens that most often cause hay fever are grass, tree, and weed pollens. Perennial allergic rhinitis is most often caused by house-dust mites, animal dander (flakes of dead skin), or mold spores.

What are the symptoms?
The symptoms of both forms of allergic rhinitis are similar, although those of the perennial type tend to be less severe. The main symptoms are:
- Initially, an itchy feeling in the eyes, nose, and throat.
- Blocked, runny nose.
- Sneezing.
- Red, sore, watery eyes.
- Occasionally, dry skin.

What can I do to help?
If the allergen is known, try to reduce or eliminate exposure to it. A child with severe hay fever should stay indoors as much as possible during the pollen season. Keep the windows closed, especially on hot, dry, breezy days, when pollen counts may be high. Animals should be kept away from a child who is allergic to animal dander. If house-dust mites are causing the problem, keep house dust to a minimum. Dust all surfaces with a damp cloth, and treat carpets with insecticide to kill mites. Enclose your child's mattress in a plastic cover, and avoid feather-filled bedding. If your child has an allergy to mold spores, make sure his or her bedroom is well ventilated, and free of mold and dust.

Oral antihistamines may help if your child's hay fever is severe or if he or she cannot avoid going outside. Antihistamines have little or no effect on perennial allergic rhinitis.

Pollen grains
Pollen from trees (shown here), grass, or weeds is the most common cause of hay fever. Tree pollens are most prevalent in the spring.

Should I consult a doctor?
Make an appointment to see a doctor if your child has severe or persistent symptoms not relieved by self-help measures.

The doctor will probably prescribe a nasal spray that contains either sodium cromoglycate or a corticosteroid drug to alleviate the symptoms of rhinitis.

What is the outlook?
In many children, allergic rhinitis becomes less severe as they grow older and eventually disappears.

ASTHMA

The most common chronic lung disease of childhood, asthma is a distressing condition in which there are recurrent episodes of wheezing, difficulty in breathing, and coughing. The disease has become more prevalent in recent years: one out of seven children in the US is affected. Most children who develop asthma have had their first attack by the age of 4 or 5 years. Untreated, asthma may slow down a child's growth and is potentially fatal.

How is it caused?

Genetic factors are involved. Many affected children have other allergic conditions, such as ALLERGIC RHINITIS (opposite) or ECZEMA (p.135). There may be a family history of asthma and other allergic disorders. Individual attacks of asthma may be triggered by infection with a virus or by allergens (see

House-dust mite
For many children who have asthma, attacks may be triggered by exposure to house-dust mites. The mites live in soft furnishings, mattresses, bedding, carpets, and soft toys.

ALLERGIES, opposite), such as house-dust mites or food. Exercising, particularly in cold air, may bring on an attack. Attacks may also be brought on or made worse by anxiety.

The symptoms of asthma are caused by narrowing of the airways in the lungs as a result of inflammation and swelling of the walls, contraction of the muscles within the walls, and an increase in the secretion of mucus.

What are the symptoms?

In young children, the first sign of asthma is often a recurring cough, especially with a cold or after exercise. Sometimes, the first sign of asthma is coughing that occurs only at night. Other symptoms, which are similar to those of BRONCHITIS, (p.154) include:
• Wheezing.
• Shortness of breath.
• Tightness in the chest.

During severe attacks of asthma, the symptoms may include:
• Difficult and noisy breathing.
• Difficulty in speaking.
• Drowsiness.
• Disturbed sleep.
• Blue lips and tongue.
• Refusal to eat or drink.

Should I consult a doctor?

If you think that your child has asthma, he or she should be seen by a doctor within 24 hours. If the symptoms are severe, call an ambulance or take your child to the nearest emergency room.

What might the doctor do?

The doctor will ask about any possible exposure to allergens and if there are factors that could be causing your child anxiety, such as difficulties at school.

To assess the severity of the disease, the doctor will use a peak-flow meter, which measures the capacity to exhale air. A chest X ray may be done to check for any associated infection.

If your child's asthma is mild, the doctor will prescribe a bronchodilator drug. The bronchodilator is inhaled to ease breathing during asthma attacks. If your child's asthma is more severe, the doctor may also prescribe an

Taking inhaled drugs
Children over 5 to 6 years old can use an inhaler. A spacer makes it easier for younger children to inhale the drug, which is usually delivered as a spray. Always supervise your child using an inhaler.

Inhaler

Spacer holds the drug for the child to breathe in when ready

Inhaler

inhaled corticosteroid. These drugs have to be inhaled regularly to help prevent attacks. Some children require oral corticosteroids or regular treatment with an inhaled, long-acting bronchodilator drug.

Children may take inhaled drugs with an inhaler (see illustration below). For infants, a nebulizer is used. This device has a pump that disperses the drug as a fine mist into a face mask.

What can I do to help?

If your child is over the age of 6 years, the doctor may suggest that you use a peak-flow meter in order to monitor the asthma; the meter should warn of an impending attack. Keep an asthma diary to chart the symptoms and the peak-flow meter readings from day to day. This record will help the doctor to modify your child's treatment as the disease changes, develops, or subsides.

You or your child should always have a bronchodilator available to use in case of an attack. If your child has a severe attack of asthma and the normal bronchodilator does not work, a repeat dose should be taken. If that fails to ease the condition, phone your doctor at once or take your child to a hospital emergency room.

How can I prevent asthma?

You cannot prevent this disease, but you may be able to reduce its severity by helping your child avoid known allergens or reducing his or her exposure to them. Help your child avoid stressful situations and be supportive during times when your child feels anxious. Some children find that taking their bronchodilator drug half an hour before vigorous exercise prevents an attack. It is important for your child to stick to the treatment recommended for him or her.

What is the outlook?

At least half the children who develop asthma before they reach the age of 5 years stop having attacks by the time they reach adulthood. If your child still has asthma at the age of 14 years, however, there is a strong chance that it will persist into adulthood.

ANAPHYLACTIC SHOCK

A rare, severe, widespread allergic reaction, anaphylactic shock causes constriction of the airways and a sudden drop in blood pressure. Without immediate medical attention, it can be fatal. Stings from insects (such as bees) and reactions to certain drugs (particularly those based on penicillin) are the most common causes. Some foods (for example, peanuts and shellfish) may also trigger anaphylactic shock (see REACTIONS TO FOOD, p.182).

What are the symptoms?
People who are sensitive to a substance usually start having a reaction a few minutes after they have been exposed to it. Initially, they may experience an itching or burning feeling in the lips, mouth, or throat. Other symptoms that soon follow may include:
- Blotchy, itchy, raised rash.
- Paleness of the skin and sweating.
- Anxiety.
- Swollen eyelids, lips, and tongue.
- Puffy face and neck.
- Difficulty in breathing.
- Abdominal pain and sometimes vomiting or diarrhea.
- Faintness, abnormal drowsiness, or loss of consciousness.
- In infants, refusal to drink and sometimes dribbling as a result of an inability to swallow.

If your child has any of the symptoms listed above, call an ambulance or take him or her to a hospital emergency room immediately.

What can I do to help?
While waiting for the ambulance to arrive, you should place your child in a semisitting position to make breathing easier (see illustration at right). Your child should not eat or drink anything. If your child starts to vomit, place him or her in the RECOVERY POSITION (p.203). If your child loses consciousness, you should follow the ABCs of resuscitation (see PRINCIPLES OF FIRST AID, p.202).

What might the doctor do?
The doctor will immediately give your child an injection of epinephrine (adrenaline) to raise low blood low pressure. He or she will check whether your child has breathing problems and may pass a tube into the windpipe for mechanical ventilation. If the heart has stopped, the doctor may give your child heart massage. To reduce swelling and relieve itching, the doctor may inject a corticosteroid or antihistamine drug. Intravenous fluids may be given to raise blood pressure.

How can I prevent anaphylactic shock?
Your child should avoid the trigger substance. The doctor will prescribe a syringe of epinephrine (adrenaline); your child should always have it handy and know how to use it. Tell the school about the allergy and have your child wear an identity bracelet.

Easing breathing
Support your child in a semisitting position to help ease breathing.

SUDDEN INFANT DEATH

Sudden Infant Death Syndrome, or SIDS, remains the leading cause of death in infants in Canada after the neonatal period (that is, among children aged between one month and 1 year). Several important factors have been identified as contributing to an increased risk of SIDS.

What are the contributing factors?
Factors associated with increased risk of SIDS include:
- Premature birth.
- Low birth weight.
- Young maternal age (under 20 years of age at first pregnancy).
- Late or no maternal prenatal care.
- Maternal smoking during pregnancy.
- Maternal smoking during first year of the baby's life.
- Substance abuse by mother.
- Room in which the baby is sleeping is kept at too high a temperature.
- Baby's temperature is too high due to excessive clothing or blankets.
- Baby sleeps on his or her stomach.

Sleeping position
Research carried out in the early 1990s found a strong association between the placement of infants on their stomachs and the incidence of SIDS, especially during sleep.
Two years after a large public campaign to place sleeping infants on their backs, SIDS rates dropped by more than half. Even placing babies on their sides to sleep was found to double the risk of SIDS.
Babies should also be placed with their feet at the bottom of the crib. If placed at the head of the crib, a baby is at risk of moving down under the covers and either overheating or suffocating.

Correct sleeping position
A baby should sleep on his or her back, with its feet at the bottom of the crib.

BRONCHIOLITIS

This acute viral infection of the lungs causes inflammation of the bronchioles (the smallest airways in the lungs). Bronchiolitis mainly affects children under 1 year and can be a serious illness, especially for infants. It usually occurs in epidemics in winter.

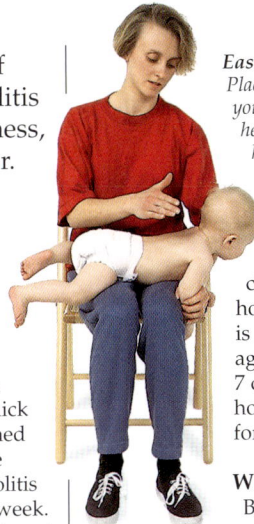

Easing the cough
Place your child across your lap and slap him or her gently on the back to help loosen thick mucus.

What are the symptoms?
Initially, your child may have symptoms resembling those of the COMMON COLD (p.148). After 2 or 3 days, the following symptoms may develop:
- Dry, rasping cough.
- Wheezing and/or rapid, difficult breathing. In some infants, long pauses (more than 10 seconds) occur between each breath.
- Reluctance to feed or eat.
- Bluish lips and tongue.
- Abnormal drowsiness.

If your child is under 1 year and is coughing and/or wheezing, phone a doctor. Call an ambulance if breathing is difficult, if the lips and tongue are blue, or if your child becomes drowsy.

What is the treatment?
For mild bronchiolitis, the doctor may prescribe a bronchodilator drug and advise you to look after your child at home. Give your child plenty of fluids and feed him or her small amounts frequently. Liquid acetaminophen can help bring down the fever. Thick mucus in the lungs may be loosened by slapping your child's back (see illustration at right). Mild bronchiolitis usually improves within about a week.

A child who needs hospital treatment may be given oxygen in a plastic head box. He or she may be fed by means of a tube inserted through the nose or, sometimes, intravenously. In severe cases, mechanical ventilation may be required. The child will be allowed home when he or she is feeding normally again, usually within 7 days. The cough, however, may persist for up to 6 weeks.

What is the outlook?
Bronchiolitis does not cause permanent damage to the lungs. For the next few years, however, many children who have had the illness tend to suffer from wheezing when they have a cold.

PNEUMONIA

Inflammation of the lungs, known as pneumonia, is usually due to a viral or bacterial infection. It is most often a complication of an upper respiratory tract infection, such as a COMMON COLD (p.148), or of an infectious disease, such as CHICKENPOX (p.120). Children with CYSTIC FIBROSIS (p.201) are particularly prone to pneumonia.

What are the symptoms?
Pneumonia may start with symptoms of a common cold, such as sneezing and a runny nose. The following symptoms then develop:
- Coughing, which in older children produces yellowish, greenish, or blood-flecked phlegm.
- Rapid, difficult breathing.
- Fever.
- Headache.
- In severe pneumonia, drowsiness, blueness of the lips and tongue, and refusal to eat or drink.

Should I consult a doctor?
Phone a doctor at once if your child is breathing fast while resting in bed, if a cough and fever last for more than a few days, or if your child seems far more ill than an ordinary cold would warrant. You should call an ambulance if your child has any of the symptoms of severe pneumonia listed above.

What might the doctor do?
The doctor will listen to your child's chest through a stethoscope and may send a throat swab or blood sample for tests to identify the cause of infection.

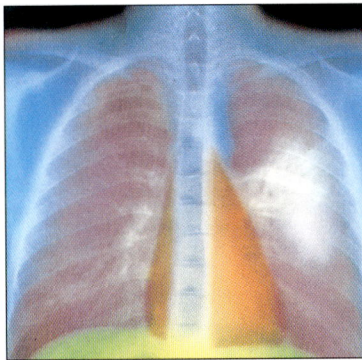

Chest X ray showing pneumonia
Pneumonia causes some of the air sacs in the lungs to fill with fluid. The affected part of the lung shows as a white shadow.

Antibiotics may be prescribed. Most children can be treated at home (see "What can I do to help?").

If your child's pneumonia is severe, he or she may be admitted to the hospital. A chest X ray will be taken to confirm the diagnosis and antibiotics will be given. Your child may receive oxygen; rarely, mechanical ventilation will be required. Your child should be able to go home after about 4 days.

What can I do to help?
Have your child drink plenty of fluids, and offer a baby frequent small feedings. Liquid acetaminophen can reduce fever and relieve a headache, but over-the-counter cough medicine is not recommended for the treatment of pneumonia. Most children recover within a week.

After discharge from the hospital, your child should not exercise vigorously for a week. Going outside will not harm your child.

What is the outlook?
A cough may continue for another 2 weeks after your child has otherwise recovered. Pneumonia does not result in any permanent damage to the lungs.

NERVOUS SYSTEM DISORDERS

MOST OF THE GROWTH AND DEVELOPMENT of the brain is complete by the age of about 5 years. Any brain injury or infection that occurs in a child's early years (or in some cases before birth), when the brain is still immature, may have serious long-term consequences. Early recognition and treatment of brain disorders is, therefore, extremely important. On the other hand, children's brains have a much greater capacity for recovery than do those of adults. However, a few nervous system disorders, such as cerebral palsy, are incurable.

FEBRILE SEIZURES

A febrile seizure is a type of seizure associated with fever – often over 39°C – that accompanies an infection in a part of the body other than the brain. The seizures may occur in children between the ages of 6 months and 7 years. Although frightening, the seizures are not usually serious.

How are they caused?
Febrile seizures are triggered by an abrupt rise in body temperature and usually occur at the onset of a febrile illness. The seizures are most often associated with upper respiratory tract infections. Children are susceptible to the seizures because their brains are not yet mature. If a child has one febrile seizure, there is an increased risk that he or she will have another.

What are the symptoms?
Some or all of the following symptoms may appear during the first 5 minutes of a febrile seizure:
• Loss of consciousness.
• Rigidity of the body.
• Cessation of breathing for up to half a minute; when it starts again, breathing may be shallow and barely detectable.
• Urinating and/or defecating.
• Twitching of the limbs and/or face.
• Rolling back of the eyes.
After 5 minutes or so, the child regains consciousness and may then fall into a deep sleep for an hour or two. He or she may be confused, sleepy, and irritable upon waking.

Should I consult a doctor?
If your child has a seizure, you should phone a doctor at once. If a seizure lasts for more than 5 minutes, you should call an ambulance.

What can I do to help?
If your child has a raised temperature, you should try to reduce it (see panel: *Bringing down a high temperature*, p.37, and illustration above right) in order to prevent febrile seizures.
Your child should be placed in the RECOVERY POSITION (p.203) if he or she has had a febrile seizure. Proceed with action to reduce your child's fever to prevent another seizure.

What might the doctor do?
The doctor will examine your child to see if he or she has any symptoms associated with MENINGITIS (p.158) or other serious infections. The doctor may also consider tests for the purpose of identifying the cause of the fever; if your child has a bacterial infection, an antibiotic drug may be prescribed for him or her. You will be given advice on how to deal with febrile seizures

Reducing your child's temperature
If your child has a fever, removing her clothes will help to reduce her temperature, but do not allow her to become cold.

in the future. If your child has had several seizures, the doctor may consider treating him or her with anticonvulsant drugs.

What is the outlook?
About a third of children who have had one febrile seizure will have a second one, usually within 6 months. Febrile seizures are common. The vast majority of children who suffer attacks have no long-term problems. A small minority of those children who have had febrile seizures later develop EPILEPSY (opposite).

EPILEPSY

Recurrent seizures (or fits), a condition called epilepsy, occur in about 1 in 200 children. During a seizure, there is chaotic and unregulated electrical brain activity, which causes an alteration in consciousness and sometimes uncontrollable movements of the limbs and/or head. There are many causes of seizures other than epilepsy (see, for example, FEBRILE SEIZURES, opposite). A child who has a single seizure is not considered to have epilepsy.

End of seizure

Start of seizure

How is it caused?

Children with epilepsy sometimes have a structural abnormality in the brain, but in most cases no obvious cause can be found. In some children, individual attacks are brought on by a trigger – for example, flashing lights; in others, the attacks have no apparent trigger.

What are the symptoms?

There are a number of different types of epileptic seizure. In children, tonic-clonic seizures are most common: more than three-quarters of children with epilepsy suffer from this type. Absence seizures are the second most common type in children. The main features of these seizures are:

Tonic-clonic seizures

• Irritability or unusual behavior for a few minutes before the seizure.

• A rigid spasm, which lasts for up to 30 seconds, during which the child usually falls unconscious to the floor and breathing becomes irregular.

• Jerky movements of the limbs or face that may last from 20 seconds to several hours. The child may bite his or her tongue and there may be loss of bladder or bowel control.

• After convulsions stop, the child may stay unconscious for a few minutes or, more rarely, for up to 10 minutes.

• When the child regains consciousness, he or she often feels disoriented and confused, may have a headache, and will probably want to sleep.

Absence seizures

• Child stops normal activities and stares into space, unaware of the surroundings, for 10 to 15 seconds, but does not fall to the floor.

• Child has no memory of the seizure.

Brain activity during a seizure
This EEG recording of the brain's electrical activity was made during an absence seizure. This type of seizure is very brief, typically lasting for just 10 to 15 seconds.

A less common form of epilepsy, called benign partial epilepsy, causes jerking of one side of the face or of one limb. The child may also lose consciousness.

In most cases, a child will have only one type of seizure. However, some children have more complex forms of epilepsy, which combine two or more different types of seizure.

What can I do to help?

If your child has a tonic-clonic seizure, place him or her in the recovery position (see photograph below right and RECOVERY POSITION, p.203) and stay until he or she has fully recovered.

For other types of seizure, sit your child down in a quiet spot, and stay until he or she is fully recovered and alert. Talk calmly and reassuringly to your child. Do not slap or shake your child in an attempt to stop the seizure.

Should I consult a doctor?

If your child has never had a tonic-clonic seizure before, phone a doctor at once. You should call an ambulance or take your child to the nearest hospital emergency room if he or she remains unconscious for longer than 10 minutes, whether the attack is the first one or not. Although other types of seizure are less serious, make an appointment to see a doctor. You should notify the doctor of any subsequent seizures.

What might the doctor do?

You will probably be asked to describe your child's behavior and symptoms before, during, and after any seizure. To identify possible triggers, the doctor may also ask what your child had been doing just before the seizure.

An electroencephalogram (EEG) is usually performed to help determine the type of epilepsy. Brain scans may be done to find out whether a structural brain abnormality might be causing the seizures. Blood may be tested to rule out other possible causes of the seizure, such as low blood sugar.

What is the treatment?

Children with epilepsy normally need regular anticonvulsant drug therapy. Anticonvulsants are usually given until 2 years have passed since the last seizure, and may then be gradually reduced over several months.

If medication does not control your child's seizures, and scans indicate a structural brain abnormality, surgery may, extremely rarely, be considered to correct the problem.

The doctor will advise you about any precautions that you or your child should take, and whether there are any activities that should be avoided.

What is the outlook?

The outlook varies, depending on the type of epilepsy. Over three-quarters of children with tonic-clonic epilepsy who have been free of seizures for 2 years do not have a recurrence. Most children with benign partial epilepsy outgrow the condition and need no medication after puberty. The outlook is less predictable for children with absence seizures. Most children, even those who do not outgrow epilepsy, have no other disability, and can go to normal schools and participate in most sports.

Dealing with a tonic-clonic seizure
Place your child on the floor in the recovery position, with the head on the same level or slightly lower than the body. You should not try to force anything into the child's mouth to prevent a bitten tongue.

MENINGITIS

Inflammation of the meninges (the membranes covering the brain and spinal cord) is known as meningitis. It is caused by infection with bacteria or viruses. The symptoms of viral meningitis are mild, but bacterial meningitis can be life threatening. Bacterial meningitis is most common in children under the age of 5 years, although it can occur at any age. It usually appears as isolated cases. Household members, if not immunized, are at increased risk for contracting the disease.

Lumbar puncture
A hollow needle is used to draw out a small amount of cerebrospinal fluid from the spinal canal for examination in the laboratory.

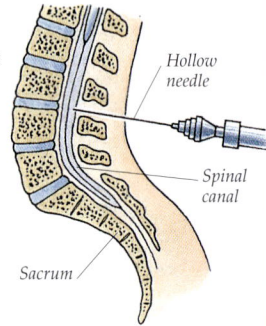

Hollow needle

Spinal canal

Sacrum

Area shown in detail
Meninges
Cerebrospinal fluid
Brain

Skull

Venous space

The meninges
Three layers of protective membranes, known as the meninges, cover the brain and spinal cord. Meningitis is caused by infection of the meninges by viruses or bacteria.

How is it caused?
Bacterial meningitis in children is most often caused by *Neisseria meningitidis* bacteria (also called meningococcal meningitis) and strep pneumonia. The *Neisseria* bacteria are normal inhabitants of the nose and throat, and usually cause no ill effects. Why they cause meningitis in some children is unknown. Immunization has reduced the incidence of meningococcal C and strep pneumonia meningitis. Another common cause of meningitis was infection with *Haemophilus influenzae* bacteria, but this has become a rare cause since the introduction of routine IMMUNIZATION (p.30) of babies in 1993.

There are many different viruses capable of causing meningitis, including those responsible for influenza, chickenpox, infectious mononucleosis ("kissing disease"), and AIDS.

Meningitis rash
Development of this rash is a serious symptom of meningitis and indicates that immediate medical treatment is vital.

What are the symptoms?
The symptoms of the bacterial and viral forms of meningitis are similar in the early stages. However, those of bacterial meningitis are usually more severe and tend to develop rapidly, sometimes within a few hours. In infants the early symptoms are often vague, and may include:
• Abnormal drowsiness.
• Fever.
• Vomiting.
• Reluctance to feed.
• Increased crying; restlessness.
In older children, the symptoms may include all of the above, as well as:
• Severe headache.
• Dislike of bright light and loud noise.
• Rigidity of muscles, particularly the muscles of the neck.
In children of all ages with bacterial meningitis, the initial symptoms may be followed by increasing drowsiness and, occasionally, by loss of consciousness or seizures. Some children with meningitis develop a characteristic rash (see photograph below) consisting of flat pink or purple spots that do not fade when pressed.

Should I consult a doctor?
If your child is abnormally drowsy or develops any two of the symptoms listed above, he or she should be seen by a doctor at once or taken to the nearest emergency room. The child will be admitted to hospital, where a lumbar puncture (see illustration above right) may be performed. This test can confirm the diagnosis of either viral or bacterial meningitis and, in some cases, enables identification of the particular infectious organisms. Blood samples may also be taken for culture in the laboratory to identify bacteria.

What is the treatment?
A course of high-dose antibiotics will be started immediately, even before the laboratory results are available.

If tests confirm viral meningitis, the antibiotics can be discontinued. No form of treatment other than painkillers is necessary, and the infection usually clears up in 5 to 14 days, depending on the particular virus involved.

If bacterial meningitis is confirmed, antibiotics will be continued (or, they may be changed, if necessary, to target the particular bacteria that have been identified). Your child may be given intravenous fluids, and anticonvulsant drugs may be prescribed if he or she is having seizures. Treatment with antibiotics may last for up to 10 days.

How can meningitis be prevented?
Routine immunization protects against *Haemophilus influenzae*, strep pneumonia meningitis, and meningococcal C meningitis. The only other way to prevent the spread of bacterial meningitis is to give antibiotics to those children who are not immunized and are in close contact with an affected child.

What is the outlook?
Viral meningitis rarely has after effects. Prompt antibiotic treatment in the early stages of bacterial meningitis usually leads to complete recovery. A few children may have some brain damage, resulting in deafness, seizures, or learning difficulties, especially if treatment is delayed. Rarely, the illness may be fatal, even if treated promptly.

ENCEPHALITIS

Inflammation of the brain is called encephalitis. A rare condition, it can be caused by any viral infection. For unknown reasons, the viruses spread through the bloodstream to the brain from sites elsewhere in the body. Encephalitis can vary in severity from being mild and harmless to a serious and life-threatening illness.

How is it caused?
In newborn babies, the herpes simplex virus (the virus responsible for cold sores) is the most common cause of encephalitis. Rarely, encephalitis can also occur after measles, rubella (German measles), or chickenpox. The live viruses contained in some vaccines (for example, the measles vaccine) may, very rarely, cause encephalitis.

What are the symptoms?
In mild encephalitis, the symptoms may be barely noticeable. Chickenpox encephalitis, for example, may cause only slight unsteadiness in walking for a few days. In more serious forms of encephalitis, the most important symptom is abnormal drowsiness that progressively worsens, possibly leading to coma. There may also be:
• Fever.
• Irritability.
• Vomiting.
• Double vision or an obvious squint.
• Weakness of a limb.
• Seizures.

Should I consult a doctor?
Phone a doctor at once if your child is abnormally drowsy or if he or she has a fever plus any two of the symptoms above. The diagnosis will be based on the child's symptoms and the results of brain scans. In the early stages of the illness, the tests may not show anything wrong, even if the child is later shown to have encephalitis. A lumbar puncture may be carried out to exclude bacterial MENINGITIS (opposite).

The antiviral drug acyclovir is used to treat herpes simplex infection. There are no drugs to treat other viral infections. Mechanical ventilation may be needed for breathing difficulties.

What is the outlook?
The outlook depends on the causative virus and the severity of the symptoms. Most children recover completely. In a few cases, there is permanent brain damage, which may cause weakness of an arm or leg, learning difficulties, behavioral problems, or epilepsy. Very rarely, encephalitis is fatal.

HEAD INJURY

Bangs or blows to the head are common in childhood and are rarely serious. Common causes include falling out of a crib or bed, falling from a tree or jungle gym, or being in a traffic accident. Even a small cut on the scalp or forehead can cause severe bleeding. The main risk of a head injury, however, is bleeding inside the skull (brain hemorrhage), which can lead to brain damage. In rare cases, a head injury can be fatal.

Blood clot

CT scan of brain
Bleeding inside the skull can result in a blood clot, which may put pressure on and damage brain tissues.

What are the symptoms?
If the head injury is mild, there may be no symptoms other than a slight headache and a bump or swelling at the site of the injury. However, if there has been a blow to the head there may be a concussion (brief unconsciousness, usually lasting a few seconds).

Common symptoms immediately after a concussion include:
• Confusion.
• Inability to remember events that occurred just before the injury.
• Dizziness.
• Blurred vision.
• Vomiting.
With more severe head injuries, there may be unconsciousness lasting for more than a few minutes or even coma.

If straw-colored fluid or watery blood trickles from your child's nose or ear, there may be a skull fracture.

Should I consult a doctor?
If your child is knocked unconscious even for only a few seconds, appears confused or abnormally drowsy, vomits continually, or there is fluid or watery blood leaking from the nose or ears, call an ambulance or take your child to the nearest emergency room.

Your child will be examined by the doctor. A cut to the scalp may need to be stitched in order to stop bleeding. An X ray of the skull may be taken if a fracture is suspected. A CT (computed tomography) scan (see photograph above) may be done. If the CT scan shows signs of a brain hemorrhage, an emergency operation may be needed to stop the bleeding and remove a blood clot. If there is a fracture of the skull or a severe concussion, your child will be observed in the hospital for 24 hours after the injury.

What can I do to help?
If your child has a minor head injury, he or she should rest at home for 2 or 3 days. You will be asked to observe your child carefully during the first 24 hours and to take him or her back to the hospital as an emergency if any of the following symptoms of a blood clot develop: abnormal drowsiness; vomiting; irritability; confusion; slurred or incoherent speech; fluid or watery blood leaking from the nose or ears.

A child with a more severe injury that required hospital treatment may need to rest at home for several weeks.

What is the outlook?
There should be no long-lasting effects from minor head injures. More severe head injuries may cause permanent brain damage, resulting in a degree of physical or mental disability.

NEURAL TUBE DEFECTS

The neural tube is the part of an embryo that develops into the brain and spinal cord, and the back of the skull and vertebrae. If normal development fails to occur, a baby may be born with defects in any of these parts. The most common type of defect is spina bifida, which affects one or more vertebrae.

What are the symptoms?
To a greater or lesser degree, the spinal cord, the brain, or their coverings (the meninges) are exposed, making them vulnerable to damage and infection. The abnormality may be so slight that it is apparent only from a dimple or a tuft of hair over the defect, or there may be a large, fluid-filled swelling, covered by a thin membrane or by skin. The symptoms, if there are any, depend on the severity of the neural tube defect and may include:
• Weakness or paralysis of the legs.
• Deformity of the legs.
• Urinary and/or fecal incontinence.
• Insensitivity to pain of the skin below the level of the abnormality.
• Sometimes, hydrocephalus (water on the brain).
• In some cases, learning difficulties (p.172).

Myelomeningocele
In this type of severe neural tube defect, part of the spinal cord and the vertebrae that normally protect it are defective. The defect appears as a fluid-filled sac covered by a thin membrane.

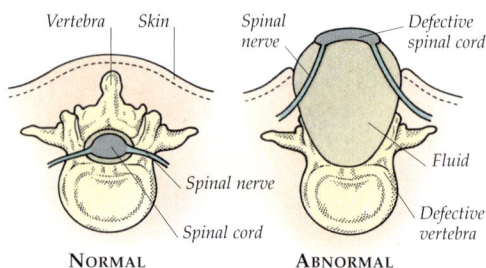

Vertebra Skin Spinal nerve Defective spinal cord

Spinal nerve

Fluid

Spinal cord Defective vertebra

NORMAL **ABNORMAL**

How can neural tube defects be prevented?
The causes of neural tube defects are unknown. However, the risk has been shown to be reduced substantially if a a woman takes a small amount of folic acid once a day for a month before she conceives and during the first month of her pregnancy. Early in pregnancy, screening tests, such as a blood test and an ultrasound examination, usually detect a neural tube defect. The parents may choose a termination if the defect is particularly severe or if there is little chance that the baby will survive.

What is the treatment?
A child with a mild defect may have no symptoms and need no treatment. Surgical treatment may be necessary for a more severely affected child; for example, in hydrocephalus, a tube may be inserted into the brain to drain off fluid. Nevertheless, the child may remain permanently disabled. He or she will receive physical therapy and help with learning to live with disability.

CEREBRAL PALSY

A general term for abnormalities of limb movement and posture, cerebral palsy results from damage to the brain in late pregnancy, at birth, in the newborn period, or in early childhood. Usually, damage occurs before or at birth. Cerebral palsy is most common in babies born prematurely or weighing less than 1.5 kg.

What are the symptoms?
Cerebral palsy may not be recognized until your child is several months old. The earliest signs are usually:
• Stiffness of the arms and legs on being picked up.
• Reluctance to use one hand or arm.
• Feeding difficulties.
• Not sitting by the age of 1 year.
In some children, the muscles of one or more limbs are stiff (spastic), making normal movements very difficult. This problem usually starts to appear from the age of 6 months onward. Other children have irregular and involuntary writhing movements of the body.

Many children with cerebral palsy have learning difficulties (p.172). Some also have epilepsy and problems with hearing and eyesight. SPEECH PROBLEMS (p.171) are common due to a variety of causes, including poor hearing, slow learning ability, and poor coordination of the muscles that are used in speech. Behavioral problems may occur as a result of a child's frustration with his or her disabilities, or can be due to family tension or to the brain damage itself.

Should I consult a doctor?
If you have any concerns that your baby is not developing properly, you should make an appointment to see a doctor.

Scans and tests may be done to make a precise diagnosis of the cause of your child's problems. Depending on the specific difficulties, your child may be seen by a consultant pediatrician, occupational and speech therapists, a psychologist, and a social worker. In some cases, deformities resulting from muscle contractures require surgery.

What is the outlook?
Although cerebral palsy is incurable, with patience and as much stimulation as possible, your child's symptoms may show improvement. Children who have mild cerebral palsy can usually attend normal schools, but those who are more severely affected may require special education. Children with mild or moderate disability should have a near-normal life expectancy.

Occupational therapy
The concentration and coordination of children with cerebral palsy can be improved by doing puzzles and playing games involving fine hand movements.

RECURRENT HEADACHES

Almost all children have occasional headaches. Some children, however, have recurrent headaches, which may be severely debilitating and interfere with schoolwork. The two main forms of recurrent headache are migraine and tension headache. Very rarely, recurrent headaches are caused by a brain disorder.

MIGRAINE

Children who suffer from migraine frequently have a family history of the disorder. The most common trigger of migraine attacks is emotional stress. Other possible triggers include certain foods, such as citrus fruits or cheese, hunger, too much sun, and tiredness.

What are the symptoms?

Attacks of migraine rarely occur more than once or twice a month. A few children have initial warning signs of seeing sparkling lights or zigzag lines. Symptoms that follow, which may last from 2 hours to 2 days, may include:
• Pain, which may affect one side of the head only or both sides of the head.
• Vomiting.
• Dislike of light and noise.
• Lightheadedness or dizziness.
• Tingling, weakness, or numbness of an arm or hand.
A doctor should see your child if the symptoms suggest migraine.

What is the treatment?

The doctor may suggest that you try to identify trigger factors, so that they can be avoided, if possible. Antiemetic medicine may be prescribed to prevent vomiting during attacks. Propranolol, a drug that prevents migraine, may be prescribed if attacks are very frequent.

Taking acetaminophen and lying down in a darkened room should help to relieve pain during a migraine attack.

What is the outlook?

Frequent attacks of migraine may be followed by long periods when there are none. If your child avoids known triggers, the number of attacks may be limited. Propranolol reduces the frequency of migraine attacks.

Stress-related headache
Migraine or a tension headache may be triggered by working too hard at school, possibly in an attempt to keep up with peers or as a result of worry over up-coming exams.

TENSION HEADACHE

The pain of a tension headache may be due to muscular tension in the face and neck – for example, from clenching or grinding the teeth. Emotional stress is the most common trigger.

What are the symptoms?

The symptoms, which may be present every day, consist of:
• Pain, affecting any part of the head.
• Sometimes, accompanying signs of tension, such as abdominal pain.

What is the treatment?

Give acetaminophen to relieve the pain, and try to identify and reduce any causes of stress. If the headaches continue, consult a doctor, who may send your child to a consultant.

BRAIN DISORDERS

The symptoms vary, but the following may point to the possibility of a brain disorder, such as a tumor:
• Headache that wakes a child up at night, is present on waking up in the morning, or is made worse by a cough.
• Seizures.
• Changes in behavior.
A doctor should see your child at once if you suspect a brain disorder. The doctor will examine your child and may arrange for tests in the hospital. The treatment and outlook will depend on the nature of the problem.

CHRONIC FATIGUE SYNDROME

This disorder consists of a collection of symptoms, of which the most important is severe fatigue that persists for months or even years. A viral illness may, for unknown reasons, be the trigger. Sometimes, the symptoms are due to unrecognized depression.

What are the symptoms?

The symptoms may include:
• Severe fatigue that prevents the child getting out of bed at the usual time.
• A feeling of weakness in the limbs.
• Pain in the head, the abdomen, or the muscles of the limbs.
• Reluctance to eat or to take part in any social activities.
• Becoming extremely exhausted after any physical or mental exertion.
• Difficulty in concentrating.

Sometimes, chronic fatigue syndrome is preceded by a sore throat or some other viral illness, such as INFECTIOUS MONONUCLEOSIS (p.124), but not always.

Should I consult a doctor?

It is normal for a child to feel "washed out" for a week or two after a severe infectious illness. If fatigue lasts for more than a month, consult a doctor. The doctor will examine your child for any physical cause for the illness and may arrange for blood tests to check for any signs of illness. In most cases, physical examination and test results are normal, although in a large number of sufferers, tests show evidence of a recent or current viral infection.

What is the treatment?

There is no specific treatment. If your child has been away from school for a long time, a gradual return should be arranged. Ask teachers about possible causes of anxiety in school that could be alleviated. Your child is considered to be cured once he or she has returned to school full time. However, if one or more relapses occur, the help of a child psychiatrist may be required.

EAR AND EYE DISORDERS

JUST AS THEY CATCH COLDS EASILY, most children have several attacks of ear and eye infections caused by either viruses or bacteria. By the time they reach the age of 7 or 8 years, they have usually become immune to the more common viruses, and infections become less troublesome; bacterial infections are usually easily treated by antibiotics. Occasionally, ear and eye infections may cause severe illness, and symptoms should never be ignored. Persistent ear infections may lead to hearing difficulties, which can delay speech and learning. Early detection and treatment of vision problems is vital to enable vision to develop normally.

OTITIS MEDIA

Inflammation of the middle ear, called otitis media, is a common cause of earache in children. Otitis media most frequently affects children up to 8 years old. It is often a painful complication of an upper respiratory tract infection, such as a COMMON COLD (p.148) or a throat infection (see SORE THROAT, p.151).

How is it caused?
When bacterial or viral infection spreads up the eustachian tube (the narrow canal that connects the middle ear to the back of the throat), the tissues that line the middle ear become inflamed and produce fluid and sometimes pus. The secretions are unable to drain away because the eustachian tube is blocked by the inflammation or by ENLARGED ADENOIDS (p.149). The accumulating secretions cause pain as they press on the eardrum, which sometimes splits.

What are the symptoms?
Earache is the main symptom of otitis media. However, in a very young child, who may have difficulty in locating the site of the pain (especially if both ears are affected), fever and vomiting may be the only initial symptoms. In children of all ages, otitis media may produce the following symptoms:
• Waking up at night, crying.
• Irritability.
• Tugging at or rubbing one ear.
• Partial deafness.
• A discharge from the ear, which relieves pain but signals that the eardrum has perforated.
Your child should be seen by a doctor within 24 hours if you think he or she has otitis media. You should phone a doctor at once if the pain is severe or if your child is very young.

What can I do to help?
To relieve the pain while waiting to see the doctor, your child should be given liquid acetaminophen and should rest the painful ear on a hot water bottle wrapped in a towel (see illustration at right). Fill the bottle with warm, not hot, water. Resting with the affected side of the head turned downward will allow any discharge to drain out. You should not use a hot water bottle to relieve earache in a baby, because he or she will not be able to push it away if it is too hot. Instead, heat a soft cloth and hold it against the baby's ear.

What might the doctor do?
The doctor will examine your child's ear with an otoscope (a viewing instrument). He or she may prescribe a course of oral antibiotics, which should bring down your child's temperature and relieve the pain within 2 days. If the earache and fever do not subside after 3 days, the doctor may prescribe a different antibiotic. Fluid sometimes remains in the middle ear for as long as 3 months. An eardrum that has perforated should heal within a week. An infection with a perforated eardrum is not any more serious than an infection with an intact eardrum.

If your child has many episodes of otitis media, or if fluid fails to drain from the ear after a reasonable period of time, your doctor will probably order a hearing test. Further treatment may include daily antibiotics or ear tubes if the problems (hearing loss, recurrent infections) do not improve.

What is the outlook?
As a child grows, the eustachian tube increases in width, allowing fluid to drain out more easily. The middle ear is therefore much less vulnerable to infection. Your child is not likely to have attacks of otitis media after he or she is about 7 or 8 years of age.

Easing earache
Lying flat may make an earache worse. Prop your child up with pillows while he or she rests the painful ear on a hot water bottle.

MIDDLE EAR EFFUSION

This condition occurs when the middle ear becomes filled with a thick, sticky, gluelike mucus that is produced by the lining of the middle ear. Hearing is usually impaired because the mucus reduces the ability of the eardrum and the small bones in the middle ear to vibrate fully and transmit sound to the inner ear.

How is it caused?
Middle ear effusion results from the overproduction of mucus by the lining of the middle ear. The excess mucus accumulates in the middle ear, especially if inflammation blocks the eustachian tube (the narrow canal that connects the middle ear to the back of the throat). This disease may develop if OTITIS MEDIA (opposite) is left untreated or is not treated adequately; it may appear even if there is adequate treatment.

What are the symptoms?
If your child has middle ear effusion, he or she may:
• Complain of partial deafness. Your child's hearing may be worse at some times than others.
• Be inattentive and slow at learning.

Pain is rarely a symptom, so the problem may be present for some time before it is detected. If you suspect middle ear effusion, have a doctor see your child.

What might the doctor do?
The doctor will examine the ears with a viewing instrument and may refer your child to an ear, nose, and throat specialist. The specialist will carry out a hearing test; he or she may also measure the movements of the eardrum. If the test results are abnormal, they will be repeated 3 months later. If the condition of the ear has not improved, treatment options include surgical drainage and tube placement. Tube placement is done by an ear, nose, and throat surgeon, who makes a small cut in the eardrum and inserts a tiny plastic tube (illustration below). The tube falls out in 2 months to 2 years; the eardrum heals a few days afterward. Consult a pediatrician before tube placement is done.

What is the outlook?
The width of the eustachian tube will increase as your child grows, and fluid will drain much more efficiently from the middle ear. This condition is unlikely to occur after 8 years of age.

An eardrum tube
A small tube is inserted into the eardrum to allow air to enter, circulate, and dry out the middle ear.

Middle ear | Tube | Eardrum | Outer ear canal

OTITIS EXTERNA

There are several causes of otitis externa (inflammation of the outer ear canal), including bacterial infection and skin conditions such as SEBORRHEIC DERMATITIS (p.134) and ECZEMA (p.135). The risk of infection is increased if the sensitive skin that lines the ear canal is exposed to water for too long – for example, during swimming; or if the lining is scratched or irritated by a foreign body, such as a cotton swab, or by long-standing wax blockage.

An infected ear canal
If your child has otitis externa, you may see a white, yellow, or honey-colored discharge coming from his or her ear canal. While the discharge sometimes relieves pain in the ear canal a little, you should still have your child examined by a doctor.

What are the symptoms?
The outer, fleshy part of the ear may be tender when it is touched or moved. However, the symptoms mainly affect the ear canal and may include:
• Itchiness, usually followed by pain.
• Discharge from the canal, which may be thick and white or yellowish.
• Partial deafness, if wax or a discharge is blocking the canal.
• Weeping, crusting blisters.
Your child should be seen by a doctor within 24 hours if he or she has an earache, a discharge from the outer ear canal, or difficulty in hearing.

What might the doctor do?
The doctor will probably examine your child's ear with an otoscope (a viewing instrument). If he or she finds a foreign body or a plug of wax, he or she will remove it, and clean and dry the canal. The doctor may prescribe antibiotic ear drops. If either eczema or seborrheic dermatitis is the cause of your child's otitis externa, the doctor may prescribe corticosteroid ear drops to relieve any itching and tenderness. With treatment, otitis externa usually clears up within 7 to 10 days.

What can I do to help?
You may give your child acetaminophen to relieve the pain. A hot water bottle filled with warm, not hot, water or a warm cloth held against your child's ear may comfort and distract him or her. If ear drops have been prescribed, have your child lie down with the affected ear facing up. Hold your child's head still while you give the ear drops, and make sure that your child lies still for a minute or two after they have been given.

Your child should not swim or get the ear wet until the otitis externa has cleared up. Keep the affected ear dry by covering it with a shower cap during a bath or shower and by sponging your child's hair clean instead of washing it. Avoid placing cotton in the ears for long periods; this may worsen the condition.

LABYRINTHITIS

The labyrinth (the inner ear) contains the fluid-filled chambers that are concerned with balance. Labyrinthitis (inflammation of the labyrinth) occurs as a complication of a viral infection and results in unpleasant feelings of dizziness and nausea.

What are the symptoms?
The symptoms of labyrinthitis occur in bouts, each of which lasts for between 5 and 15 minutes. Several bouts a day may occur. The main symptoms are:
• Vertigo, which is the sensation that the surroundings are spinning around and around uncontrollably.
• Unsteadiness and falling down. Your child has to lean on a wall or hold on to furniture to steady him- or herself.
• Nausea and vomiting.
Your child will probably feel extremely distressed by the condition. He or she should see a doctor within 24 hours of the symptoms developing.

What might the doctor do?
The doctor will examine your child and will ask whether he or she has had any illnesses recently. A special type of anti-histamine syrup may be prescribed to relieve the vomiting and dizziness. No other treatment is required.

What is the outlook?
Labyrinthitis usually clears up within 1 to 3 weeks, but it sometimes lasts for several months. Although labyrinthitis can be a frightening experience, it does not lead to any permanent disability.

ALTITUDE TRAUMA

This condition consists of temporary blockage of the eustachian tube (the passage that connects the middle ear and the throat) and bulging of the eardrum as a result of abrupt changes in atmospheric pressure. It is usually brought on by air travel.

How is it caused?
Air flow through the eustachian tube normally maintains equal air pressure inside and outside the middle ear. When an airplane ascends, the air pressure in the cabin falls, and so does the pressure inside the middle ear. When the airplane descends, pressure outside the middle ear increases, causing the eustachian tube to shut and pushing the eardrum inward. An upper respiratory tract infection (such as a COMMON COLD, p.148), hay fever (see ALLERGIC RHINITIS, p.152), or an ear infection (see OTITIS MEDIA, p.162) makes this trauma more likely.

What are the symptoms?
The symptoms of altitude trauma are:
• Pain as the eardrum bulges in.
• Partial hearing loss.
• Ringing in the ears.
The symptoms usually disappear within 3 to 5 hours and do not cause any lasting damage. Liquid acetaminophen relieves the pain.

How can I prevent this trauma?
When an airplane descends, sucking on candy, swallowing, chewing gum, or using the method shown at right (called the Valsalva maneuver) all open the eustachian tube, allowing air to flow freely into the middle ear. In babies, bottle- or breast-feeding during descent prevents altitude trauma. A child with an upper respiratory tract infection, hay fever, or an ear infection should avoid air travel.

Preventing altitude trauma
When your child begins to feel the pressure changing in the ear during descent in an airplane, he or she should pinch the nose while keeping the mouth closed, and blow down the nose until the ears "pop."

IRITIS

Inflammation of the iris and the muscular ring that surrounds it (the ciliary body) is known as iritis. Serious attacks are rare in childhood, but children with JUVENILE RHEUMATOID ARTHRITIS (p.132) may suffer from a persistent or recurrent form of iritis.

What are the symptoms?
Iritis may affect one or both eyes at the same time. The main symptoms are:
• Pain (which may be dull or severe) in the affected eye.
• Redness of the white of the eye, particularly of the part around the edge of the iris.
• Acute sensitivity to light.
• Blurred vision.
• A swollen iris that has lost its normal color and looks muddy.
• An irregularly shaped pupil, which (if only one eye is affected) is smaller than the pupil of the unaffected eye.
• Watering of the affected eye.
If you think your child may have iritis, you should phone a doctor at once.

What is the treatment?
The doctor may prescribe eye drops or an ointment containing a corticosteroid to reduce the inflammation. You may be able to relieve the symptoms by holding a ball of cotton dipped in warm water to the affected eye. Make sure that you boil the water first.

What is the outlook?
Treated promptly, iritis often clears up within 1 to 2 weeks and has no long-term ill effects. If iritis is not treated, or if it is persistent or recurrent, it can permanently damage vision.

PINK EYE

Inflammation of the thin, transparent membrane (conjunctiva) that covers the whites of the eyes and lines the eyelids is called pink eye, or conjunctivitis. A newborn baby may develop pink eye as a result of infection by bacteria normally found in the birth canal; rarely, infection is transmitted by a mother who has gonorrhea, genital herpes, or a chlamydial infection. In older children, the usual cause of pink eye is viral infection. Pink eye may also be a symptom of hay fever (see ALLERGIC RHINITIS, p.152).

What are the symptoms?
One or both eyes may be affected. The main symptoms are:
• Redness of the white of the eye and the inside of the eyelid.
• Itchiness and irritation of the eye.
• In bacterial conjunctivitis, yellow, sticky pus in the corner of the eye and on the eyelashes. Sticky lashes may make it hard for your child to open the affected eye in the morning.
• In allergic conjunctivitis, swollen eyelids and a clear discharge from the eye that is not sticky.

Should I consult a doctor?
Conjunctivitis affecting a baby may be detected and treated in the hospital soon after birth. However, in some cases, the symptoms do not appear for

Appearance of bacterial conjunctivitis
The whites of the eyes are bloodshot and the eyelashes are gummy with yellow pus. Pus has also collected in the corners of the eyes.

several weeks. If symptoms develop, contact your doctor at once. Although viral conjunctivitis in older children is not serious, you should get medical advice so that the possibility of a serious eye disorder can be excluded.

What is the treatment?
Bacterial infection is treated with an antibiotic ointment or eye drops and usually clears up within a week. Oral or intravenous antibiotics may be given for severe bacterial infection, which may take up to 6 weeks to get better.

Viral conjunctivitis clears up without treatment within a week. To relieve the discomfort of allergic conjunctivitis, anti-inflammatory eye drops may be used. Some preparations are available over the counter; others are prescribed.

What can I do to help?
Remove pus from eyelashes with a towel soaked in cooled, boiled water and squeezed out. Keep this towel on the eye for a few minutes every 2 to 3 hours. Prevent infection by washing hands and not sharing towels and washcloths. With eye drops, tilt back the head and place a few drops along the nasal side of the eye. The drops will leak in if the head is tilted back.

What is the outlook?
With prompt treatment, a baby infected at delivery should recover. Infectious and allergic conjunctivitis never affect vision permanently in older children.

BLOCKED TEAR DUCT

The tear ducts are narrow passages that drain excess fluid from the eyes to the inside of the nose. Sometimes one or both ducts are partially blocked by dead cells at birth so that tear fluid cannot drain away. As a result, the baby's eye waters continually.

What are the symptoms?
The main symptoms are:
• Continual watering of the eye, even when the baby is not crying.
• If the eye is infected, pus in the inner corner of the eye, and swelling of the side of the nose just below the eye's inner corner.

Should I consult a doctor?
In almost all cases, a blocked tear duct opens naturally by the age of 1 year. However, with treatment, the duct may open sooner than this. Therefore, make an appointment to see a doctor if your baby's eyes water continually. If there are signs of infection, your baby should be seen by a doctor within 24 hours.

What is the treatment?
The doctor will examine your child's eyes and, if there are no signs of an infection, he or she may suggest that you gently massage the upper part of the duct (see illustration at right).

If the eye is infected, the doctor may prescribe an antibiotic ointment. Once the infection has cleared up (usually in a week, but check with the doctor to make sure), you may start the massage treatment to unblock the duct.

If the duct has not opened by the age of 6 to 8 months, the doctor may refer your baby to an ophthalmologist. Under general anesthesia, the specialist will clear the obstruction from the tear duct using a thin metal probe.

Use your index finger to massage the duct gently with a circular motion

Unblocking a tear duct
After washing your hands, massage the skin just below the inner corner of the eye gently with your index finger. Repeating this procedure three or four times a day for a week or two may force a blocked tear duct to open.

What is the outlook?
Once the duct is unblocked, the eyes should stop watering and your baby will be less susceptible to eye infection.

EYELID DISORDERS

Styes and blepharitis are common disorders affecting the eyelids in children. A stye is a pus-filled swelling that forms at the base of an eyelash. Blepharitis is inflammation of the eyelid edges. Although they cause discomfort, these disorders are not serious.

STYES

A stye results from an infection, usually by bacteria. Styes sometimes develop as a complication of blepharitis.

What are the symptoms?
The main symptoms of a stye are:
- A yellow head of pus on the eyelid around the base of an eyelash.
- Swollen and inflamed eyelid skin surrounding the head of pus.
- Pain or tenderness to the touch.

What is the treatment?
A stye usually clears up in a few days. Pressing a warm cloth to the infected area for about 20 minutes every hour may help to relieve the pain, and it also encourages the discharge of pus, which hastens healing. Avoid touching the stye to prevent spreading the infection.

A child with recurring styes should be seen by a doctor, who may prescribe an antibiotic ointment. Applying the ointment three or four times daily can prevent styes from recurring.

BLEPHARITIS

In many cases, blepharitis is associated with dandruff and most often affects children who suffer from SEBORRHEIC DERMATITIS (p.134). Less commonly, it is due to viral or bacterial infection.

What are the symptoms?
The main symptoms of blepharitis are:
- A burning sensation, redness, and itching of the eyelid margins.
- Scales at the roots of the lashes. The scales in the seborrheic form of blepharitis are yellow and greasy.

Infectious blepharitis
The eyelids are red and swollen, and crusted with scales. The white of the eye is red, indicating accompanying conjunctivitis.

- Sometimes, eyelashes that grow in the wrong direction or fall out.

In some cases infectious blepharitis is accompanied by PINK EYE (p.165). Your child should be seen by a doctor if you think he or she has blepharitis.

What is the treatment?
The doctor will show you how to wipe off any crusting scales from the eyelid margins using a cotton ball moistened with warm water. He or she may take a swab from the lid margins for tests to determine the cause. If the eyelid is infected, the doctor may prescribe an antibiotic ointment, which you can apply after you have removed any scales. Infectious blepharitis usually clears up within 2 weeks; the ointment should be used for at least another 2 weeks to prevent a recurrence. Seborrheic blepharitis tends to be persistent. Washing the eye with tear-free baby shampoo will clear the problem.

STRABISMUS

An abnormality in the direction of the gaze of one eye is known as strabismus. Most young babies appear cross-eyed occasionally up to the age of 2 to 4 months, but persistence beyond the age of 4 months or constantly crossed eyes at any age is abnormal.

How is it caused?
Strabismus usually occurs because the mechanism that coordinates the eyes is not fully developed. In older children, it is often due to severe farsightedness (see REFRACTIVE ERRORS, opposite), which causes the eyes to accommodate (adjust for near focus) too strongly, forcing one eye inward. It can also be due to unequal refraction, which causes the two eyes to produce conflicting images. The weaker eye's image is suppressed, and the eye is poorly controlled.

What are the symptoms?
The main symptoms of strabismus are:
- An eye that turns too far in or out (convergent or divergent strabismus), or up or down (vertical strabismus), when a child looks at an object.

Convergent strabismus
This child has a convergent strabismus of the left eye. The normal eye looks straight ahead, while the left eye is focused inward.

- Poor vision in the affected eye.
- Double or blurred vision, which the child may try to remedy by closing or covering the affected eye.

To prevent the double vision produced by strabismus, the brain ignores the image from the weaker eye. Because the eye is not used, its vision eventually may become permanently impaired.

If strabismus develops after your child is 4 months old or if the condition is persistent, consult a doctor, who may send your child to an ophthalmologist.

What is the treatment?
The ophthalmologist will evaluate your child's vision. He or she may prescribe glasses if your child is farsighted or has another refractive error. Treatment may also involve covering the normal eye with a patch, which forces your child to use the affected eye. In some cases, the position of the deviating eye may be corrected by an operation. After the operation, your child will be given a series of eye exercises that encourage normal development of vision.

What is the outlook?
If treatment for strabismus is provided within a few weeks, a child's vision should develop normally.

REFRACTIVE ERRORS

Problems with the focusing mechanism of the eyes are known as refractive errors. There are three types of refractive error, all of which cause blurred vision to some degree. The three errors are nearsightedness (myopia), farsightedness (hypermetropia), and astigmatism. Refractive errors tend to run in families. Farsightedness and astigmatism are often present from birth. Nearsightedness is often not apparent until puberty, although it starts to develop a few years before a child reaches adolescence.

How are they caused?
Nearsightedness and farsightedness result from an incorrect relationship between the eyeball's length and the focusing power of the cornea, the front part of the eye (see illustrations below).

In nearsightedness, the images of distant objects are brought into focus in front of the retina and appear blurred.

In farsightedness, images of objects are focused behind the retina instead of on it. However, children who are mildly or moderately farsighted are able to see clearly because, in young eyes, accommodation (the process by which the eyes adjust for near focus) is strong enough to enable the focusing point to be brought forward onto the retina.

Astigmatism occurs when the curve of the cornea is uneven. It results in an inability to focus on all the parts of an object at the same time; for example, horizontal lines may be in focus, while vertical lines appear blurred.

What are the symptoms?
If your child is nearsighted or has an astigmatism, he or she will probably not be aware that anything is wrong. However, your child may:
- Sit too close to the television set.
- Have problems with schoolwork, or appear not to be interested, because he or she cannot see what is going on at the front of the classroom.
- Complain that objects at a distance appear blurred.

If your child is severely farsighted, he or she may:
- Develop STRABISMUS (opposite).
- Complain that nearby objects appear blurred.

Should I consult the doctor?
Your child should be seen by a doctor or an optometrist if you think that there is a focusing problem. A doctor who suspects a refractive error will probably refer your child to either an optometrist or an ophthalmologist.

What might the optometrist or ophthalmologist do?
Your child's eyes will be tested one at a time. The method chosen for testing visual acuity (sharpness of vision) will depend on the age and reading ability of your child. Children who can read are usually tested using the standard adult vision-testing charts. A child who is unable to read may be tested with a chart showing the capital letter E in decreasing sizes and turned in various directions. He or she may be asked to show the orientation of the letter with a finger. A very small child's sight may be tested with charts showing images of familiar objects. Alternatively, a small child's vision may be examined using retinoscopy, which involves observing the movement of a light shone into the eye and reflected from the retina.

Once your child's visual acuity has been assessed, the severity of his or her refractive error will be established. To make sure of an accurate result, your child may be given atropine eye drops to paralyze the strong accommodation mechanism temporarily. A series of lenses is held in front of the eye, and the child is asked whether the vision improves with each lens. Once the combination of lenses that gives good vision has been found, the results are checked using retinoscopy.

The optometrist or ophthalmologist prescribes glasses based on the figures obtained by retinoscopy. Contact lenses can, alternatively, be prescribed. They usually give better corrected vision than glasses and are often preferred by teenagers. The need for proper hygiene and disciplined wearing time makes them unsuitable for young children.

What is the outlook?
In most cases, refractive errors do not become any worse once body growth is complete. However, because the power of accommodation decreases with age, farsightedness that earlier did not produce any symptoms may become apparent during middle age.

NEAR- AND FARSIGHTEDNESS
For vision to be clear, the focusing power of the cornea and the distance from the cornea to the retina must be in the correct relationship, so that the image of an object is brought into focus on the retina. Near-sightedness occurs when the cornea is too steeply curved and/or the eyeball is too long. Farsightedness occurs when the curve of the cornea is too flat and/or the eyeball is too short.

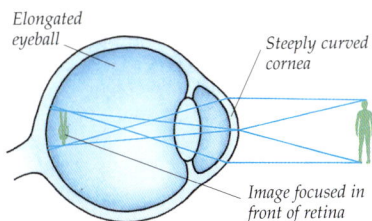

Normal vision
The shape of the eyeball and the focusing power of the cornea are correctly related. The image of an object is focused on the retina and can be seen clearly.

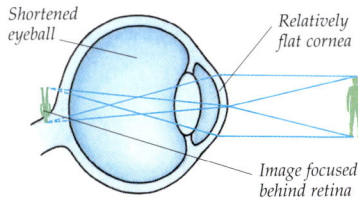

Nearsightedness
The eyeball is too long, and the focusing power of the steeply curved cornea is too strong. The image of a distant object is brought into focus in front of the retina, and appears blurred.

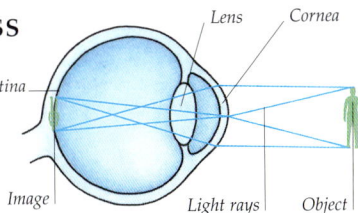

Farsightedness
The eyeball is too short and the focusing power of the relatively flat cornea is too weak. The image of an object is focused behind the retina, and appears blurred.

BEHAVIORAL AND EMOTIONAL PROBLEMS

WHEN A CHILD BEHAVES in a way that causes concern, parents want to know whether the problem behavior is likely to last. Children usually grow out of upsetting or odd habits, but some require professional help. An early consultation with a doctor can help to relieve anxiety and determine whether treatment is likely to be needed.

SLEEP PROBLEMS

Children up to the age of 5 years are the group most commonly affected by sleep problems, although some older children may also be affected. The problems discussed below are usually temporary. Rarely, they are signs of anxiety (see ANXIETY AND FEARS, p.170) or, very rarely, of serious behavioral problems.

WAKEFULNESS AT NIGHT

Most children normally sleep through the night by the age of 1 year. If a child older than a year fails to settle down at night or wakes up during the night, you should try to identify the cause. Possible causes are lack of a fixed bedtime or a bedtime that is too early. Your child might also be afraid of the dark.

Imposing a sensible bedtime routine and being firm with your child might help him or her to settle down at night. If your child is afraid of the dark, a night light might help. Older children may respond to a reward system.

Wakefulness
Problems in going to sleep at night or waking up during the night are most common in young children between the ages of 1 and 2 years.

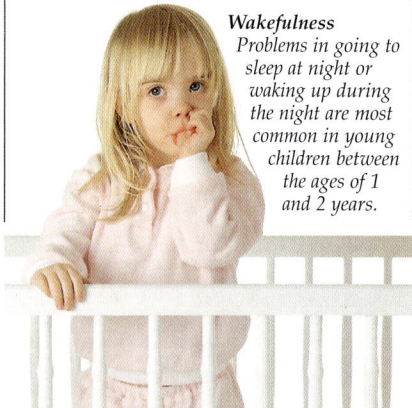

Should I consult a doctor?

Consult a doctor if the wakefulness is becoming unbearable. You may be asked to monitor your child's bedtime routine and sleep patterns, then make changes in order to establish a regular sleep pattern. This approach usually succeeds in establishing a normal sleep routine within a few weeks.

NIGHTMARES

Frightening dreams are most common in children 5 to 6 years of age. Usually, nightmares are triggered by disturbing experiences – for example, a frightening movie. Sometimes, they indicate anxiety.

What can I do to help?

When your child is woken up by a nightmare, comfort him or her until sleep returns. Sometimes, nightmares can be prevented by screening what your child watches on television. It may help to leave the bedroom door open or a light on. For some children, discussing the nightmares is helpful. If nightmares are persistent or frequent, discuss this with your child's doctor.

Nightmares usually occur less often after the age of 6 years, but people of all ages have them occasionally.

NIGHT TERRORS

Children aged 4 to 7 years seem most susceptible to night terrors, which tend to occur about 2 hours after falling asleep. Before a terror, the child becomes increasingly restless. During a terror, he or she seems to be awake and terrified, and is likely to scream, shout, and moan. However, the child is not awake and cannot be woken easily; he or she does not respond to comforting.

If you know when a night terror is likely to occur, wake your child in the restless period that precedes it or about 15 minutes before. Once a terror is under way, staying with your child provides comfort and reassurance, but do not wake him or her at this time.

Should I consult a doctor?

Consult a doctor if night terrors occur more than a few times a week. He or she will help pinpoint any household stresses contributing to the upset. Your child will outgrow night terrors.

SLEEPWALKING

This problem occurs most commonly in children 6 to 12 years of age. The child gets out of bed and wanders around, often finding his or her own way back to bed in a few minutes. There is no need to do anything except ensure his or her safety. Gently guide your child back to bed without waking him or her.

Most children outgrow sleepwalking by puberty, but a minority continue to have episodes throughout their lives.

HABITUAL BEHAVIOR

Many childhood habits are so common that they should be seen as normal. Habits may provide comfort for stress or anxiety or may be a means of expressing anger, frustration, or boredom. The most common habits of infancy are thumb-sucking, head-banging, and breath-holding attacks. Tics and compulsions mainly affect schoolchildren. Nail-biting and twirling or pulling hair can affect children of any age. Most habits do little harm.

THUMB-SUCKING

A child may suck his or her thumb when bored, nervous, or in need of comfort. Thumb-sucking is most common in children up to 3 years old and is harmless. Some children continue until they are 6 or 7 years old. In these cases, discuss trying to stop with your child. A reward system may help your child to give it up.

Comforting habit
Thumb-sucking is the most common childhood habit. About half of all 3-year-olds suck their thumbs.

NAIL-BITING

About a third of all children bite their nails. The habit usually starts during a child's early years at school and may persist into adulthood. Nail-biting may make the nails unsightly and painful. A young child may give up the habit if distracted when nail-biting occurs; older children may respond to a gift of a nail file and clippers or scissors.

HEAD-BANGING

A frustrated, angry, or bored child may bang his or her head against a hard surface. Such behavior occurs in a small number of preschool children, and usually disappears by the age of 4 years. Although alarming, it seldom harms the child. You may offer the child a cushion or pillow to soften the impact, but otherwise it is usually best to ignore the habit. If head-banging is severe or persistent, consult a doctor.

BREATH-HOLDING ATTACKS

A small number of preschool children habitually hold their breath for periods of up to 30 seconds. A child may pass out as a result. An attack may be brought on by pain or frustration and may be used as a way of manipulating parents. You should ignore the attacks as much as possible. They usually disappear by the age of 4 years, but if you are concerned, consult a doctor.

TICS

Repetitive, involuntary movements, tics mainly affect schoolchildren and often involve the head and face; for example, rapid, repetitive blinking may occur.

Tics are often due to stress and are usually temporary. If a tic is severe or is accompanied by disturbing behavior such as loud verbal noises or outbursts, consult a doctor. Your child may be referred to a child psychiatrist or neurologist for evaluation and possible treatment of Tourette's syndrome.

COMPULSIONS

Schoolchildren often have compulsions, in which they feel the need to perform a particular action such as avoiding cracks in the sidewalk. Compulsions usually disappear if ignored. If they continue or get worse, consult a doctor.

TWIRLING OR PULLING HAIR

Children of all ages may twirl or pull their hair from frustration or anxiety. In most cases, this habit is not a cause for concern. Rarely, serious emotional disturbance may result in such severe hair-pulling that bald patches develop. Consult a doctor if your child is pulling out his or her hair.

Bald patch
The large, bald patch on this child's scalp was caused by repetitive hair-pulling.

SOILING

Most children achieve bowel control by the age of 3 years. An occasional accident after this age is usually nothing to worry about. However, persistent soiling or soiling that starts after a child has been toilet-trained indicates a problem.

What are the causes?

Soiling is most often a result of chronic CONSTIPATION (p.181). Hard stool cannot be passed, and fecal liquid leaks out. Some illnesses occasionally cause soiling due to diarrhea. Slowness in achieving bowel control, poor toilet-training, or stress are other causes. Soiling in which the child passes stool in inappropriate places (encopresis) may be a sign of serious emotional disturbance.

Should I consult a doctor?

Consult a doctor if your child is soiling after the age of 3 years, if he or she starts soiling after having achieved bowel control, or has encopresis. The doctor will examine your child and treat him or her for any physical causes of soiling. For other cases of soiling, the doctor may suggest the measures on the right. A child with encopresis may be referred to a child psychiatrist.

What can I do to help?

Punishing your child for soiling may make the problem worse. Gently but firmly encourage frequent defecation. Your child should sit on the toilet after every meal for about 5 minutes; give him or her a book to read. Every time your child defecates into the toilet, give praise and perhaps a treat. To prevent relapse, you may need to continue this treatment for 3 to 6 months after soiling has stopped. Try to identify sources of anxiety for your child and remove or alleviate them as much as possible.

With appropriate treatment, most soiling problems disappear within a few weeks. If they persist, see a doctor.

ANXIETY AND FEARS

All children experience anxiety and fears. Some degree of anxiety is normal in many situations; for example, a child may cry for a few minutes when separated from a parent. Short-lived specific fears of the dark, animals, thunder, or places, such as school, are also common. Anxiety and fears only become a cause for concern when they last longer than a few months, are so severe that they amount to a phobia, and/or disrupt a child's life.

Separation anxiety
Preschool children often feel frightened and anxious when they are separated, even briefly, from their parents, especially their mothers.

What are the symptoms?
In children, the presence of anxiety or specific fears may be indicated by:
• Prolonged or persistent crying.
• Irritability and temper tantrums.

• Poor appetite and sleep disturbance.
• BED-WETTING (p.192) and SOILING (p.169).
• Unexplained physical symptoms, such as recurrent stomach pains, headaches, and limb or joint pains.
• Tics and compulsions (see HABITUAL BEHAVIOR, p.169).

What are the causes?
Insecurity often causes anxiety and fears. Obvious triggers or causes of distress are being parted from a parent (separation anxiety), problems at school or at home, or peer group difficulties. Children may pick up anxiety or specific fears from other people. For example, fear of loud noises or insects may develop because a child is aware that his or her mother dislikes them.

What can I do to help?
Talking to your child about his or her worries and fears may help. If possible, take steps to remove or limit the causes.

Making a fuss about fears may only increase them. In general, it is best to adopt a calm and reassuring attitude, acknowledging and accepting a child's concern. Try to help your child gain the confidence to deal with his or her particular fear. For example, you may cuddle your child while you both look at pictures of animals he or she fears.

Should I consult a doctor?
There is no need to worry about short-lived episodes of anxiety or fearfulness, especially in toddlers. However, if a child's anxieties or fears persist, or are so intense that they interfere with daily life, consult a doctor. He or she will try to identify underlying problems, and may suggest using reward systems and relaxation techniques. If a problem is particularly troublesome, your child may be referred to a child psychiatrist.

Anxiety and fears usually disappear within a few months. However, a child who has experienced severe problems may have recurrences later in life.

ADHD (ATTENTION DEFICIT HYPERACTIVITY DISORDER)

Young children are normally very active and, in most cases, nothing is likely to be wrong. However, a child who is restless, impulsive, and unable to concentrate may have attention deficit hyperactivity disorder (ADHD). As a result, his or her school performance may be poor. About 4 percent of primary school children are affected. Diagnosis of ADHD is best made by a pediatrician.

What are the causes?
The cause of ADHD is often uncertain, but in many cases there is a genetic component.

The condition occurs more often in boys than girls, and tends to appear when the child is between the ages of 3 and 7 years.

What are the symptoms?
Symptoms of attention deficit hyperactivity disorder may not be noticed until a child goes to school and his or her behavior is seen in comparison with that of other children.

A child with ADHD may be:
• Unable to concentrate.
• Excessively restless.
• Impulsive and excitable.
• Destructive, disruptive, and accident prone.
• Irritable and aggressive.
Consult a doctor if you are concerned that your child's behavior is abnormal.

What is the treatment?
The doctor may refer your child to a child psychologist, a child psychiatrist, or a pediatrician for assessment. If ADHD is diagnosed, treatment will depend on its severity and the impact it has on your child's life. You may receive advice about giving your child opportunities to expend energy. Some children need special education. Diet is rarely helpful (see p.182). ADHD may be treated with stimulant drugs which, oddly, are calming and improve concentration.

What is the outlook?
Most children with ADHD improve with treatment and as they get older. In a few cases, antisocial behavior appears later in childhood.

Hyperactive child
A child who has ADHD is very restless and tends to change activities frequently.

AUTISM

This disorder affects a child's ability to relate to others, delays language development, and causes repetitive behaviors. Autism is usually noticeable by the age of 2 years and tends to affect boys more than girls. In Asperger's syndrome, which is at the mildest end of the autism spectrum, intelligence is normal.

What are the symptoms?
Autism varies in severity, but a child with the disorder may:
- Fail to make eye contact or point to objects in order to draw people's attention to them.
- Engage in repetitive behavior, such as flapping the hands or moving a toy.
- Be later than expected for his or her age in developing speech or language skills (see SPEECH PROBLEMS, below).
- Appear indifferent to other people.
- Prefer solitary activities.
- Show no interest in creative play.
- Be upset by changes in routine.
- Have LEARNING DIFFICULTIES (p.172). You should consult a doctor if you are concerned about your child's speech or language development, or if he or she is having learning difficulties or seems to have difficulty relating to others.

What is the treatment?
If autism is suspected, your child may be referred to a child psychologist or psychiatrist, or a developmental pediatrician for assessment. There is no curative treatment for autism. Your child may be helped by communication and language therapy and special education. Most autistic children attend schools for children with learning difficulties, but a few can go to ordinary schools, where they receive special support. Parents can help by teaching as many self-help skills as possible.

What is the outlook?
Autistic children who receive early treatment tend to improve gradually throughout childhood and adolescence. Although some achieve a degree of independence as adults, almost all remain disabled to a certain extent and continue to find relating to other people difficult throughout their lives.

SPEECH PROBLEMS

Speech problems are common in childhood, especially in boys. The most common problem is delay in speaking, which may result from a problem with understanding language or with speech production. Other difficulties are stammering, stuttering and lisping. Specific speech or language problems are common in children whose development is normal. In some cases, they are associated with LEARNING DIFFICULTIES (p.172) or AUTISM (above).

DELAY IN SPEAKING

Diminished hearing, which can result from recurrent ear infections (see OTITIS MEDIA, p.162) or MIDDLE EAR EFFUSION (p.163), is one cause of speech delay. There may be a familial tendency to speak late or a physical disorder, such as CEREBRAL PALSY (p.160), that makes it difficult for a child to control the parts used in speech. A child may learn to speak later than other children if there is little conversation or interaction with parents. Children from bilingual families or who are left-handed or ambidextrous are sometimes late in speaking.

Should I consult a doctor?
If, by the age of 2 years, your child has not spoken any words or is not able to follow even simple commands, consult a doctor. The doctor will probably ask questions about the family background and will arrange for a hearing test. A speech therapist or child development team may be asked to assess your child.

Speech production
Air from the lungs vibrates the vocal cords to produce noise. Controlled and coordinated by the brain, movements of the mouth, lips, and tongue modify the noise to produce speech; contact of the tongue with the teeth or palate allows articulation of certain sounds.

Language and speech centers of the brain

Nasal cavity (amplifies sound)

Palate

Lips

Teeth

Tongue

Site of vocal cords

What is the treatment?
A hearing problem will be dealt with first. The speech therapist may give you advice on techniques for encouraging your child to speak and may also work directly with your child. A child who has learning difficulties or a permanent hearing problem will probably require special education. Many provinces have a speech and language program.

What is the outlook?
Children with verbal skills only slightly below those expected for their age, and who are not slow in other areas, tend to catch up with their peers. Those who are more delayed should improve with treatment, but some may later develop reading and writing difficulties.

SPEECH DIFFICULTIES
Children who are learning to speak often lisp or leave out consonants because they are not yet physically able to articulate sounds, and many children aged 2–4 go through a period of stammering. These problems often disappear before a child starts school. If they are persistent (over 4 months) and severe, consult a doctor. Speech therapy may be needed and will usually help to cure the problem. In a few cases, speech difficulties continue into adult life.

LEARNING DIFFICULTIES

A child with learning difficulties functions at a level below that expected for his or her age. Difficulties that affect all aspects of learning are known as general learning difficulties. A difficulty that affects only one particular sphere of learning, such as reading or writing, is termed a specific learning difficulty.

GENERAL LEARNING DIFFICULTIES

Skills are acquired over a wide range of ages, and DEVELOPMENTAL MILESTONES (pp.24–25) indicate where development may be delayed.

What are the causes?

The known causes of generalized difficulties include genetic disorders, such as DOWN SYNDROME (p.198), PHENYLKETONURIA (p.201), and FRAGILE X SYNDROME (p.199); impaired hearing or vision; and brain damage that occurred before, during, or shortly after birth. A physical disability, such as CEREBRAL PALSY (p.160), is sometimes associated with learning difficulties. For many children, no specific cause can be identified. In rare cases, severe emotional problems are the cause.

What are the symptoms?

There is a wide range of disability so the symptoms are varied. A child may have been diagnosed at birth with a disorder, such as Down syndrome, that includes learning difficulties. It may become clear early in life that a seemingly normal child has learning difficulties, or no signs may appear until a child starts school. A child with general learning difficulties may:

- Sit up and walk later than expected for his or her age.
- Be slow in developing speech (see SPEECH PROBLEMS, p.171).
- Fail to notice and respond to sounds and so appear to be deaf.
- Fail to make progress at nursery of school.

There may also be signs of ANTISOCIAL BEHAVIOR (p.174) or ATTENTION DEFICIT HYPERACTIVITY DISORDER (p.170).

What is the treatment?

Treatment is aimed at helping a child achieve his or her maximum potential. A specialist will assess your child by using a series of psychological and/or developmental tests. Your child may be offered educational assistance (either in

Special educational help
Children who have general learning difficulties need special educational help to enable them to achieve their maximum potential. They are often taught individually or in small classes.

a normal school or in special classes or units), speech therapy, occupational therapy, and/or psychotherapy.

What is the outlook?

With appropriate support, a child with mild or moderate general learning difficulties may achieve some degree of independence by adulthood. A child with more severe learning difficulties will benefit from special help but may never be completely independent.

SPECIFIC LEARNING DIFFICULTIES

A child whose general development is normal for his or her age, but who is 2 or more years below the expected level in one area of learning, is said to have a specific learning difficulty. The difficulty may be with reading and/or writing (sometimes called dyslexia), or with arithmetic.

What are the causes?

Specific learning difficulties may be due to impaired hearing or vision or minor brain damage. In most cases, the cause is unknown.

What are the symptoms?

A child with a specific learning difficulty may not show any signs of the problem until the

time when speech, language, and math skills would normally have developed. Comparison with peers or siblings at a similar age is helpful. A child who has a specific learning difficulty may:

- Be slow in developing speech.
- Find spatial tasks, such as doing jigsaw puzzles, difficult.
- Have below-average drawing ability.
- Read from back to front, and reverse letters or symbols when writing.
- Find spelling particularly hard.
- Have difficulty counting objects or recognizing numerical symbols.
- Show antisocial behavior.

If you believe your child has a specific learning difficulty, consult a doctor.

What is the treatment?

Your child's hearing and vision will be tested. A psychoeducational evaluation is helpful. Besides receiving any required medical treatment, your child may be given special educational help and, if he or she has behavioral problems, psychotherapy. To improve your child's confidence, encourage him or her in areas where reading, writing, and arithmetic are not so important.

What is the outlook?

The outlook depends on the severity of the problem and the age of your child when it was first detected. Children whose learning was delayed as a result of a physical problem, such as impaired hearing, tend to catch up quickly once the problem has been treated. Most children who need special educational help show improvement, and a number make good progress. Some children continue to experience difficulties in a particular area throughout their lives.

Testing a child's hearing
A child with a learning difficulty is given a hearing test. Sounds of varying pitch and loudness are played into one ear. The child presses a switch to indicate when and in which ear he or she has heard the sounds.

EATING DISORDERS

Most common in adolescents, especially girls, anorexia nervosa and bulimia nervosa are eating disorders in which there is a fear of becoming fat and a preoccupation with body shape. Another type of eating problem is overeating, which may lead to a child's being overweight or obese. Obesity (weighing 20 percent or more than expected for a person's height and sex) is common in developed countries and can lead to serious health problems.

ANOREXIA AND BULIMIA

These disorders may develop because a teenager feels insecure and associates thinness with attractiveness. The desire to avoid growing up by staying thin and undeveloped may also be a cause. Anorexia and bulimia are dangerous illnesses that must be taken seriously.

What are the symptoms?
An adolescent suffering from anorexia or bulimia may:
- Be fussy about food and eat little.
- Binge and purge (a more prominent feature of bulimia than anorexia).
- Feel guilty, anxious, and depressed about his or her eating behavior.
- Use a large amount of laxatives.
- Exercise excessively.
- Avoid eating with the family.
- Wear clothes that conceal thinness.
- In girls, menstrual periods may fail to begin, become irregular, or stop.

A child with long-standing anorexia becomes thin, weak, and lethargic; fine hair may grow on the face and trunk;

Bingeing and purging
Bouts of overeating followed by self-induced vomiting are the main features of bulimia. These activities are often carried out in secret.

and skin becomes dry. Rarely, a child may starve to death. A child who has bulimia is at risk of dehydration.

Your child should be seen by a doctor if you think that he or she might be suffering from anorexia or bulimia.

What is the treatment?
Treatment consists of a program of supervised eating and psychotherapy to help modify eating habits. A stay in the hospital may be needed. Sometimes, long-term psychotherapy is required.

If treated promptly, most adolescents who have anorexia or bulimia make a full recovery. However, some continue to have eating problems throughout life. A very small number of those with anorexia die, often by suicide.

OVEREATING AND OBESITY

The main cause of obesity is probably a family pattern of overeating, although there may also be a genetic factor. To help your child lose weight, set a good example by eating healthfully yourself and encouraging him or her to do the same. Consult a doctor if there is no improvement within a few months.

What is the treatment?
Your child will be measured, weighed, and examined to exclude any physical disorders. The doctor will ask about your child's intake of food at mealtimes and between, and whether there are any emotional or behavioral problems. Treatment consists of a low-calorie diet; behavior therapy may be considered to help alter a child's eating patterns.

The earlier a child is given treatment, the better the outlook for establishing and maintaining a normal weight.

DEPRESSION

Most people feel sad sometimes. In true depression, however, there are intense feelings of hopelessness, lack of self-worth, and guilt that last longer two weeks. In children, depression most often affects teenagers and is an important cause of suicide.

What are the causes?
The reasons for depression are varied. Grief over the loss of a loved one may develop into depression. Some types of depression run in families, and there may also be a biochemical factor. Stress is sometimes an aggravating factor.

What are the symptoms?
A child who is depressed may:
- Look unhappy most of the time.
- Have frequent bouts of crying.
- Be irritable, listless, and inattentive.
- Complain of feeling anxious, bored, sad, or tired most of the time.
- Perform badly at school.
- Wake very early in the morning or sleep excessively.
- Lose weight or gain too much weight.
- Have headaches, or stomach pain and diarrhea, with no apparent cause.

What can I do to help?
You may be able to end a mild bout of depression by talking to your child and trying to identify the reason for his or her feelings. Offer emotional support and try to remove or limit any sources of anxiety. Taking up a sport or hobby, or mixing with others may also help.

Should I consult a doctor?
If the depression deepens or persists for more than a few weeks, or if grief over a bereavement has lasted for more than a few months, consult a doctor. Treatment may consist of psychotherapy or cognitive behavioral therapy, and/or, for severe cases, antidepressant drugs.

Most children improve soon after receiving treatment, although some remain depressed for several months before showing improvement. In a minority, depression recurs or persists and occasionally leads to suicide.

ANTISOCIAL BEHAVIOR

Behavior that has a negative impact on others or their property may be termed antisocial. Almost all children behave antisocially at some point; it is only when the behavior becomes persistent, recurrent, or extreme that it is a cause for concern.

What forms does it take?

Although characterized by aggression and disobedience at all ages, antisocial behavior tends to take different forms in different age groups.

Preschool children:
• Physical attacks on other children and/or on parents.
• Deliberately destroying objects.
• Temper tantrums.

Schoolchildren and adolescents:
• Bullying or fighting with others.
• Cruelty to other children or animals.
• Stealing and lying.
• Being disruptive in class.
• Truancy and vandalism (these occur mainly in adolescents).

What are the causes?

Antisocial behavior is often a reflection of an emotional problem, such as unhappiness at home or at school. Other causes include LEARNING DISABILITIES (p.172), oppositional defiant disorders, and conduct disorders. Aggression is usually learned by example, from parents, the media, or a peer group.

What can I do to help?

Provided that temper tantrums are ignored, they usually stop within a few months. With an aggressive child of any age, be consistent, firm, and loving. Talk with an older child or teenager to find out the causes of the behavior.

If antisocial behavior is persistent or severe, you should consult a doctor, who may refer you and your child to a child and family therapy center.

What is the outlook?

Antisocial behavior can be curtailed if dealt with before it is entrenched and forms a vicious cycle with low self-esteem. It is often outgrown after the age of 15 years. Children who have severe and prolonged behavioral problems may become antisocial adults.

SUBSTANCE ABUSE

The use of a drug or chemical to alter the way the mind works is termed substance abuse. It is rare before adolescence and more common in boys than girls. Substances most frequently abused are alcohol, tobacco, solvents (such as glue, lighter fluid, or paint thinner, which are inhaled), marijuana (cannabis), amphetamines ("speed," including Ecstasy), and LSD. Abuse of hard drugs, such as heroin or cocaine, does not usually occur in this age group.

What are the causes?

Children experiment with substances in order to have enjoyable, exciting, or new experiences, to "fit in" with their peer group, or to feel grown up. Some may use substances to relieve anxiety and depression caused by problems at school or at home. For a minority of children, the abused substance becomes the focal point of their life: a physical and/or psychological dependence on it develops. Dependence is more likely when a drug is used to relieve emotional problems.

Using solvents
Inhaling solvents is most common among younger teenagers. It can lead to brain, liver, and/or kidney damage.

How can I prevent it?

A child is less likely to drink too much if others in the family do not drink or drink only moderately. If people in the family do not smoke, your child is less likely to take up the habit.

Prohibition of drugs is not helpful. Discuss with your child the drugs he or she may be offered and explain honestly the harm that drugs can cause. Point out the legal risks that may be involved. Your child will almost certainly be less vulnerable to substance abuse if he or she has other interests to occupy his or her time. Spend time with your children so that they know and trust you.

What are the signs?

Alcohol use and cigarette smoking are usually easy to detect. It may be hard to tell if your child is abusing another substance unless he or she is doing so on a regular basis. Although different substances have different effects, there are some general changes in behavior that may indicate that your child is abusing a substance on a regular basis:
• Changes in sleeping patterns.
• General lack of energy or drowsiness.
• Unusual moodiness, irritability, or aggressiveness.
• Changes in appetite.
• Increased time spent away from home.
• Lies and secretiveness about activities.
• Dropping school grades.

What can I do to help?

If you think that your child is abusing a substance, do not overreact. Try to find out why the abuse has taken place so that you can give appropriate help. For example, if your child is taking drugs because of emotional problems, extra attention and support may give your child the self-confidence to stop.

Consult a doctor if you think your child may be becoming dependent on a drug. Advice on support and treatment is also available from many self-help groups, counseling centers, and hotlines.

What is the outlook?

Most children who abuse substances do so only occasionally, and after some experimentation, give them up entirely. Some, however, progress to hard drugs. A substance-dependent child can usually be helped provided that he or she has recognized the problem and positively wants help in giving up the habit.

MOUTH AND TEETH DISORDERS

YOUNG CHILDREN USE THEIR MOUTHS for exploring the world around them. Most of the body is protected by tough skin, but the mouth is more vulnerable: the tongue and lining of the mouth are exposed to infections and are damaged easily by chewing coarse food or other objects. Although a child's first teeth are replaced by permanent teeth, which begin to emerge around 6 years of age, both sets must be carefully taken care of to avoid tooth decay and gum problems.

MOUTH ULCERS

Ulcers, which are open sores, may develop on the lining of the mouth or the margins of the tongue. Aphthous ulcers are the most common type of mouth ulcer; they develop for no known reason and tend to recur. Although they may make your child's mouth painful, they are not serious and usually heal on their own. Mouth ulcers may also be due to minor injury – from a jagged tooth, for example – or, rarely, to an underlying disorder.

Appearance of an aphthous ulcer
An aphthous ulcer is seen here at the base of the gums of the lower jaw. It has a hollowed-out gray center, with a raised, paler rim. The area surrounding the ulcer is inflamed.

What are the symptoms?
A child with mouth ulcers may have the following symptoms:
- A single ulcer or a cluster of ulcers inside the cheeks or lips or on the margin of the tongue. Each ulcer has a gray center with a pale white or yellow rim and a red border.
- Painful, tender mouth, which may make your child reluctant to eat and to brush his or her teeth.

For 1 or 2 days before aphthous ulcers appear, there may be a sore or burning sensation of the lining of the mouth, the insides of the lips, or the tongue.

Most ulcers heal without treatment within 4 to 10 days. Mouth ulcers that are less than 2 mm in diameter heal quickly; other, larger mouth ulcers may take longer to heal.

What can I do to help?
Your child may find that rinsing out his or her mouth with a diluted solution of baking soda helps to relieve pain or tenderness. To make up the solution, dissolve ¼ teaspoon of baking soda in 3.5 fl. oz (100 ml) of warm water. Another means of relieving discomfort is to apply an anesthetic ointment or gel (available over the counter) to the ulcers. You may also give your child liquid acetaminophen to relieve pain.

Avoid offering food or drinks that are acidic, spicy, hot, or salty because they can irritate the ulcers. If chewing is very painful, offer your child soft foods or liquify his or her meals. Drinking through a straw may help because it prevents liquid from bathing the ulcers.

Should I consult a doctor?
If the ulcers are causing your child a great deal of pain, fail to heal within 10 days, or recur frequently, make an appointment to see a doctor. If an ulcer recurs in the same place, your child should be seen by a dentist because a sharp tooth may be the cause.

If you notice that your child is experiencing considerable pain, avoid feeding him or her acidic substances such as the fruit or juice of oranges, grapefruits, and lemons, tomatoes, and condiments containing vinegar. A mild anesthetic of xylocaine in a solution may be painted on the ulcers; this provides pain relief only, and has no effect on healing. Too much of the xylocaine solution acts as a sedative, and overuse may even cause seizures, so exercise caution in giving it to small children. If the sores are the result of an oral herpes infection, acyclovir solution, taken by mouth within 24 to 36 hours of the onset, may be effective in shortening the course of healing.

If the doctor thinks that your child's mouth ulcers point to the presence of an underlying disease, he or she may arrange for your child to undergo tests.

What is the outlook?
Attacks of aphthous ulcers are usually infrequent, minor, and short-lived, and cause little distress. In some children, attacks occur frequently or are severe. The outlook is unpredictable, but most children grow out of the problem.

ORAL THRUSH

A yeast infection of the mouth, oral thrush occurs most commonly in babies during the first year of life. The infection is caused by an abnormal growth of the yeast *Candida albicans*, which occurs naturally in the mouth.

Appearance of oral thrush
Here, oral thrush has caused raised, white spots to appear inside the mouth. They occur on the gums and soft palate, and merge to form a foamlike coating on the tongue.

How is it caused?
The amount of *Candida* in the mouth is usually small, but the balance between *Candida* and oral bacteria (which keep it in control) may be upset by a course of antibiotics or by general illness.

What are the symptoms?
The main symptoms of oral thrush are:
• A sore mouth, which may make your baby reluctant to feed.
• Creamy yellow or white spots on the tongue, gums, and lining of the mouth (see photograph at right).
Have a doctor see your child within a few days if you suspect oral thrush.

What is the treatment?
The doctor will examine your child and may send scrapings from the mouth for analysis. He or she may prescribe antifungal gel or drops to apply to the white patches on the inside of your baby's mouth. To help prevent reinfection, be meticulous when sterilizing baby bottles and nipples. If you are breast-feeding, the doctor may prescribe an antifungal cream to treat your nipples.

GINGIVOSTOMATITIS

This quite common illness causes painful ulcers to appear in the mouth. It results from a first infection by the herpes simplex virus, which also causes COLD SORES (p.139). Gingivostomatitis occurs most often in children between 6 months and 4 years old.

What are the symptoms?
Gingivostomatitis usually starts with a fever and sore mouth. Infants are often irritable, restless, and unwilling to eat or drink anything. The following more distinctive symptoms soon develop:
• Painful, shallow ulcers on the gums, tongue, and palate.
• Red swollen gums that bleed easily.
• Swelling of lymph nodes in the neck.
A child with these symptoms should be seen by a doctor within 24 hours.

What is the treatment?
If necessary, follow the advice given in the panel: *Relieving a sore mouth* (p.105). To prevent dehydration and provide energy, you should offer frequent, small drinks of cool milk, ice pops, or rehydrating solution (see panels: *Preventing dehydration in babies*, p.38, or *Preventing dehydration in children*, p.53).

The doctor may prescribe a course of the antiviral drug acyclovir. If the child is very sick or has been refusing fluids, he or she may be sent to the hospital so that acyclovir and rehydrating fluids can be given intravenously.

Without treatment for the infection, full recovery usually occurs in about 10 days. If given acyclovir within 3 days of the onset of severe symptoms, your child should recover more quickly.

GINGIVITIS

Inflammation of the gums is known as gingivitis. It may develop if a child does not clean his or her teeth and gums thoroughly. The condition is caused by the irritant effect of bacteria that live in plaque, a sticky deposit of food debris and saliva that collects on and around the teeth, and at the gum margins.

What are the symptoms?
The main symptoms of gingivitis are:
• Red, swollen, and tender gums.
• Tendency of the gums to bleed when they are brushed.
Gingivitis itself is a minor, reversible problem. However, if it is not checked, it may progress to a serious infection, with the risk that teeth may be lost. Your child should be seen by a dentist if you think he or she has gingivitis.

Signs of plaque
Disclosing agents reveal plaque. The stained areas show the places where plaque has accumulated.

What is the treatment?
If the gingivitis is mild, the dentist may just give your child instructions about how best to care for his or her teeth properly (see TOOTH DECAY, opposite, for advice on oral hygiene). For more advanced gingivitis, the dentist may also recommend that your child use an antibacterial mouthwash to relieve inflammation and tenderness. When the gums are less tender, the dentist may scale (scrape) the teeth to remove plaque and calculus (hardened plaque).

What is the outlook?
With good oral hygiene, your child's gums should return to normal in a few months. Continued attention to proper oral hygiene, with regular visits to the dentist for checkups and plaque removal, will help to prevent gingivitis from recurring.

TOOTH DECAY

Also known as dental caries, tooth decay was formerly the most common childhood disease. However, over the past 15 years, its prevalence and severity in children have greatly declined, mainly because of the addition of fluoride to water and toothpastes. This decline has now come to a halt, and in some areas, especially socially deprived ones, tooth decay is becoming more common again. Research has shown that the increase in tooth decay is due to the consumption of too much sugary food and drink.

Position yourself slightly behind your child

Tilt your child's head back

Brushing your child's teeth
Until the age of 6 or 7 years, most children cannot brush their teeth effectively. Using a pea-sized amount of toothpaste, gently scrub all surfaces of your child's teeth thoroughly.

Enamel

Decay

Dentin

Pulp

Tooth decay
A cavity forms when acids produced by the bacterial breakdown of food erode the tooth's hard outer surface of enamel. The softer layer of dentin beneath is exposed, and as it, too, is eroded, the cavity gradually enlarges.

How is it caused?
Tooth decay results from the action of the bacteria that live in plaque, a sticky coating of saliva and food debris that forms on the surface of the teeth. The bacteria use components of food and drinks (mainly sugars) for energy and, in breaking them down, produce acids. These acids, which are held in close contact with the teeth by plaque, cause calcium and phosphate to be lost from the tooth's enamel (demineralization). If this process continues unchecked, the enamel and eventually the dentin beneath is destroyed (see illustration above). If tooth decay is not treated at this stage, the pulp at the center of the tooth may become infected, resulting in permanent damage to the nerves and blood vessels that it contains.

What are the symptoms?
Early tooth decay does not usually cause any symptoms. The main symptoms of established decay are:
• Sensitivity of the tooth to hot, cold, and/or sweet foods or liquids.
• In very advanced decay, the tooth may be brown, have visible pits or holes in the enamel surface, and may also be very painful.

Should my child see a dentist?
Your child should be visiting a dentist every 6 months so that tooth decay can be detected at an early stage. However, if any symptoms of tooth decay develop between regular checkups, you should make an appointment for your child to see a dentist within a few days.

What might the dentist do?
The dentist will examine your child's teeth and may also take X rays. If the dentist finds signs of early decay, he or she may just clean the teeth and scrape them to remove plaque. This treatment allows the surface of the teeth to come into contact with saliva, which has a natural ability to remineralize enamel. A fluoride gel may also be applied.

For more advanced decay, the dentist may remove the decayed portion of the tooth, using a drill, and then insert a filling. If the nerve of the tooth has been irreversibly damaged or destroyed by infection, it may need to be removed. The entire tooth may need to be taken out if tooth decay is very advanced.

How can I prevent tooth decay?
A diet low in sugar, good oral hygiene, and regular visits to the dentist are the keys to preventing tooth decay.

The amount of sweet food and drink that your child has, and the frequency with which he or she consumes them, should be limited. Discourage sugary snacks and drinks between meals. Your child should avoid having acidic food and drinks, including fruit juice and all carbonated drinks (diet and regular), frequently; ideally, he or she should have them only with a meal. Fruit juice should be diluted to half strength with water and drunk through a straw (as should carbonated drinks). Do not give a baby sweet drinks in a bottle; the liquid will bathe the teeth and lead to rapid decay. Ask the dentist whether your water supply is fluoridated, and if fluoride treatment is advisable for your child.

Your child's teeth should be brushed twice a day with a fluoride toothpaste, after breakfast and especially right before bedtime. If brushing after a meal is not convenient, it is a good idea to chew sugar-free gum, which stimulates the flow of saliva. Saliva neutralizes acid and helps to remineralize tooth enamel.

From the age of about 2½ years, your child should visit a dentist regularly for checkups as often as the dentist advises, usually once every 6 months.

Visiting the dentist
At your child's routine dental examination, the dentist will examine the teeth for signs of tooth decay. X rays may also be taken to detect areas of decay that may be hidden in the crevices of the teeth's biting surfaces.

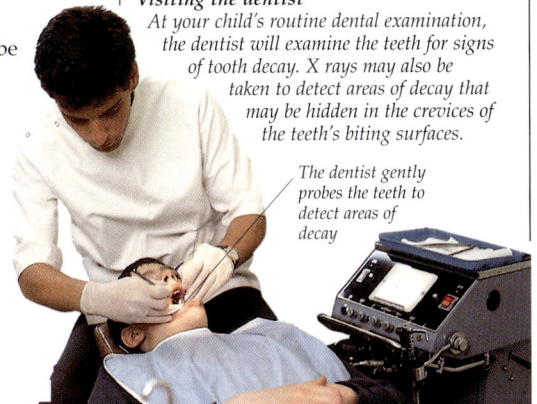

The dentist gently probes the teeth to detect areas of decay

DENTAL ABSCESS

A dental abscess is a collection of pus around the root of a tooth. An abscess results when the pulp (the tooth's sensitive core, containing nerves and blood vessels) is invaded and destroyed by bacteria. Bacteria can enter the pulp cavity only if the tooth has been badly damaged or has become severely decayed.

What are the symptoms?
The main symptoms of an abscess are:
- A persistent and throbbing toothache.
- Severe pain in the tooth when biting or chewing on it, or when consuming hot foods or liquids.
- Tenderness, redness, and swelling of the gum around the affected tooth.
- Occasionally, a discharge of foul-tasting pus through an opening in the gum, after which the pain tends to subside.
- Looseness of the affected tooth.

Swelling caused by a dental abscess
Infection that has spread from a dental abscess has caused the right side of this girl's face to swell. There is usually little pain at this stage.

If the infection spreads into surrounding tissue, the face and lymph glands in the neck may swell. Eventually, the child might develop symptoms of general infection, such as fever and headache.

Should my child see a dentist?
You should take your child to see a dentist within a few hours of any of the symptoms appearing.

If possible, the dentist will try to save the affected tooth. He or she will drill into your child's tooth to release the pus and relieve the pressure. The dead and dying pulp is removed, and the cavity washed, dried, and filled, a procedure known as root canal treatment. The dentist may extract the tooth if it is severely affected or if it is a primary ("baby") tooth. A course of antibiotics may be prescribed to clear up any remaining infection.

What can I do to help?
To relieve the pain while waiting to see the dentist, you may give your child liquid acetaminophen. A well-wrapped hot water bottle held against the affected side of the face may also provide relief.

How can I prevent a dental abscess?
The tooth decay that sometimes results in a dental abscess can be prevented by good oral hygiene (see TOOTH DECAY, p.177), sensible eating habits (such as avoiding sweet foods), and by regular visits to the dentist every 6 months.

What is the outlook?
After root canal treatment, a tooth usually functions as well as a healthy tooth. If a tooth has been removed, the other teeth often move into the space.

MALOCCLUSION

A poor fit between the upper and lower teeth when they bite together is called malocclusion. Treatment is necessary only if the teeth are so crooked or out of position that they look ugly or are difficult to clean, which increases the risk of tooth decay (see TOOTH DECAY, p.177) or gum problems (see GINGIVITIS, p.176).

How is it caused?
Malocclusion is most commonly caused by overcrowding of teeth. About two out of three 12-year-old children have overcrowded teeth. The condition is usually inherited and appears as the child's jaws and teeth develop. It may also occur when primary ("baby") teeth are lost early, because of either decay or injury. Early loss of this kind may lead to the remaining teeth moving into the gaps so that there is insufficient room for the permanent teeth. Teeth that are overcrowded may grow to be crooked, overlapping, or too prominent.

Another less common, inherited cause of malocclusion is misalignment of the jaws so that the upper or lower set of teeth is too far forward or too far back.

Should my child see a dentist?
Regular 6-monthly visits to the dentist will allow the growth of the teeth and jaws to be monitored. However, if you are worried about your child's teeth or if your child is concerned about his or her appearance, make an appointment with the dentist as soon as possible. The dentist may recommend waiting to see if the malocclusion corrects itself as the jaws grow. If treatment is needed, your child will be referred to an orthodontist.

What is the treatment?
Orthodontic treatment is usually done at 11 to 13 years of age. If the teeth are overcrowded, the orthodontist may remove some of them and/or fit an orthodontic appliance (braces). Braces may be fixed (see photograph below) or removable. The braces exert pressure on the teeth to move them into the right position. In another type of treatment, a device called a bioblock, which the child bites into, is used to guide the growth of the jaws. Orthodontic treatment may take up to 2 years. Misalignment of the jaws may be corrected by surgery.

Fixed braces
This type of appliance is used most often to correct malocclusion. Brackets are cemented to the teeth; flexible wires are attached to the brackets and exert pressure to move the teeth.

DIGESTIVE SYSTEM DISORDERS

PROBLEMS AFFECTING THE digestive system are second only to colds and sore throats in frequency as causes of illness in childhood. Infections of the digestive system resulting in diarrhea and/or vomiting are especially common. Although these symptoms may be upsetting for parent and child, they are rarely persistent enough to be a threat to health. Other digestive disorders are less common, but some may cause chronic illness that can affect growth if not treated.

APPENDICITIS

The appendix is a small, worm-shaped tube that branches off the first part of the large intestine. It has no known function, yet for no apparent reason, it sometimes becomes infected and inflamed (appendicitis). Appendicitis is a common cause of abdominal pain requiring surgery in children under 16 years old.

What are the symptoms?
The main symptoms are:
- A dull pain in the lower abdomen (see illustration below). Slight pressure on the painful area, movement, or deep breathing increase the pain, and a child with appendicitis often lies still.
- Nausea, which may or may not be accompanied by vomiting.
- Fever.
- Constipation or diarrhea.

Should I consult a doctor?
If the pain is so severe that it makes your child cry out or if the pain continues for 3 hours, phone a doctor at once. Call an ambulance or take your child to a hospital emergency room if the pain has been continuous for more than 6 hours. If appendicitis is not treated promptly, the appendix may perforate (burst). Pus is then able to pass into the abdominal cavity, causing infection, and leading to a potentially fatal condition called peritonitis (inflammation of the lining of the abdominal cavity). If the appendix bursts, the pain affects the whole abdomen and is present continuously.

Pain of appendicitis
Abdominal pain usually begins around the navel. The pain gradually becomes more severe and migrates to the lower right-hand side of the abdomen during the next few hours. In some children, the pain is in the lower right abdomen from the beginning.

Usual first site of pain

Usual site of pain after a few hours

What can I do to help?
When an episode of abdominal pain occurs, it may be difficult to know at first whether it could be a serious problem. A hot water bottle wrapped in a towel may be held against the site of the pain. Do not give your child acetaminophen or other painkillers because they may make the diagnosis more difficult for the doctor. The child should not eat or drink anything in case an operation may be necessary.

What might the doctor do?
The doctor will examine your child. If appendicitis is suspected, your child will be admitted to the hospital. If further examinations, such as a CT scan, indicate that appendicitis is likely, an operation to remove the appendix will be performed.

Your child may be given painkillers for about 24 hours after the operation. If the appendix did not burst, your child should be able to go home after 3 to 4 days. If the appendix did burst, your child will be given antibiotics and will need to stay in the hospital until the infection has cleared up, which can take about 7 days.

After leaving the hospital your child will be able to eat a normal diet. Strenuous physical activities should, however, be avoided for about a month.

GASTROENTERITIS

Attacks of gastroenteritis (inflammation of the stomach and intestines), causing diarrhea and/or vomiting, are common in children. Although gastroenteritis is usually a mild illness, it can be serious, especially in infants. The most common cause of the illness in children is infection with viruses that are transmitted through the air or by contact with infected feces. Bacteria transmitted in food or drinks may also cause gastroenteritis.

Rehydrating solution
To prevent your child from becoming dehydrated, offer him or her a rehydrating solution such as Rehydralyte. Alternatively, give your child a sports drink or any other clear liquid.

Micrograph of rotaviruses
A group of spherical viruses, rotaviruses are responsible for most cases of gastroenteritis in children under 2 years of age.

What are the symptoms?
Some or all of the following symptoms appear 1 to 5 days after infection:
• Diarrhea.
• Vomiting.
• Loss of appetite.
• Abdominal pain.
• Lack of energy.
• Fever.

What are the complications?
Dehydration due to diarrhea and/or vomiting is a serious complication of gastroenteritis. Young babies are at the greatest risk of becoming dehydrated.

Should I consult a doctor?
Phone a doctor at once if your child is under 2 months old and you suspect gastroenteritis. You should also phone a doctor at once if your infant or child has any symptoms of dehydration (see *Danger signs*, pp.38 or 52). In other cases, you may try self-help treatment (see "What can I do to help?"). If the gastroenteritis has not improved after 24 hours, you should phone a doctor, even if the symptoms are mild.

What can I do to help?
To replace fluids lost through vomiting and/or diarrhea, it is vital to give a child drinks of rehydration fluid (see panel: *Preventing dehydration in babies*, p.38 or *Preventing dehydration in children*, p.53 for quantities to give).

If your baby is entirely breast-fed, give the rehydrating solution first and then breast-feed. If the symptoms subside, gradually reduce the amount of solution over a period of 5 days.

For how to treat bottle-fed babies and older children, see the table below. For an infant who already eats solid food, follow the instructions given in the table for a bottle-fed baby. In addition,

give no solids on Day 1. From Day 2 to Day 4, give a gradually increasing amount of rice and puréed vegetables and fruit, followed by a light diet. The early introduction of solids and milk speeds up recovery from gastroenteritis.

What might the doctor do?
The doctor will examine your child and decide whether treatment at the hospital or at home is needed. If your child is to be treated at home, you will be advised about how to care for him or her.

In the hospital, your child may need to have blood tests to determine how severe the dehydration is. Rehydrating solution may be given intravenously and he or she may not be allowed to eat or drink for 24 hours. Rehydrating solution will then be given orally and ordinary food will soon be reintroduced.

How can I prevent gastroenteritis?
Your child cannot be prevented from becoming infected with the viruses that cause gastroenteritis. However, after infection your child will be immune to the particular virus that caused it.

The spread of gastroenteritis due to bacterial infections is prevented more easily. For example, avoid keeping turtles and other reptilian pets (they may carry *Salmonella* bacteria), sterilize a baby's eating utensils and pacifiers, be sure family members are scrupulous about personal hygiene, and always store food at the correct temperatures. To reduce the risk of infection with *Salmonella*, hardboil eggs for 6 minutes and make sure chicken is well cooked.

An infected child will be infectious to others until the stool returns to normal and may continue to be so for several weeks. Be very careful about personal hygiene; wash hands meticulously.

TREATING BOTTLE-FED BABIES		TREATING OLDER CHILDREN	
DAY 1	Feed 2 to 3 teaspoons of rice and rehydrating solution at regular intervals.	DAY 1	Instead of milk, give your child rehydrating solution; alternatively, give unsweetened clear fluids.
DAY 2	Add small amounts of bananas and toast and offer rehydrating solution throughout the day.	DAY 2	You may add rice, vegetables, and unsweetened fruit purée to your child's diet.
DAY 3	Add apple sauce; give clear liquids and offer 2 to 3 tablespoons of foods throughout the day.	DAY 3	You may add chicken and/or soups to your child's diet. You may also reintroduce milk.
		DAY 4	You may add bread, biscuits, eggs, meat and/or fish to your child's diet.
		DAY 5	Your child should have recovered completely and may return to his or her normal diet.

Treating gastroenteritis in babies
The diet of bananas, rice, cereal, apple sauce, and toast, given to bottle-fed babies who eat solid food, is called the BRAT diet. You should consult your doctor about reintroducing milk or formula. In some circumstances, you can do this on Day 1.

TODDLER'S DIARRHEA

Children between the ages of 1 and 3 years may be affected by toddler's diarrhea. With this form of diarrhea, a child who is healthy passes watery stools that often contain recognizable pieces of food, such as raisins, carrots, peas, or beans.

How is it caused?
The cause of toddler's diarrhea is not certain, but the problem may be due to insufficient chewing of food.

What are the symptoms?
Apart from passing watery stool with pieces of food in it, your child will probably feel well. A persistent DIAPER RASH (p.136) may be a problem.

Should I consult a doctor?
Although toddler's diarrhea is not a cause for concern, your child should be seen by a doctor to make sure that the condition is not the result of an infection or another disorder. The doctor will check whether your child's growth is normal by measuring his or her height and weight. Toddler's diarrhea does not affect growth, so failure to grow usually suggests another disorder. As a precaution, the doctor may send out a stool sample for laboratory analysis.

What can I do to help?
No treatment is necessary, and dietary restrictions do not have any effect on the condition. It may help, however, if you mash or purée the foods that your child has difficulty chewing and digesting. A lactose-free milk may help.

What is the outlook?
Your child will grow out of toddler's diarrhea by 3 years of age and will not suffer any lasting adverse effects.

CONSTIPATION

A child who is constipated passes hard, dry stool infrequently. Infrequent defecation by itself does not indicate constipation since children differ in their bowel habits: the normal frequency for passing stool may vary from four times a day to once every 4 days. Constipation is usually short-lived but sometimes persists.

How is it caused?
Temporary constipation is commonly caused by dehydration that results from illness involving vomiting and fever. Some medicines may also have a dehydrating effect. From 1 to 2 years of age, the changes that are made in a child's diet (for example, from formula or breast milk to cow's milk) may cause constipation. Insufficient fiber in the diet is the most common cause of constipation in older children.

A child's constipation may become chronic if a painful anal fissure (see illustration above right) develops as a result of passing hard stool. Chronic constipation can also develop if a child deliberately withholds stool during toilet-training (which is most likely if training is started too early) or because he or she has emotional problems.

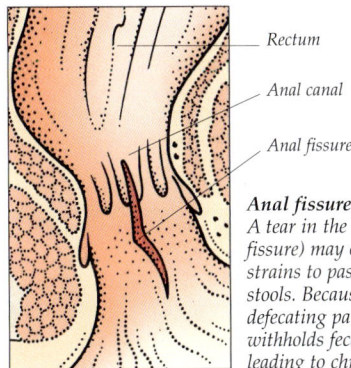

Rectum

Anal canal

Anal fissure

Anal fissure
A tear in the anal canal (anal fissure) may occur if a child strains to pass large, hard, stools. Because the tear makes defecating painful, the child withholds feces deliberately, leading to chronic constipation.

What are the symptoms?
The symptoms of constipation include:
• Infrequent defecation.
• Pain on defecation.
• Hard, dry stool.

In chronic constipation, there may be:
• Liquid stool trickling from the anus, which may soil underwear.
• Pain on trying to defecate.
• Loss of appetite.
• Blood in the stool.

What can I do to help?
Constipation can usually be alleviated and prevented by giving your child plenty of fluids and (if the child is 6 months old or more) more fiber in the form of fruit and vegetables. Wholegrain cereals are another source of fiber. If constipation is a problem, a child should not drink more than 2 cups (500 ml) of milk a day: milk aggravates the problem.

Your child should be seen by a doctor if constipation lasts for more than a week, if there is pain on defecation, or if you suspect chronic constipation.

What might the doctor do?
After examining your child, the doctor will ask about his or her diet and any recent illnesses. Usually, dietary advice (see "What can I do to help?") is all that is required.

Your doctor will confirm a diagnosis of chronic constipation by feeling the child's abdomen; he or she may also do a rectal examination. Your child will be put on a high-fiber diet with plenty of fluids, and laxatives and stool softeners will be prescribed. You will be asked to have your child sit on the toilet at the same time each day to reestablish regular bowel habits. After about 3 months, when regular bowel habits are regained, the drug dose is gradually reduced. No local treatment is needed for an anal fissure; the softened stool produced by laxatives allows it to heal on its own, usually within 6 weeks.

If the cause of the constipation is not clear and dietary advice and medicines do not relieve it, your child may be sent to a pediatrician or a child psychiatrist to look further for causes.

What is the outlook?
Temporary or chronic constipation in childhood does not increase the risk of bowel problems later in life.

REACTIONS TO FOOD

Certain foods can cause an adverse reaction. Some children may experience food intolerance, a digestive disorder that has some of the same symptoms as food allergies but a different cause. A child with food allergies (see ALLERGIES, p.152) has a reaction to food due to an inappropriate response by the immune system. Children who are thought to have the disorder should be seen by a doctor; a baby should be seen within 24 hours of the onset of symptoms.

COW'S MILK PROTEIN ALLERGY

Cow's milk protein is the most common cause of an adverse reaction to food. The problem initially appears in the first year of life, between a week and several months after starting cow's milk formula. The allergy usually disappears by the age of 3 years. The cause is unknown.

Milk substitutes
Children under 1 year who are allergic to cow's milk protein may be given a soy-based formula or a milk substitute, made by breaking down cow's milk protein into smaller, more easily absorbed components.

What are the symptoms?
Symptoms develop soon after drinking milk and include:
• Diarrhea.
• Vomiting.
• Wheezing.
• Rarely, ANAPHYLACTIC SHOCK (p.154).
• Dry skin patches.

What might the doctor do?
If cow's milk protein allergy is suspected, your doctor will recommend that all products containing cow's milk be avoided for 2 weeks. If your child's symptoms disappear, a small amount of cow's milk will be given under medical supervision. The diagnosis is confirmed if symptoms recur.

What can I do to help?
Under the supervision of a dietitian, your child will follow a diet free of products containing cow's milk. Children under 1 year may need a milk substitute. The cow's milk trial will be repeated every 3 months, until your child no longer has an adverse reaction to the protein. The amount of milk given can then be increased gradually.

LACTOSE AND SUCROSE INTOLERANCE

Children can be intolerant of the sugar lactose (found in milk) or of sucrose (a sugar present in many fruits). They may also be intolerant to other foods.

How is it caused?
Intolerance occurs when there is a deficiency of the enzyme that breaks down lactose or sucrose in the small intestine. Both lactose and sucrose intolerance may develop as a result of an infection (see GASTROENTERITIS, p.180) or another intestinal disorder, such as CELIAC DISEASE (p.183), and are usually temporary. Some children with an allergy to cow's milk protein are also lactose intolerant.

Permanent lactose intolerance of genetic origin is common in people of African or Asian descent. Children up to the age of 2 or 3 years tolerate an unlimited amount of milk, but when older suffer from diarrhea after ingesting only a small amount.

Sucrose intolerance also occurs occasionally as an inherited, permanent disorder.

What are the symptoms?
Symptoms appear within 6 hours of drinking milk or eating foods containing lactose or sucrose and may include:
• Diarrhea and abdominal pain.
• Vomiting.

What might the doctor do?
The child is given a test dose of lactose or sucrose in water. The stool is then examined to see if an excessive amount of the sugar has passed through the intestines without being absorbed.

If your child is intolerant of lactose, a dietitian can design a lactose-free diet. Lactose-free milk and fermented milk products, such as yogurt, may be tolerated. A sucrose-free diet is used to treat sucrose intolerance.

SPECIFIC FOOD ALLERGIES

The foods, apart from milk, to which allergies most frequently occur in children are shown in the illustrations below. The reason why an allergy to a specific food occurs is not known.

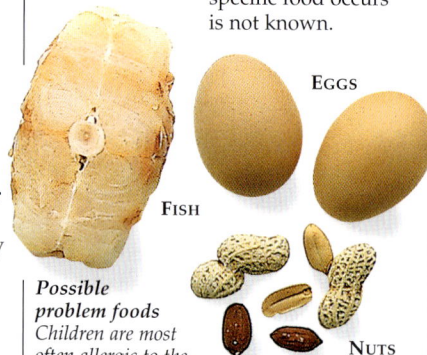

EGGS

FISH

NUTS

Possible problem foods
Children are most often allergic to the foods illustrated here. Sometimes a child can tolerate a food when it is cooked, but not raw.

What are the symptoms?
Symptoms, which appear soon after a particular food is eaten, may include:
• Rashes, including HIVES (p.138).
• Swelling of the lips and mouth.
• Diarrhea and abdominal pain.
• Vomiting.
• Breathing difficulties.

What might the doctor do?
The doctor will examine your child and may carry out tests to exclude other causes. A dairy-free diet may be tried to rule out allergy to cow's milk protein or intolerance to lactose. If symptoms continue, one of two methods may be used to find out if your child is allergic to another specific food.

One method involves comparing symptoms when the suspected food is included or excluded from the diet. In another method, the child is given a "few foods" diet, consisting of specific foods known to be unlikely to induce symptoms. Within 2 weeks, symptoms usually stop. One new food is given every 3 days until symptoms occur or the diet has returned to normal.

The doctor may prescribe an Epi-Pen.

What is the outlook?
In many children, no specific cause can be found and the problem often clears up with a "few foods" diet. In others, the symptoms disappear with the exclusion of one to three foods. Most children outgrow reactions to food.

CELIAC DISEASE

This rare but serious disease is caused by a sensitivity of the small intestine to a protein (gluten) present in the cereals wheat, rye, barley, and oats. Eventually, the lining of the small intestine becomes abnormal (which is reversible). As a result, absorption of food is impaired, a condition known as MALABSORPTION (below).

Fingerlike villi   *Flattened villi*

NORMAL   ABNORMAL

Damage to the small intestine
The lining of the small intestine has millions of fingerlike projections, called villi, which absorb nutrients. In celiac disease, the villi become flattened and absorption is impaired.

What are the symptoms?
Symptoms occur a few months after a baby starts on solids. They may include:
• Weight loss or failure to gain weight.
• Very pale, floating stool that has an unpleasant smell.
• Pale skin, breathlessness, and lack of energy due to ANEMIA (p.145).

Foods containing wheat, such as bread, breakfast cereals, and crackers, are most likely to cause symptoms.

Should I consult a doctor?
Symptoms usually develop gradually, so your baby is not likely to get sick suddenly. However, if your child has any of the symptoms listed above, he or she should be seen by a doctor.

What might the doctor do?
The doctor will check to see whether your baby's weight is less than would be expected for his or her age and birth weight. Blood tests to look for anemia and antibodies to gluten may then be done. If these tests indicate that celiac disease is likely, your child may be sent to the hospital for a biopsy of the lining of the small intestine. A biopsy involves removal of a minute sample of tissue for analysis. If the biopsy shows changes in the intestinal lining (see micrographs above left), the diagnosis of celiac disease is confirmed.

What can I do to help?
Keeping to a diet free of gluten is the most important factor for the health of a child affected by celiac disease. Many specially produced substitute foods are available, including gluten-free bread, crackers, flour, and pasta. Other foods, such as dairy products, eggs, meat, fish, vegetables, fruit, rice, and corn, can be eaten as normal. You should make sure that everyone concerned with the care of your child knows that he or she can eat only certain foods.

As your son or daughter grows up and becomes increasingly independent, you will need to make sure he or she is aware of the importance of sticking to the diet. Children vary in how they react to renewed exposure to gluten, and you will soon learn how much gluten is likely to cause a reaction and how severe the reaction might be.

The symptoms of celiac disease will clear up within a few weeks of your child starting a gluten-free diet, and he or she should begin to put on weight.

What is the outlook?
Your child will remain in good health and grow as expected, provided that he or she sticks to a gluten-free diet. Your child will, however, have to adhere to a gluten-free diet throughout life.

MALABSORPTION

Failure of the small intestine to adequately absorb nutrients from food is termed malabsorption. The disorder is always associated with an underlying condition, such as CELIAC DISEASE (above), Crohn's disease (see INFLAMMATORY BOWEL DISEASE, p.184), CYSTIC FIBROSIS (p.201), or REACTIONS TO FOOD (opposite).

How is it caused?
Malabsorption sometimes results from damage to the intestinal lining, which interferes with the intestine's ability to absorb nutrients. It may also be due to a deficiency of digestive enzymes, which prevents the breakdown of food into units small enough to be absorbed.

What are the symptoms?
The main symptoms are:
• Very pale, floating stool that has an unpleasant smell.
• Weight loss or failure to gain weight.
• Listlessness.

In severe cases, malabsorption results in vitamin and mineral deficiencies. These deficiencies may, in turn, lead to malnutrition and ANEMIA (p.145).

Your child should be seen by a doctor if there are symptoms indicating that he or she might have malabsorption.

What might the doctor do?
Your child will be examined and his or her weight checked. Tests may then be carried out to determine the underlying cause of malabsorption. The doctor may ask a dietitian to assess whether your child's intake of food is adequate.

Malabsorption is treated by attention to the underlying cause and also by modifying or supplementing the diet, which in most cases will ensure that your child grows and gains weight normally. Your child may, however, need to stay on a special diet for life.

Checking weight
Malabsorption is a possible reason for a child's failing to put on weight normally.

INFLAMMATORY BOWEL DISEASE

The term inflammatory bowel disease includes Crohn's disease and ulcerative colitis, both of which cause chronic inflammation of the intestine. Ulcerative colitis and Crohn's disease are rare under the age of 7 years and are more common in adolescents. The causes are unknown, but the diseases tend to run in families.

CROHN'S DISEASE

Once a rare disorder, Crohn's disease is becoming more common. Although it can cause inflammation of any part of the digestive tract, the condition most often affects only the last section of the small intestine (the ileum). As a result of chronic inflammation, the intestinal wall becomes extremely thick, and deep, penetrating ulcers may form. Crohn's disease reduces the ability of the small intestine to absorb nutrients from food (see MALABSORPTION, p.183).

What are the symptoms?

The symptoms of Crohn's disease often develop gradually and consist of:
• Diarrhea. Occasionally, the stool contains blood, pus, or mucus if the colon is affected.
• Spasms of abdominal pain.
• Fever.
• Nausea.
• Poor growth and/or delayed puberty.
• Loss of weight and reduced appetite.
• Sometimes, ulceration of the anus.

What are the complications?

Thickening of the intestinal wall may narrow the inside of the intestine to such an extent that the bowel becomes obstructed (see INTESTINAL OBSTRUCTION, opposite). Complications in other parts of the body may include arthritis and inflammation of the eye (see IRITIS, p.164).

Should I consult a doctor?

Your child should be seen by a doctor if symptoms persist for more than a few days. Crohn's disease is less likely to be the cause of the symptoms than some other disorder, such as intestinal infection. However, if Crohn's disease is suspected, diagnostic tests, which may include barium X ray, endoscopic examinations, and biopsy of the intestines, will likely be performed in the hospital to look for evidence of the disease.

What is the treatment?

If your child has Crohn's disease, anti-inflammatory drugs may be prescribed. As an alternative to drugs, your child may be given a liquid diet containing proteins that have been broken down into smaller components, making absorption easier.

In severe cases, and if your child is badly malnourished, he or she may receive drugs and nutrients intravenously. A blood transfusion may also be needed. If the condition does not improve with medical treatment or if complications occur, damaged parts of the intestine may need surgical removal.

What is the outlook?

Crohn's disease is a long-term condition, and some children continue to suffer from flare-ups of the disease for many years; the symptoms may recur at intervals of a few months or a few years. For others, Crohn's disease may subside after only one or two flare-ups.

ULCERATIVE COLITIS

In this condition, the colon and rectum become inflamed and ulcerated. The initial attack of ulcerative colitis is often the worst, and then the symptoms may fluctuate over a long period of time.

What are the symptoms?

Bloody diarrhea is the main symptom. It may be accompanied by:
• Abdominal pain and tenderness.
• A feeling of fullness in the bowel.
• Fever.
• Nausea.
• Loss of appetite.
• Poor growth.
• Weight loss.

Ulcerated lining of colon

Diseased colon

Ulcerative colitis
In the barium X ray (at left), areas affected by disease are distinguished by loss of the folds found in a healthy colon. In the endoscopic view (above), ulcerated areas of the lining of the colon are seen as whitish patches.

Repeated blood loss may cause ANEMIA (p.145). Another possible complication is an abnormally enlarged colon, which may become life threatening.

Should I consult a doctor?

Your child should be seen by a doctor within 24 hours if he or she has bloody diarrhea and abdominal pain. Bacterial infection is the most common cause of these symptoms; but, if ulcerative colitis is suspected, tests like those for Crohn's disease may be done.

What is the treatment?

Anti-inflammatory drugs may have to be taken indefinitely. If drugs do not control the symptoms, or if the colon is badly damaged, the affected part may be removed surgically. If a large part is removed, your child may be left with an ileostomy (an opening through the abdominal wall for elimination of stool).

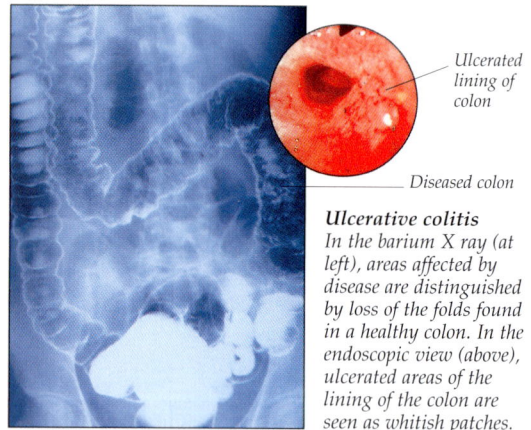

Ulcerated lining of small intestine

Narrowed area

Crohn's disease
The barium X ray (at right) shows narrowing of the last part of the small intestine due to Crohn's disease. The endoscopic view (above) reveals a thickened lining punctuated with ulcers, which appear as yellow or whitish patches.

IRRITABLE BOWEL SYNDROME

An uncommon disorder in children, irritable bowel syndrome consists of recurrent bouts of abdominal pain accompanied by either diarrhea or constipation and often both. The condition may be triggered by anxiety or, in some cases, an allergy to a specific food, such as cow's milk protein, nuts, or eggs.

What are the symptoms?
The main symptoms are:
- Abdominal pain, which is relieved by a bowel movement or passing gas.
- A persistent sense of fullness and distension of the bowel.
- Gas and diarrhea or constipation, or bouts of diarrhea alternating with periods of constipation.
- Sometimes nausea, headache, and general lack of energy.

Your child should be seen by a doctor if you think that he or she could have irritable bowel syndrome.

What is the treatment?
The diagnosis is usually made on the basis of the symptoms and a physical examination. Sometimes investigations are carried out in the hospital to exclude another disorder, such as GIARDIASIS (p.187), REACTIONS TO FOOD (p.182), or INFLAMMATORY BOWEL DISEASE (opposite). A high-fiber diet is helpful in many cases, especially if constipation is the predominant symptom. Certain foods may make the symptoms worse, and you may find it helpful to keep a diary of your child's diet so that the problem foods can be identified and avoided. Stress sometimes increases the severity of symptoms. Try to identify situations that make your child feel anxious, and if they cannot be avoided, give your child additional support.

What is the outlook?
Irritable bowel syndrome is a condition that often persists, and symptoms may recur periodically throughout life.

INTESTINAL OBSTRUCTION

A partial or complete blockage of the small or large intestine is known as an intestinal obstruction. The passage of food through the intestine is blocked, which results in abdominal cramps. Treatment is usually needed for intestinal obstruction. Complete obstruction of the intestine may be fatal without treatment.

How is it caused?
In children under 2 years, obstruction is most often due to a disorder called intussusception (see illustration at right). However, a blocked intestine in infants may be due to a strangulated HERNIA (p.187) or to a congenital abnormality of the intestine. Other possible causes of intestinal obstruction in children of any age include Crohn's disease (see INFLAMMATORY BOWEL DISEASE, opposite) and volvulus (twisting) of the intestine.

What are the symptoms?
The symptoms may include:
- Intermittent attacks of severe pain in the abdomen.
- Vomiting, which may produce greenish yellow fluid and occur at increasingly frequent intervals.
- Gas and failure to pass stool. In partial obstruction, passing gas and defecating usually bring temporary relief from pain.
- Bloodstained, jellylike mucus in the stool, in cases of intussusception.
- Fever and swelling of the abdomen, if treatment is delayed.

There is a chance that the blocked part of the intestine may rupture, leading to

Intussusception
A condition in which part of the intestine telescopes in on itself, intussusception tends to occur in the area where the large and small intestines meet.

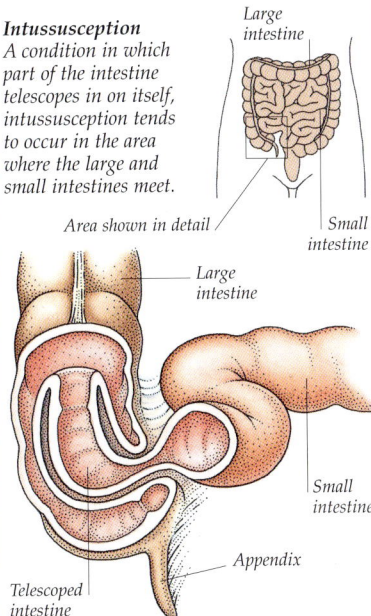

Large intestine

Area shown in detail

Small intestine

Large intestine

Small intestine

Appendix

Telescoped intestine

peritonitis (inflammation of the lining of the abdominal cavity), or that it may die and become gangrenous, which is a potentially fatal complication. Another serious complication that may develop as a result of frequent vomiting attacks is dehydration (see *Danger signs*, p.38, for signs of dehydration).

Should I consult a doctor?
Call an ambulance or take your child to to the nearest hospital emergency room if you think that he or she might have an intestinal obstruction. A doctor will examine your child, and fluids may be given intravenously to prevent dehydration. To confirm the diagnosis and to find out the cause of the obstruction, an X-ray examination may be performed. If intussusception is suspected, a special X-ray examination that involves the use of an air or a barium enema may be carried out. Pressure exerted by the enema often forces the displaced intestinal tissue back into the correct position. If the enema does not resolve the problem, an operation is necessary. Other types of intestinal obstruction require surgery, which sometimes involves removing the obstructed part of the intestine.

What is the outlook?
Normal growth and development occur once the obstruction has been treated, even if only a short section of bowel has been surgically removed. However, if the intestinal obstruction was due to an underlying condition (such as Crohn's disease), the blockage may recur unless the disorder that caused it is effectively treated.

GASTROESOPHAGEAL REFLUX

Gastroesophageal reflux is a common problem in the first year of life, usually starting a few weeks after birth. The contents of the baby's stomach pass back into the esophagus because the muscle at the entrance to the stomach is weak. In most cases, gastroesophageal reflux is a temporary problem.

What are the symptoms?

The main symptoms of reflux are:
- Persistent vomiting; the vomit may be bloodstained.
- Regurgitation of feedings, which may dribble continuously from the mouth.
- A cough, if regurgitated milk or formula is breathed into the lungs.
- Crying and irritability.
- Failure to gain weight, if the reflux is prolonged and severe.

Phone a doctor at once if your baby's vomit is bloodstained. Otherwise, you should make an appointment for your baby to be seen by a doctor.

What might the doctor do?

The doctor will examine your baby. In addition, he or she may send samples of urine and blood for testing so that any other cause of the vomiting, such as GASTROENTERITIS (p.180) or PYLORIC STENOSIS (below), may be ruled out.

What is the treatment?

Altering your baby's normal sleeping position may help to reduce reflux (see illustration right). If he or she is old enough, your child should also spend more time sitting in a baby chair. If the symptoms of reflux are severe, make your baby's formula thicker with rice cereal. If your baby is eating solids, you should reduce the amount of liquid in his or her diet and introduce more solids. You should try to avoid giving your child anything to drink without offering solids as well.

If your baby continues to be irritable and persistently cries despite self-help treatment, the doctor will probably refer him or her to a pediatrician who may prescribe a drug that reduces the amount of acid in the stomach. Most babies outgrow gastroesophageal reflux by the age of 1 year whether or not they receive treatment.

Treating gastroesophageal reflux
Your baby should sleep on his or her side with the head higher than the feet. This position will help to reduce gastroesophageal reflux.

PYLORIC STENOSIS

An uncommon condition that occurs in babies who are less than 2 months of age, pyloric stenosis is a narrowing of the outlet (pylorus) from the stomach into the small intestine. A severely narrowed outlet allows only a small amount of food to enter the intestine; the rest is vomited, causing the baby to lose weight.

Narrowed pylorus
In pyloric stenosis, the pylorus is narrowed as a result of thickening of the surrounding muscle. The cause of the thickening is not known, but it is more common in boys.

Stomach

Area shown in detail

Small intestine   Narrowed channel   Thickened muscle

Normal muscle

Pylorus

What are the symptoms?

The main symptoms of pyloric stenosis usually appear between 2 and 6 weeks after birth. They are:
- Persistent projectile vomiting (vomit that is produced forcefully, reaching some distance from the baby).
- Constant hunger: the baby often accepts another feeding immediately after vomiting.
- Infrequent bowel movements.
- Weight loss and listlessness if symptoms have been present for more than a few days.

Your baby may become dehydrated from persistent vomiting. Phone a doctor at once if your baby has any of the symptoms listed above or if there are any signs indicating that he or she might be dehydrated (see *Danger signs*, p.38). Until you are able to see the doctor, feed your child small amounts frequently, so that there is not too much undigested food in his or her stomach.

What might the doctor do?

The doctor will examine your baby's abdomen, while the baby is feeding, to feel for a swelling in the area of the pylorus. If pyloric stenosis seems likely, your child will be hospitalized, where another physical examination and an abdominal ultrasound will probably be done to confirm the diagnosis.

Intravenous fluids are given if your baby is dehydrated. The obstruction is relieved by a surgical operation to widen the pylorus. Your baby can probably leave hospital the next day.

After the operation, gradually increase the amount of your baby's feedings until feeding is normal again (usually within 48 to 72 hours).

What is the outlook?

Once pyloric stenosis has been treated, the condition will not recur and there are no permanent ill effects. It does recur in families, especially in boys.

HERNIA

A hernia is a weakness of the abdominal wall through which a part of the intestine may protrude. Umbilical and inguinal hernias are the most common types of hernia in children. In an umbilical hernia, the intestine bulges through the muscle wall at or above the navel (umbilicus). In an inguinal hernia, the intestine protrudes into the inguinal canal (the passage in the groin through which, in boys, the testis descends into the scrotum before birth).

UMBILICAL HERNIA

This type of hernia occurs as result of a gap in the muscles of the abdominal wall and usually appears a few weeks after birth. In most cases, an umbilical hernia disappears without treatment before 2 years of age but it may last up to the age of 5 years.

What are the symptoms?

Appearing as a soft swelling, usually at the navel, an umbilical hernia:
• Is often not present in the morning but may reappear during the day.

Umbilical hernia
Usually, an umbilical hernia is at the navel (umbilicus); sometimes, it appears just above.

• May increase in size if the child cries or tenses the abdominal muscles.
• Is painless.
Your child should be seen by a doctor if the hernia is particularly large or if it has not disappeared by the time the child has reached the age of 5 years.

What is the treatment?

A minor operation may be required to replace the intestine in the abdominal cavity and stitch together the gap in the muscles of the abdominal wall. Hernias above a child's navel more often require surgery. An umbilical hernia is unlikely to recur after it has been treated.

INGUINAL HERNIA

Boys under the age of 1 year are most commonly affected by inguinal hernia. The hernia occurs when the inguinal canal, which normally closes shortly after birth, remains open, forming a space through which a loop of intestine can pass into the groin or scrotum.

What are the symptoms?

An inguinal hernia appears as a soft swelling just above the groin crease or in the scrotum. The hernia:
• Is often not present in the morning but may reappear during the day.
• May increase in size if the child cries.
An incarcerated hernia is a complication that occurs when a loop of intestine becomes trapped in the canal so that its blood supply is reduced or cut off. If a hernia is strangulated, the swelling in the groin or scrotum will become hard, tender or painful, and discolored, and your child may vomit.

If there is a painless swelling in the groin or scrotum, your child should be seen by a doctor within 24 hours. If the swelling is painful or tender, however, you should call an ambulance or take your child to the nearest hospital emergency room.

What is the treatment?

An inguinal hernia will not disappear without treatment, so an operation is needed. If the hernia is painful or tender, your child may be admitted to the hospital immediately for emergency surgery. The intestine is replaced in the abdominal cavity and the inguinal canal is stitched closed. An inguinal hernia is not likely to recur once your child has had surgery to reposition the intestine and close the inguinal canal.

GIARDIASIS

Swallowing food or water contaminated with the single-celled parasite *Giardia lamblia* can lead to giardiasis, an infection of the small intestine. Once confined to the tropics, giardiasis now also occurs in temperate countries, where it mainly affects preschool children.

What are the symptoms?

About two-thirds of children who are infected have no symptoms. When they do occur, the symptoms start 1 to 3 days after the parasite has entered the body. The symptoms of giardiasis are:
• Violent attacks of diarrhea accompanied by gas.
• Very pale, floating, unpleasant-smelling stool, resulting from MALABSORPTION (p.183).
• Abdominal discomfort and cramps.
• Swollen abdomen and nausea.

What is the treatment?

The majority of cases of giardiasis are mild and clear up on their own within 2 weeks. A doctor should see your child if he or she has been suffering from diarrhea for more than 2 weeks or from severe diarrhea for over 48 hours. Stool samples will be sent to the laboratory for microscopic

Lining of the intestine

Parasite

The cause of giardiasis
The parasite Giardia lamblia *clings to folds in the lining of the intestine and absorbs nutrients from the fluid in the intestine.*

examination. If *Giardia lamblia* is found, the doctor will prescribe a week-long course of an antiparasitic drug.

You should make sure that your child drinks plenty of fluids to replace those he or she has lost through diarrhea.

Being scrupulous about handwashing after going to the bathroom and before preparing food helps prevent the disease from spreading to other members of your family.

PINWORMS

The most common parasitic worms in temperate countries, pinworms live in the intestines. The threadlike parasites primarily affect children. Often, several members of a household are infested at the same time (although some may have no symptoms), so all family members should be treated together.

Collecting worms' eggs
Eggs may be collected for microscopic examination by pressing a piece of sticky tape to your child's anal area. You should do this in the morning before your child bathes or uses the toilet.

How is infestation caused?
Children catch pinworms by sucking objects or eating foods that have been contaminated with worms' eggs. The swallowed eggs develop into adults in the intestine. The female worms emerge from the rectum at night to lay their eggs on the skin around the anus.

What are the symptoms?
The main symptoms of infestation are:
• Itching in the anal region, especially at night when the worms lay eggs.
• An itchy vulva in girls.
• Inflammation of the anus as a result of constant scratching.
Sometimes, tiny white worms can be seen wriggling in the stool.

Should I consult a doctor?
If you suspect pinworms, take your child to a doctor, who may have you collect eggs for microscopic examination (see photograph at right). The family will be treated with antiparasitic drugs as well. There are a number of options for treatment that you can discuss with your doctor. To prevent reinfection, doctor will ask you to wash bed linens and bath towels in hot water, and may treat the family again in 2 weeks.

HEPATITIS

The most common cause of hepatitis (inflammation of the liver) is viral infection. Several strains of virus can cause the infection. The hepatitis B virus causes some cases among newborn babies, who may be infected during birth if their mothers are carriers of the virus. However, most babies who are thought to be at risk are immunized against hepatitis B. The strain that most often causes hepatitis in children is the hepatitis A virus.

How is it caused?
The hepatitis A virus is usually caught by swallowing water or food that has been contaminated with infected feces. Immunization against the hepatitis A virus may be recommended if you and your family are planning to visit one of a number of developing countries where the disease is most prevalent.

Jaundice
In hepatitis, a build-up in the blood of the waste product bilirubin may cause jaundice, yellowing of the whites of the eyes and skin.

What are the symptoms?
In preschool children, most hepatitis A infections are mild and do not produce any symptoms. Older children usually do have symptoms. The symptoms are rarely severe and may include:
• Flulike symptoms of fever, headache, and weakness.
• Poor appetite.
• Nausea and vomiting.
• Tender upper right abdomen (where the liver is located).
About a week after the other symptoms have appeared, your child may develop jaundice (see photograph left), often accompanied by dark urine and pale stool and, sometimes, by diarrhea. Jaundice may last for up to 2 weeks.

Should I consult a doctor?
Make an appointment to see a doctor within 24 hours if your child has any symptoms of hepatitis. Hepatitis A cannot be treated with drugs, but the doctor will advise you on how to care for your child at home. Rarely, an attack may be serious enough for your child to be admitted to the hospital, where he or she can be monitored closely.

The doctor may recommend that all family members should be immunized against hepatitis to prevent the spread of the disease. A child with hepatitis A is infectious for 2 weeks before and for 1 week after the onset of jaundice.

What can I do to help?
Your child should be allowed to stay in bed if he or she wishes to. While your child is vomiting or his or her appetite is poor, small volumes of rehydrating fluid (see panel: *Preventing dehydration in children*, p.53) flavored with fruit juice should be given hourly during the day. As the jaundice increases, your child's appetite should improve and he or she may be given a fully mixed diet.

The spread of the hepatitis A virus between members of the family can be prevented by scrupulous handwashing and by boiling food utensils.

What is the outlook?
Your child should feel well enough to go back to school from 2 to 6 weeks after the onset of symptoms.

Hepatitis A rarely causes permanent damage to the liver and, after the first attack, your child should be immune to further attacks of the disease.

HORMONAL DISORDERS

HORMONES IN THE BLOOD CONTROL growth, production of energy, biochemical activities such as digestion, and sexual development and function. They also help the body deal with stress, danger, and fatigue. A fault in the production of hormones may affect physical and/or mental development.

HYPOTHYROIDISM

The thyroid gland manufactures hormones essential for normal physical and mental development. Hypothyroidism (underactivity of the thyroid gland) is a condition that results in insufficient production of hormones. Untreated hypothyroidism may adversely affect a child's growth and learning abilities.

How is it caused?
Hypothyroidism may be present from birth, usually as a result of a small thyroid gland. The incidence of congenital hypothyroidism is 1 in 2,500. The condition may also develop later as a result of disease of the thyroid gland or underactivity of the pituitary or hypothalamus gland (both of which stimulate the thyroid gland to produce thyroid hormones).

What are the symptoms?
All babies have their blood tested for hypothyroidism within a week of birth. Treatment for the disorder will be given before any symptoms appear.

Thyroid cartilage

Thyroid gland

Trachea

Location of the thyroid gland
The thyroid gland is located at the base of the neck in front of the trachea. The gland helps to regulate the body's energy levels and growth.

The symptoms in older children who develop hypothyroidism are:
• A noticeable reduction in the child's growth rate.
• LEARNING DIFFICULTIES (p.172).
• Lack of energy, poor appetite, and weight gain.
• Goiter (enlarged thyroid gland).

Should I consult a doctor?
Your child should be seen by a doctor. The doctor will probably take a sample of your child's blood to measure his or her hormone levels. A synthetic form of thyroxine (the principal hormone produced by the thyroid gland) will be prescribed if the tests confirm that your child has hypothyroidism.

What is the outlook?
Provided a baby who is born with the condition or a child who develops it is treated promptly, physical and mental development will probably be normal. However, the child will have to take thyroxine for the rest of his or her life.

GROWTH HORMONE DEFICIENCY

In order to grow normally, children and adolescents need growth hormone, which is produced by the pituitary gland at the base of the brain. A congenital fault in the pituitary gland, disease of the pituitary gland, or a head injury may lead to a deficiency of the hormone, resulting in a slow rate of growth.

What are the symptoms?
Growth hormone deficiency in a child is usually indicated by:
• Slow rate of growth (see GROWTH CHARTS, pp.17–21).
• Short stature and chubbiness.
• Delayed development of sexual characteristics in older children.

Make an appointment for your child to be seen by a doctor if you are worried about his or her rate of growth.

What might the doctor do?
Your child's height will be measured at regular intervals and plotted on a chart. If the doctor finds that your child's rate of growth is slower than normal, your child will probably be sent to a hospital for tests. If growth hormone deficiency is diagnosed, the doctor may prescribe synthetic growth hormone. Treatment includes growth hormone injections, 5 times a week, until your child has completed puberty.

What is the outlook?
Treatment improves a child's growth rate. However, your child may reach the normal adult height expected for your family only if treatment begins by about the age of 6 years.

DIABETES MELLITUS

In childhood diabetes (Type 1), cells in the pancreas gradually stop making insulin, a hormone that enables body cells to use and store the sugar glucose. The lack of insulin causes a build-up of glucose in the blood and a disturbance of the body's chemical processes. The unused glucose is passed out in large volumes of urine, causing frequent urination and thirst. Children with diabetes mellitus need daily insulin injections throughout life.

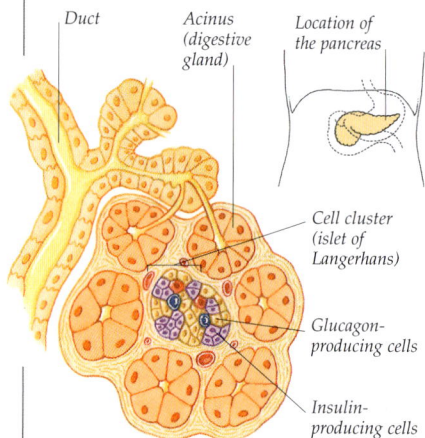

Duct Acinus (digestive gland) Location of the pancreas

Cell cluster (islet of Langerhans)

Glucagon-producing cells

Insulin-producing cells

Cells in the pancreas
The pancreas, a digestive gland, has several types of cells arranged in clusters. Some cells secrete insulin to lower the blood glucose level; others secrete glucagon to raise it. In diabetes mellitus, insufficient insulin is produced.

What are the symptoms?
In diabetes that has not been treated or that is poorly controlled, the amount of glucose in the blood is greatly raised (hyperglycemia). The body also uses fats and protein as alternative energy sources because the cells are not able to use glucose for energy. This upset of internal biochemistry typically causes:
• Frequent passing of urine (which sometimes causes bed-wetting in children previously dry at night).
• Excessive thirst.
• Tiredness and lack of energy.
• Poor appetite.
• Severe weight loss.
In more severe cases of biochemical upset, there may also be:
• Vomiting.
• Abdominal pain.
• Dehydration.
• Abnormally fast breathing.
• Drowsiness and confusion, which, without treatment, may be followed by loss of consciousness and coma.

What are the complications?
People with diabetes mellitus, especially those in whom the disease is not well controlled, are at risk of developing complications that affect the heart and circulation, the kidneys, the eyes, and the nervous system. Complications do not appear during childhood; typically, they develop about 10 to 15 years after the onset of the disease.

Should I consult a doctor?
Phone a doctor at once if you think that your child might have diabetes mellitus.

If your child has been diagnosed as having diabetes mellitus, you should consult the doctor if you ever have any worries about your child's condition. You should consult the doctor without delay if your child has an infection or an attack of gastroenteritis, because these conditions may make it difficult to control the blood glucose level.

What might the doctor do?
If the doctor suspects that your child might have diabetes mellitus, he or she will arrange for a sample of urine to be tested for the level of glucose. Blood may also be tested for the glucose level. If the level of glucose is abnormally

high, the doctor will probably arrange for your child to be admitted to the hospital immediately. Usually, several days' stay in the hospital is necessary at this time for tests and for the start of insulin treatment. The length of your child's hospital stay will depend on his or her age and condition. If your child is dehydrated from excessive urination, intravenous rehydrating fluids may be given as well as insulin.

The long-term control of your child's diabetes mellitus will be carried out under medical supervision. The aim of treatment is to provide sufficient insulin to keep your child's blood glucose level within the normal range, so that he or she is able to lead a normal life. Keeping the blood glucose level normal requires eating regular, balanced meals and having injections of insulin twice and, sometimes, three times a day.

Your child's blood glucose level may sometimes fall too low, resulting in a hypoglycemic attack. Hypoglycemia may be triggered by too high a dose of insulin, missing a meal, or a sudden burst of exercise. You will be told how to recognize hypoglycemia and what action you should take if your child has an attack (see "What should I do if my child has a hypoglycemic attack?"). The doctor will prescribe glucagon, which can be injected to stop an attack.

What can I do to help?
You will need to learn how to test for the amount of glucose in your child's blood, and how to record the results. The measurements obtained from the tests allow adjustments to be made to the amount of insulin your child is to be given by injection. You will also need to learn how to give injections, and how to store and dispose of used insulin bottles and syringes.

Another important aspect of caring for a child with diabetes mellitus is to make sure he or she has the right kind of diet. A dietitian will be available to give you advice. Meals will need to be planned with extra care and to be served at regular times. Your child should eat a normal, balanced diet that

WEIGHT LOSS DUE TO DIABETES

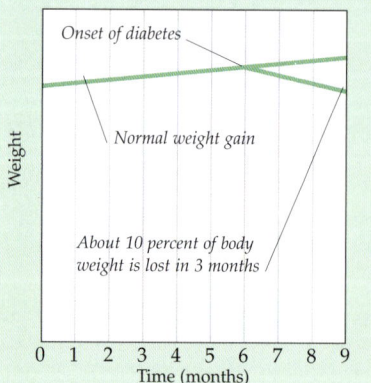

Onset of diabetes

Normal weight gain

About 10 percent of body weight is lost in 3 months

Weight

0 1 2 3 4 5 6 7 8 9
Time (months)

Example of severe weight loss
A typical symptom of diabetes is rapid and severe weight loss. A child may lose as much as 10 percent of his or her total body weight over a period of just 3 months.

contains consistent proportions of fats, protein, and carbohydrates. The daily energy intake should be constant. For a child over 5 years of age, just over a third of the diet should be made up of fats, about 15 percent should consist of protein, and the remainder should be carbohydrates. Children younger than 5 years may eat more fats. Your child's diet should also be high in soluble and insoluble fiber. Soluble fiber is found in beans and oat-based dishes, such as oatmeal; foods containing insoluble fiber include wholegrain breads, pasta, and cereals. You do not have to make special meals for a diabetic child. A similar healthy, well-balanced diet will benefit all members of the family.

If your child has a poor appetite for any reason, it is important that he or she get the same amount of energy in the form of glucose drinks as he or she would be getting in a healthy diet. Make sure that you give your child the normal amount of insulin.

Exercise can trigger a hypoglycemic attack, so your child's diet and dosage of insulin may need adjustment if he or she is participating in a sports event or will be doing strenuous exercise. Ask the doctor who is supervising your child's treatment for advice.

Your child should carry a medical identification card or bracelet indicating that he or she has diabetes mellitus and showing the medication that he or she is taking. It is essential that everyone involved in caring for your child, such as teachers, knows what to do if the child has a hypoglycemic attack.

As your child gets older, he or she should be encouraged to take as much responsibility as possible for control of his or her own diabetes mellitus. In fact, even quite young children can soon learn to inject themselves, to test and record their own blood glucose levels, to understand the need to eat regularly, and to watch for and treat symptoms of hypoglycemia.

What should I do if my child has a hypoglycemic attack?

The main signs of hypoglycemia are abdominal pain, sweating, dizziness, and/or confusion. If your child shows any of these signs, give a sweet drink or sweet food, such as chocolate or a cookie, immediately. If your child will not eat or drink, or blood glucose drops so low that he or she becomes drowsy or even loses consciousness, give an injection of glucagon in order to bring the glucose level back to normal.

What is the outlook?

A well-controlled blood glucose level should allow your child to live a normal life, with a normal amount of exercise, and should reduce the chance of any complications developing. However, your child will need to monitor his or her blood glucose level and to have injections of insulin daily for life.

TESTING FOR GLUCOSE

Blood glucose levels can be checked by two methods. For each method, a finger is pricked (which can be done using an automatic device) to obtain a drop of blood. The blood is applied to a special strip that chemically reacts with glucose.

Container with color chart

Strip

Color-match method
The strip changes color and is compared with a color chart provided on the side of the strip container. The blood glucose level is given underneath the relevant color.

Strip inserted into slot

Blood glucose level displayed

Glucometer

Glucometer method
In this more precise method, the strip does not change color, but the chemical reaction can be read automatically by a glucometer, which displays the blood glucose level on a screen.

DIABETES INSIPIDUS

The main symptoms of diabetes insipidus – frequent, copious urination and excessive thirst – are similar to those of diabetes mellitus (opposite). However, diabetes insipidus is due to a deficiency of an entirely different hormone and has nothing to do with the sugar glucose, or with energy use.

What are the causes?

In most cases, diabetes insipidus is the result of failure of the pituitary gland to secrete antidiuretic hormone (ADH). ADH normally acts on the kidneys to cause them to concentrate the urine and thus restrict the amount of fluid that is excreted from the body. Failure of the pituitary gland to produce ADH may be the result of injury to the gland or, less commonly, a tumor.

In rare cases, diabetes insipidus occurs because the kidneys fail to respond to normal levels of ADH.

What are the symptoms?

The symptoms of diabetes insipidus are:
• Excessive thirst.
• Frequent passing of large quantities of very dilute urine.
Dehydration can occur as a result of the excessive fluid passed as urine.

Should I consult a doctor?

Phone a doctor at once if your child has any of the symptoms listed above or if he or she has any of the following signs of dehydration: sunken eyes, abnormal drowsiness, or weight loss.

What might the doctor do?

The doctor will arrange for a sample of urine to be analyzed. If the urine is not adequately concentrated, diabetes insipidus is a possibility. More tests will probably be carried out in the hospital to confirm the diagnosis and determine the cause. If the pituitary gland is not producing ADH in sufficient quantities, your child will need to take synthetic ADH. If your child's kidneys are failing to respond to normal levels of ADH, the treatment is a low-sodium diet and, paradoxically, a diuretic drug.

What is the outlook?

A damaged pituitary gland may return to normal. In other cases, the condition is lifelong. However, treatment enables the person to live a normal life. There are no long-term complications.

URINARY AND GENITAL DISORDERS

URINARY TRACT INFECTIONS are common in childhood, but they affect many more girls than boys. Most of these infections clear up quickly with treatment, but all urinary infections and any other disorders affecting the kidneys, the bladder, or the genitals require investigation to check for a possible structural defect present from birth. Serious kidney disorders today are mainly treatable, including glomerulonephritis, which affects more children than adults.

BED-WETTING

Bed-wetting (enuresis) is a common problem. The age at which children become dry at night is extremely variable. Few children can control their night-time bladder function before they are 3 years old. Reliable control day and night may be gained any time between 3 and 7 years of age. There is usually no cause for concern unless your child is still bed-wetting after 7 years of age or has started bed-wetting after a prolonged dry period (6 to 12 months).

How is it caused?
In most cases, bed-wetting probably results from delayed maturation of the parts of the nervous system that control the bladder. Bed-wetting may also occur if a child has a URINARY TRACT INFECTION (opposite) or is anxious (see ANXIETY AND FEARS, p.170). Rarely, a congenital defect of the urinary tract or DIABETES MELLITUS (p.190) is responsible.

Should I consult a doctor?
Make an appointment to see a doctor if you are concerned about your child's bed-wetting, especially if he or she is 7 years of age or over. Your child should also be seen by a doctor if the problem starts after your child has been dry at night for a prolonged period. The doctor will examine your child and will test a urine sample for infection or diabetes.

If a physical cause for the condition is identified, treatment will be given; for example, antibiotics may be prescribed to treat a urinary tract infection. If no physical reason can be found, follow the advice given here (see also panel: *Toilet-training tips*, p.63).

What can I do to help?
Bed-wetting may be less likely to occur if a child forms the habit of urinating at regular times during the day and just before going to bed. Avoiding drinking liquids before bedtime may also help.

Do not punish your child if he or she does wet the bed; you may increase his or her anxiety and make the problem worse. Always give praise for dry nights. A chart on which your child can stick a star after each dry night may provide motivation (see photograph at right). Some children become completely dry after using a star chart for a few weeks with no other treatment. If your child becomes discouraged because the chart reflects poor results, discontinue the method.

If methods involving praise and encouragement are not successful, you could try using an enuresis alarm. This device has a detector (which is placed under the bottom sheet) that activates a buzzer when urination occurs. The alarm wakes the child up, who stops the urine stream, and gets up to go to the toilet. The amount of urine passed before the child wakes up becomes less and less. After a few months, most children wake up before the alarm starts or sleep through the night without wetting the bed. If your child has been dry at night for 6 weeks, remove the alarm. If bed-wetting recurs, however, the alarm may be used to treat your child again.

What is the outlook?
Most children stop bed-wetting without treatment. Those who are treated often improve within a few months. The older a child is, however, the longer it may take for the condition to improve.

Chart made by the child

Star chart
Sticking a star on a chart after each dry night is a satisfying way for your child to mark progress. The chart also allows family members to see how well the child is doing and to give praise for good results.

URINARY TRACT INFECTIONS

Infections of the urinary tract are common in children, especially in girls. However, newborn male babies are more susceptible to urinary tract infections than female babies. An infection may affect the urethra (urethritis), the bladder (cystitis), and/or the kidneys (pyelonephritis). Prompt treatment of urinary tract infections is important to prevent scarring of the kidneys, which is most likely to occur in children under 5 years of age.

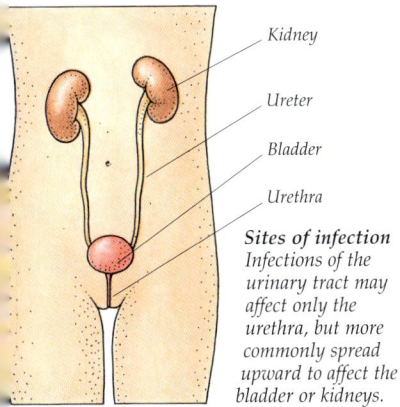

Kidney

Ureter

Bladder

Urethra

Sites of infection
Infections of the urinary tract may affect only the urethra, but more commonly spread upward to affect the bladder or kidneys.

How are they caused?

Urinary tract infections are most often caused by bacteria from the rectum that enter the urethra. Bacteria sometimes spread to the urinary tract through the bloodstream. Girls are more prone to infections of the urinary tract than boys because they have shorter urethras.

Children who have urinary reflux are especially vulnerable to infection. In this congenital condition, when the bladder empties, some urine passes backward toward the kidneys. Children who have congenital malformations of the urinary tract, suffer from chronic CONSTIPATION (p.181), or have kidneys scarred from previous infection are also more susceptible to infection.

What are the symptoms?

Children under the age of 2 years tend to have symptoms of general infection, which may include the following:
• Fever.
• Diarrhea.
• Vomiting.
• Lack of energy or irritability.
In older children, symptoms are usually more specific, and may include:
• Burning sensation on urination.
• Urinating increasingly often.
• Pain affecting the lower back or one side of the abdomen.

• Bed-wetting after being dry at night.
• Urine that is red, pink, or smoky in color, due to the presence of blood.
• Fever.
Scarring of the kidneys from recurrent infections may lead to high blood pressure or kidney failure in adult life.

Should I consult a doctor?

Your child should be seen by a doctor within 24 hours if there are symptoms of a urinary tract infection.

What might the doctor do?

The doctor may collect a urine sample from your child or may ask you to do so (see "What can I do to help?"). A baby may be seen at the hospital or in the doctor's office to have urine withdrawn from the bladder via the urethra (with a catheter) or through the abdominal skin (with a small needle). The urine is tested to rule out an underlying disorder and to confirm that infection is the cause of the symptoms.

If infection is confirmed, the doctor may prescribe oral antibiotics. A seriously ill child may be treated in the hospital with intravenous antibiotics for up to a week. A day or two after treatment for infection has finished, the urine may be tested again. If infection is still present, your child may be given more antibiotics.

Further tests may be done to see if your child has scarred kidneys or a structural abnormality of the urinary tract. Special tests for urinary reflux may be done in some children. Because children with these conditions are often prone to recurrent infections, antibiotics may be prescribed for several years, as a preventive measure.

What can I do to help?

If the doctor asks you to collect a urine sample, you will be given a sterile container and an adhesive bag (for an infant). Collect the sample after your child has had a bath or after washing the genital area with plain water. For an infant, a urine sample can be caught in the container, without letting the container touch the child (to avoid contamination), or in an adhesive bag applied around the genitals. Soon after urination, pour a small amount of the sample into the container.

After washing the genitals, an older child should collect a midstream sample by urinating, stopping, and starting again, directing the stream into the sterile container. The child should stop when the container is full and then complete emptying the bladder. If you are unable to take the urine sample to the doctor right away, you may keep it in the main compartment of your refrigerator for up to 48 hours. While your child has an infection, he or she should drink plenty of fluids. A high fluid intake dilutes the urine, easing pain and discomfort when urinating, and helps to get rid of bacteria.

Collecting a sample
After bathing, your child should urinate a little and discard it before collecting a sample.

How can the infections be prevented?

Children should urinate at least every 4 hours or before each meal, and at bedtime. After using the toilet, your child's bottom should be wiped from front to back. Your child should have a bath or shower every day, avoiding the use of irritants, such as scented soaps or bubble bath, and should be dried thoroughly afterward. Constipation should always be treated.

What is the outlook?

Recurrences are common, but prompt treatment should prevent permanent kidney damage. Scars of the kidneys become smaller as your child grows. A tendency to reflux usually disappears without treatment by 9 years of age.

GLOMERULONEPHRITIS

Inflammation of the glomeruli, the filtering units in the kidneys, is known as glomerulonephritis. The condition usually affects both kidneys. The inflamed glomeruli are not able to process wastes efficiently, resulting in decreased urine production and loss of blood and protein into the urine. Sometimes, the cause of glomerulonephritis is not known. Usually, the condition may follow an infection by streptococcal bacteria or by viruses.

What are the symptoms?
In postinfective glomerulonephritis, the symptoms begin about a week after the infection. Whatever the cause, the main symptoms are:
• Urine that is red, pink, or smoky in color, caused by the presence of blood (see photographs right).
• Urinating in smaller amounts than usual.
• Sometimes, a headache.
Fluid may accumulate in the tissues, leading to swelling, particularly of the face and legs. High blood pressure is a rare complication.

Should I consult a doctor?
You should phone a doctor at once if you suspect that your child might have glomerulonephritis. Your child will be examined by the doctor and will probably be admitted to the hospital for diagnostic tests. A sample of urine will be examined, and your child's intake and output of fluid may be measured.

NORMAL ABNORMAL
URINE   URINE

Blood in urine
The presence of blood gives urine an abnormal appearance. It looks darker and cloudier than normal clear, pale yellow urine.

What is the treatment?
If the diagnosis is confirmed, your child will need to stay in the hospital for treatment. He or she may be put on a diet that is low in sodium and protein, and his or her intake of fluids may be restricted. This regimen alleviates the strain on the kidneys and prevents the accumulation of fluids. Your child does not need to stay in bed if he or she feels like walking around.

Your child may be given antibiotic drugs if the glomerulonephritis was caused by a bacterial infection. If he or she has high blood pressure, this condition may be treated for several days until it returns to normal.

With treatment, glomerulonephritis usually clears up within a week.

What is the outlook?
In most cases, glomerulonephritis does not have any lasting effect on a child's kidneys and does not often recur. Very rarely, it may be followed by NEPHROTIC SYNDROME (below), a chronic disease that may require prolonged treatment.

NEPHROTIC SYNDROME

In this condition, a large amount of protein is lost through the kidneys from the bloodstream into the urine. Reduced levels of protein in the blood lead to edema (accumulation of excess fluid in body tissues). Nephrotic syndrome is an uncommon disorder, mainly affecting children between 1 and 6 years of age.

What are the symptoms?
The main symptoms are:
• Gradual swelling of parts of the body (see photograph at right) over several weeks.
• Reduction in the quantity of urine.
• Weight gain.
• Sometimes, diarrhea, loss of appetite, and unusual tiredness.
Children who have nephrotic syndrome are susceptible to infections and to the formation of blood clots in veins.

Should I consult a doctor?
Your child should be seen by a doctor within 24 hours if parts of his or her body are swollen. The doctor will examine your child and test the urine for protein. If results suggest nephrotic syndrome, your child will be admitted to the hospital for further tests. If the

Swelling around the eyes

Pale, puffy face

Distended abdomen

Swollen scrotum

Swollen legs (particularly ankles)

Effects of nephrotic syndrome
In nephrotic syndrome, little fluid is passed in the urine. Instead, the fluid collects in body tissues, causing them to swell.

diagnosis is confirmed, your child will be treated in the hospital with corticosteroids. (Be aware of stomach pain and low-grade fevers while your child is on steroids.) Within 10 days, as the excess fluid in the body is excreted by the kidneys, edema should improve and there should be a rapid decrease in weight. Your child may be kept in the hospital until tests show that there has been a marked reduction in the amount of protein being lost in the urine.

What can I do to help?
After your child leaves the hospital, you may be asked to test a sample of urine every day, using strips that change color when protein is present. If the test shows that there is protein in the urine, phone the doctor for advice.

What is the outlook?
Your child may make a full recovery and have no further problems. However, some children have one or more relapses. If your child suffers from frequent relapses, he or she may be given steroids for a year or more.

HEMOLYTIC UREMIC SYNDROME

Typical hemolytic uremic syndrome (HUS), an uncommon but serious disease, mostly occurs in children under 4 years old. Caused by eating undercooked beef tainted with *Escherichia coli*, it can result in kidney failure if left untreated.

What are the symptoms?
Symptoms of typical HUS include:
- Diarrhea, often watery and/or bloody, lasting 3 to 12 days.
- Severe abdominal pain.
- Decreased urination.

Other signs are listlessness, irritability, swollen hands and feet, and vomiting.

Atypical HUS is rarer and occurs in children over 4 years old. After a respiratory illness, irritability, lethargy, and decreased urination follow. High blood pressure or seizures can result.

How is it caused?
Typical HUS is caused by consuming undercooked meat or unpasteurized dairy products. It also can be transmitted by personal contact. Atypical HUS may be caused by certain drugs or viral infections, and can be inherited.

How can I prevent HUS?
Wash hands after using the bathroom, changing diapers, or handling meat. Refrigerate or freeze all meat within 2 hours. Wash kitchenware thoroughly.

Should I consult a doctor?
Call the doctor at once if symptoms appear. An office examination may include blood or urine tests. If HUS is suspected, hospitalization is necessary.

What is the treatment?
Supportive care will be given. Your child will receive intravenous fluids. Seizures or high blood pressure will be treated with medication. Kidney dialysis, or a blood transfusion for severe anemia, may be needed.

What is the outlook?
Typical HUS usually results in a full recovery and rarely recurs. Atypical HUS usually does not have as good an outlook, but results vary.

VULVOVAGINITIS

Inflammation of the vulva and vagina is called vulvovaginitis. The problem is common in young girls and is usually minor. Vulvovaginitis may be caused by irritation of the delicate genital tissues (for example, by bubble baths) and, in this case, usually clears up with self-help treatment. Sometimes, the cause is a bacterial or yeast infection, and medical treatment is required. Frequently, however, vulvovaginitis has no obvious cause.

Micrograph of **Candida** *yeast*
The yeast Candida albicans *is responsible for the infection known as yeast. Although* Candida *normally lives in the vagina, an overgrowth of the yeast causes vulvovaginitis.*

How is it caused?
Common causes of irritation include poor hygiene, tight clothing, bubble baths, or scented soap. In some girls, there may be no obvious cause for the symptoms; the vulva and vaginal lining are just particularly sensitive.

Bacteria from the rectum may infect the vulva and vagina if your child's bottom is wiped from back to front after a bowel movement. Less often, a bacterial infection may be due to the presence of a foreign body (such as a crayon or a forgotten tampon) in the vagina. A possible cause in young girls may be an infestation by PINWORMS (p.188). After puberty, yeast (see micrograph at left) is a common cause.

What are the symptoms?
The symptoms of vulvovaginitis are:
- Inflammation, soreness, and itchiness affecting the genital area.
- Pain on urination.
- Greenish or grayish yellow vaginal discharge, if bacterial infection is the cause. The discharge may be foul-smelling if the infection is caused by a foreign body in the vagina.
- Thick white vaginal discharge, if a yeast infection is the cause.

Should I consult a doctor?
If your daughter is very uncomfortable, has a vaginal discharge, or experiences pain when urinating, she should be seen by a doctor within 24 hours. Consult a doctor if other symptoms have lasted for more than 2 weeks.

The doctor will examine your child. If it is likely that a foreign body is in the vagina, your child will be sent to the hospital; if an object is found, it will be removed under general anesthesia. A vaginal smear may be taken to check for infection. An antibiotic cream or oral antibiotics may be prescribed for a bacterial infection. An antifungal cream or suppositories (put into the vagina) may be given for a yeast infection.

For persistent irritation when there is no infection, the doctor may prescribe an estrogen cream, which thickens the skin of the vulva and the vaginal lining.

What can I do to help?
Vulvovaginitis that is not caused by an infection usually clears up with self-help treatment. Twice a day for a week, your child should sit in a bath to wash the area, without using scented soaps or bubble baths. After washing, a barrier cream (for example, zinc cream) may be applied. Your child should wear loose-fitting cotton underwear, which should be changed daily. If possible, the genital area should be exposed to the air for a little while each day.

To keep the vulva and vagina free of irritating fecal material, make sure that your child's bottom is wiped from front to back after a bowel movement.

PENIS AND TESTIS DISORDERS

Disorders of the penis affecting boys include a tight foreskin, paraphimosis (a tight foreskin stuck in the retracted position), balanitis (inflammation of the head of the penis and foreskin), and hypospadias (an abnormally positioned urethral opening). The most common disorders of the testis in young boys are a hydrocele (an abnormal collection of fluid around a testis) and an undescended testis. Adolescent boys are prone to the painful disorders of testicular torsion (in which the testis twists around in the scrotum) and orchitis (inflammation of the testis).

TIGHT FORESKIN

In the first year of life, a boy's foreskin cannot usually be pulled back over the head of his penis (glans). You should never attempt to retract the foreskin by force. You are likely to injure the tissues, resulting in bleeding and the formation of scar tissue. In most boys, retraction becomes possible during the second year of life, but in some boys may not occur until the age of 4 years. After this age, inability to pull back the foreskin over the glans is abnormal.

Should I consult the doctor?

Your child should be seen by a doctor if he is older than 4 years and his foreskin cannot be retracted and/or he is having problems urinating.

The doctor will examine your son. If your son has phimosis, the doctor may recommend circumcision, an operation to remove the foreskin. If the foreskin is attached to the glans and the outlet is of normal diameter, the tissues may be separated surgically. Both operations are performed under general anesthesia.

NORMAL — Loose foreskin, Opening in foreskin

ABNORMAL — Tight foreskin, Small opening in foreskin

Phimosis
An abnormally small opening in the foreskin is known as phimosis. The condition makes the foreskin tight and hard to retract over the glans. Urinating may also be difficult.

What are the causes?

A tight foreskin may simply be due to persistence of the strands of tissue that attach it to the glans at birth. It may also be due to phimosis, a narrowed outlet in the foreskin (see illustrations above). Phimosis may be congenital, or is sometimes due to scarring caused by recurrent balanitis (right) or by forceful attempts to retract the foreskin.

What are the symptoms?

The only symptom may be difficulty in retracting the foreskin. If phimosis is present, the narrowed opening may cause the following symptoms:
• Ballooning of the foreskin when the child urinates.
• A narrow stream of urine.
A boy with phimosis is at increased risk of URINARY TRACT INFECTIONS (p.193).

PARAPHIMOSIS

Forcible retraction of a foreskin that is affected by phimosis may result in a condition known as paraphimosis. In this disorder, the retracted foreskin is stuck behind the glans and constricts the penis, causing swelling and pain.

Should I consult a doctor?

If your child's retracted foreskin has become stuck, you should take him to the nearest emergency room at once. Your son will be sedated or anesthetized, after which the doctor gently compresses the penis and returns the foreskin to its normal position. In some cases, the doctor may make an incision in the foreskin to free it. Paraphimosis will probably recur unless circumcision is performed to correct your son's phimosis.

BALANITIS

Infection by bacteria or fungi, usually as a result of inadequate cleaning of the penis, is the most common cause of balanitis. Phimosis tends to make cleaning difficult and so may increase the likelihood of balanitis occurring. Balanitis may appear as a reaction to chemicals in detergents or soaps or to irritating materials such as wool.

What are the symptoms?

The main symptoms of balanitis are:
• Swelling of the glans and foreskin (in uncircumcised boys).
• Pain or itching.
• White discharge from the penis.
• Redness of the genital area.

What can I do to help?

In most cases, balanitis clears up with improvements in hygiene. You should make sure your son washes his penis and genital area twice daily. After the inflammation has disappeared, the penis should be washed thoroughly every day to prevent recurrence.

If the balanitis is due to irritation, make sure that your son wears cotton underwear and that his clothes are thoroughly rinsed after washing. He should avoid using scented soaps.

Should I consult a doctor?

If balanitis does not clear up with self-help treatment within 3 days, make an appointment to see a doctor. He or she will probably prescribe an antifungal or antibiotic cream or oral antibiotics, which usually clears up the infection within a week. If your son suffers from recurrent attacks of balanitis, the doctor may recommend circumcision.

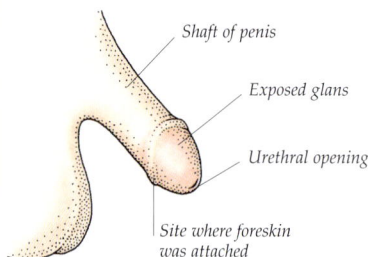

Shaft of penis

Exposed glans

Urethral opening

Site where foreskin was attached

Penis after circumcision
Circumcision involves removing the foreskin so that the glans is exposed. The operation may be recommended if the foreskin is tight or a boy suffers from recurrent infections.

HYPOSPADIAS

In this congenital abnormality, affecting about 1 in 300 male babies, the opening of the urethra is located on the underside of the penis rather than at the tip. The opening is usually on the glans, but may be anywhere along the shaft of the penis. The lower half of the foreskin may be absent, and the upper half may form a hood over the end of the penis. In some babies, the shaft curves downward. Hypospadias is detected during the routine physical examination that is done on all newborn babies.

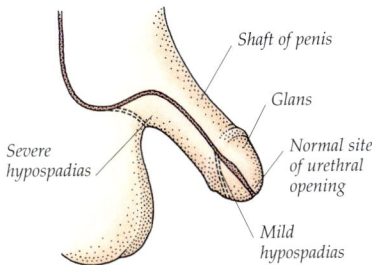

Degrees of hypospadias
In mild hypospadias, the urethral opening is on the glans. The opening may also be on the shaft of the penis; in the most severe cases, it is located well back toward the scrotum.

What is the treatment?

Hypospadias is usually corrected by an operation that is performed before a boy is 2 years of age. The surgeon may construct an extension for the urethra out of a tube of skin (made from the foreskin) so that it is able to reach the tip of the penis. A curved penis shaft is straightened during the same operation. A child should not be circumcised before hypospadias has been surgically repaired because the foreskin is needed at the operation.

What is the outlook?

Once your son has received treatment for hypospadias, his penis should look normal and he should not have any difficulties with urination, or, in adult life, with sexual intercourse.

HYDROCELE

This painless swelling of the scrotum occurs when fluid accumulates in the space around a testis. Hydroceles are common in newborn babies, and they usually disappear without treatment by the age of 6 months. The sudden appearance of a hydrocele in an older boy may be the result of an injury.

Should I consult a doctor?

Your child should be seen by a doctor if a scrotal swelling continues beyond the age of 6 months, or if it makes its first appearance after this age. In these cases, the hydrocele may be associated with an inguinal hernia (see HERNIA, p.187), and will require surgical treatment. A hydrocele that suddenly appears in an older boy should also be assessed by a doctor. It is likely to be caused by an injury and will probably get better without treatment. However, tests, including ultrasound, will be done to exclude damage to the testis.

UNDESCENDED TESTIS

Sometimes one or, less frequently, both testes fail to descend into the scrotum before birth. All newborn male babies are examined to determine whether the testes have descended normally. If not, a further examination is done at 3 months because descent often occurs naturally up to this age. If the testis has still not descended, an operation will probably be performed to move the testis into the scrotum, usually when your child is 2 or 3 years old.

What is the outlook?

As long as the operation is done at the right time, your child's sexual development and fertility should not be affected. There may, however, be a slightly increased risk of testicular cancer developing later in life.

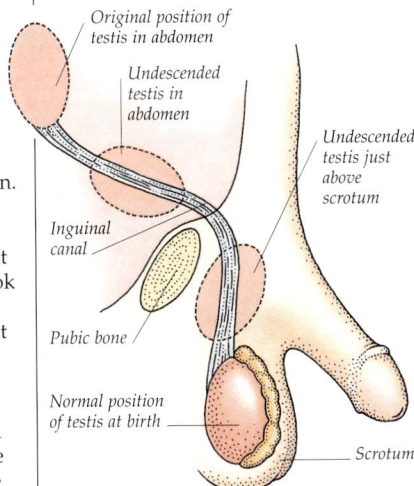

Possible sites of an undescended testis
The testes normally move down the inguinal canal into the scrotum before birth. A testis that fails to descend may stop anywhere, from high in the abdomen to just above the scrotum.

TESTICULAR TORSION

This condition occurs when a child's spermatic cord (the cord from which the testis is suspended) becomes twisted, cutting off or reducing blood supply to the testis. Testicular torsion causes acute pain. If the torsion is not corrected within hours, the affected testis may be permanently damaged.

What are the symptoms?

The main symptoms of torsion are:
- Sudden, severe pain in the abdomen.
- Severe pain in the testis.
- The affected testis may be noticeably higher than normal in the scrotum.
- Possibly, nausea and vomiting.
- After a few hours, the scrotum may become swollen, red, and tender.

If your son has pain in a testis, call an ambulance or take him to the nearest hospital emergency room immediately.

What is the treatment?

An operation is done to untwist the spermatic cord, and both the testes are stitched to the scrotum to prevent torsion recurring. A testis that has been irreversibly damaged is removed.

What is the outlook?

Provided that treatment is done in time, your child's testis should function normally. If a testis has been removed, the remaining testis should be sufficient for normal sexual development and fertility in your son.

ORCHITIS

This inflammation of a testis most often occurs as a complication of mumps. Orchitis is also occasionally caused by a bacterial infection. It is not serious, and usually disappears within a week.

What are the symptoms?

The main symptoms of orchitis are:
- Pain in the testis.
- Sometimes, fever.

If your son has not had mumps within the past 2 weeks, call an ambulance or take him to a hospital emergency room immediately in case he has testicular torsion (above). If your son has had mumps recently, he should be seen by a doctor within 24 hours.

What is the treatment?

You may give your child acetaminophen to relieve the pain. If your child has a bacterial infection, the doctor may prescribe antibiotic drugs for him.

GENETIC DISORDERS

ALL THE INFORMATION needed for growth and development is carried on around 30,000 pairs of genes packaged in 23 pairs of chromosomes. Abnormalities of these genes (or of whole chromosomes) may cause birth defects, or symptoms that may not appear until later. Genetic analysis allows couples with a family history of an inherited disease to estimate their chances of having an affected child. Tests during pregnancy can reveal whether a fetus is affected.

DOWN SYNDROME

The most common chromosomal abnormality, Down syndrome affects about 1 in every 700 babies. Children with the condition have a characteristic physical appearance combined with slow mental development. The diagnosis is usually suspected at birth. The risk of giving birth to a Down syndrome baby increases sharply in women over 37 years old; a third of all babies with Down syndrome are born to women in this age group. The risk is also greater in women who have already had an affected child.

What are the symptoms?
The characteristics of children affected by Down syndrome include:
- Upward-sloping eyes, which have prominent skin folds at the inner corner of the eyelids.
- Small, round face and full cheeks.
- Large tongue that tends to protrude.
- Flat back to the head.
- Floppy limbs.
- Slow physical development.
- LEARNING DIFFICULTIES (p.172).
- Short stature.

What are the complications?
Many children with Down syndrome are born with a heart defect, and some have an intestinal abnormality. Down syndrome children are at greater than average risk of developing an under-active thyroid gland and acute LEUKEMIA (p.146), and have an increased frequency of instability of the neck joints (which may mean restricting some sports activities). They may have hearing problems and tend to be susceptible to infections.

What might the doctor do?
The doctor will examine your child for typical features of Down syndrome. He or she will arrange for chromosome analysis of blood samples to confirm the diagnosis. Most parents are offered genetic counseling to discuss the risks of other children being affected.

Ultrasound examination of the heart may be done in the hospital to look for defects, and X rays of the abdomen may be taken if an intestinal defect is suspected. Surgery may be required to correct any defects that are found.

Follow-up care from specialists, such as speech and occupational therapists, and special educational help will be arranged for your child.

Abnormal chromosomes
In the usual form of Down syndrome, body cells have an extra chromosome 21. Each cell normally has 22 pairs of identical chromosomes and two sex chromosomes.

Normal pair of identical chromosomes

Extra chromosome 21

What can I do to help?
You may want to contact a support group for Down syndrome to get advice and suggestions of pamphlets and books. Your child's therapists and teachers may suggest ways to stimulate and help your child to develop his or her capabilities as much as is possible.

How can Down syndrome be prevented?
Pregnant women who have already had an affected child or who are over the age of 37 years will be offered chorionic villus sampling (removing a sample of tissue from the edge of the placenta) or amniocentesis (removing a sample of the fluid around the fetus). Extracted fetal cells are analyzed for chromosomal abnormalities. If the results indicate the fetus has Down syndrome, the parents may opt to terminate the pregnancy.

Pregnant women of all ages should be offered a blood test that determines whether they are at increased risk of having a baby with Down syndrome. Women shown to be at increased risk are offered amniocentesis.

What is the outlook?
Many children with Down syndrome survive into early middle age, but up to 20 percent die before the age of 5 years, often because of severe heart problems. Adults with Down syndrome are susceptible to Alzheimer's disease and atherosclerosis (hardening of arteries). As a result of educational advances, the outlook for the achievement of potential has improved and the majority of children with Down syndrome receive their education at normal schools.

FRAGILE X SYNDROME

This inherited chromosomal abnormality is a relatively common cause of LEARNING DIFFICULTIES (p.172) and also results in a slightly abnormal physical appearance. It affects about 1 in 1,000 boys and 1 in 2,500 girls. A woman with no symptoms can carry the defective chromosome and pass it on to some of her children.

What are the symptoms?
Features of fragile X syndrome include:
- Relatively large head.
- Delay in mental development, which is usually slight in girls and moderate to severe in boys.
- Delayed speech development, which is usually more severe in boys.
- Hyperactivity and ATTENTION DEFICIT HYPERACTIVITY DISORDER (p.170).

- Features of AUTISM (p.171).
- Square jaw, long face, large ears, and large testes in boys at puberty.

Fragile X syndrome may be suspected only after puberty, when the physical features become more apparent. By this time, your child will probably already be receiving special education. Consult your doctor, however, so that a definite diagnosis of the disorder can be made.

What might the doctor do?
The doctor will examine your child and assess his or her learning ability. If the doctor suspects fragile X syndrome, he or she will arrange for chromosome analysis of a blood sample. If the tests show that your child has the defective chromosome, you will be referred for genetic counseling to discuss the risks of further children being affected. Prenatal diagnosis is possible by DNA analysis of cells taken at amniocentesis.

There is no specific treatment. If your child is not already receiving special help for speech or learning difficulties, the doctor may refer him or her to a speech therapist and/or psychologist.

SICKLE-CELL ANEMIA

Most commonly affecting people of African descent, sickle-cell anemia is a serious, inherited blood disease in which red blood cells become distorted into a sickle shape. The "sickle" cells can block narrow blood vessels. The cells are also destroyed more easily than normal red blood cells, producing ANEMIA (p.145).

How is it caused?
The distortion of red blood cells occurs because the cells contain an abnormal type of hemoglobin (oxygen-carrying pigment) known as hemoglobin S. If a child inherits the abnormal gene from each parent, the child will have sickle-cell anemia. If a child inherits the abnormal gene from one parent and a normal hemoglobin gene from the other, the child will have sickle-cell trait. Children with sickle-cell trait have no symptoms but are able to pass on the abnormal gene to their children.

What are the symptoms?
The main symptoms are:
- Lack of energy and breathlessness.
- Episodes of jaundice (yellowness of the skin and whites of the eyes).
- Attacks of severe pain in the bones, chest, or abdomen, resulting from blockage of narrow blood vessels (which reduces the oxygen supply to tissues). Dehydration, cold, or severe infection makes attacks more likely.

Children who have sickle-cell anemia are at increased risk of pneumococcal pneumonia. Occasionally, blood supply is reduced to the kidneys, spleen, or brain, causing damage to these organs.

Should I consult a doctor?
Affected babies are identified by blood tests at birth. Consult a doctor if you are unsure whether your child might be at risk or if he or she has any of the symptoms listed above.

The diagnosis can be confirmed by blood tests. Treatment includes folic acid supplements to reduce the severity of anemia, penicillin given regularly to prevent infections, immunization against pneumococcal infection, and painkillers to be taken as necessary.

What can I do to help?
In order to reduce the likelihood of painful attacks, you should make sure that your child drinks plenty of fluids (to prevent dehydration) and that he or she does not become chilled.

Phone a doctor at once if your child has a painful attack accompanied by a fever, sudden paleness, persistent vomiting or severe diarrhea, difficult or fast breathing, drowsiness, or lack of energy. You should call an ambulance if your child has severe abdominal pain or tenderness.

Your child may need to be admitted to the hospital for pain relief and to treat dehydration or any infection.

Normal red blood cell   Sickle cell

Red blood cells in sickle-cell anemia
Seen through a microscope, blood taken from a person affected by sickle-cell anemia shows distorted, sickle-shaped red blood cells.

How can sickle-cell anemia be prevented?
People at risk of sickle-cell anemia are advised to have a blood test to find out whether they have the abnormal gene. A couple who both have the abnormal gene should have genetic counseling before starting a family. Tests can be carried out during early pregnancy to find out whether a fetus has sickle-cell anemia; if the fetus is affected, the parents may opt for termination.

What is the outlook?
With good medical care, most affected children survive into adulthood. If symptoms are severe, a child with sickle-cell anemia may be considered for bone marrow transplantation if a suitable donor is found. If successful, a transplant provides a complete cure.

THALASSEMIA

An inherited form of ANEMIA (p.145), thalassemia occurs most commonly among people of Mediterranean, African, and Asian origin. There are two types: thalassemia major is a serious disorder that, untreated, causes slow growth and deformity of the skull; thalassemia minor does not usually cause symptoms.

How is it caused?
Thalassemia results from a defect in the gene that codes for the production of hemoglobin (the oxygen-carrying pigment in red blood cells). A child who inherits the faulty gene from both parents has thalassemia major, which causes an inability to produce normal hemoglobin. Red blood cells are small and fragile and are rapidly broken up, leading to severe anemia. If the faulty gene is inherited from only one parent, the result is thalassemia minor. Red cells are slightly smaller than normal.

What are the symptoms?
Children with thalassemia major have symptoms of anemia, beginning in infancy. These symptoms include:
• Pale skin.
• Chronic tiredness.
• Shortness of breath.

If your child has symptoms of anemia, you should make an appointment for him or her to see a doctor.

What is the treatment?
Thalassemia is diagnosed by blood tests. Thalassemia major is treated by monthly blood transfusions, from the age of a few months. Frequent blood transfusions may, however, eventually cause damage to internal organs, such as the heart and the liver, because they become overloaded with iron. This problem can be prevented by regular infusions of a compound known as desferrioxamine. Thalassemia minor does not require any treatment.

How can thalassemia be prevented?
The parents or other close relatives of a child with thalassemia, and any prospective parent with thalassemia

Healthy red blood cell   *Pale red blood cell*

NORMAL   ABNORMAL

Blood cells in thalassemia major
A microscopic view of blood from a person with thalassemia major shows abnormally pale red blood cells. The cells are fragile and rapidly broken up, causing severe anemia.

may benefit from genetic counseling to establish the risk of having an affected child. Prenatal tests are available in specialized centers. Parents may opt for termination if the fetus is affected.

What is the outlook?
Children with thalassemia major who receive regular blood transfusions and desferrioxamine have a good prospect for normal growth and development, and many survive into middle age.

HEMOPHILIA

A genetic disorder that causes episodes of spontaneous bleeding, hemophilia affects about 1 in 10,000 boys. The condition is due to deficient activity of factor VIII, a clotting factor in the blood. Girls who carry the hemophilia gene have no symptoms, but some of their sons may be affected by the disorder.

What are the symptoms?
The symptoms of hemophilia include:
• Prolonged bleeding after an injury or even a minor surgical operation, such as tooth extraction.

Swollen knee joint
Bleeding due to hemophilia has caused this child's right knee to become swollen. Joints can become damaged and painful as a result of recurrent episodes of internal bleeding.

• Painful swelling of muscles and joints as a result of internal bleeding.
The extent and frequency of bleeding in hemophilia vary greatly from one person to another. Some people suffer from only occasional episodes of minor bleeding. When the condition is severe, there is a risk of damage to muscles and joints from recurrent internal bleeding.

Should I consult a doctor?
If your child has any signs of abnormal bleeding, he or she should be seen by a doctor. The doctor will ask about your son's symptoms, and if he or she thinks that hemophilia is a possibility, will arrange for blood tests to assess the blood's ability to clot. The results of the tests confirm the diagnosis.

What is the treatment?
Treatment may consist of injections of factor VIII, given by parents, to treat bleeding episodes. Severe bleeding may require admission to the hospital. If bleeding is frequent, factor VIII can be given regularly by parents via a drip in order to prevent bleeding. Factor VIII in current use is free of viruses, such as HIV (the AIDS virus).

How can hemophilia be prevented?
Women who have a family history of hemophilia can be tested to find out if they have the hemophilia gene and can seek genetic counseling to assess the risk of having an affected child.

What is the outlook?
Children with hemophilia are advised to avoid hazardous activities, such as contact sports. As long as factor VIII is given promptly when bleeding occurs, or regular infusions are given, muscles and joints may not be damaged, and life expectancy should be normal.

PHENYLKETONURIA

In this inherited condition, a defect in body chemistry causes a build-up of phenylalanine (a constituent of protein) in the blood. Untreated, phenylketonuria causes brain damage. The disorder affects about 1 baby in 15,000 in Canada. Babies are routinely screened for phenylketonuria by a blood test soon after birth.

What are the symptoms?
At birth, affected babies show no signs of abnormality. If phenylketonuria is not treated, however, the child may develop the following symptoms:
• Severe LEARNING DIFFICULTIES (p.172).
• A tendency to have seizures.
• A characteristic musty odor.
• Rash like that of ECZEMA (p.135).

What is the treatment?
Phenylketonuria is treated by a special diet. Phenylalanine, which is present in most protein foods, must be restricted while ensuring that the child receives sufficient protein for growth. The diet is mainly vegetarian; supplements may also be prescribed. A baby needs to be given special milk substitutes.

How can phenylketonuria be prevented?
If a couple have an affected child, there is an increased risk that other children will also be affected. Prenatal diagnosis is available, and the parents may opt for termination if the fetus is affected.

What is the outlook?
The majority of children with treated phenylketonuria attend normal schools and have normal intelligence. A small proportion have behavioral problems and learning difficulties. It is usually recommended that the special diet be continued throughout life.

CYSTIC FIBROSIS

A serious inherited disease, cystic fibrosis causes recurrent chest infections and inability to absorb nutrients from the intestines (see MALABSORPTION, p.183). The repeated chest infections result in progressive lung damage. Although cystic fibrosis is present from birth, the condition sometimes goes undetected for many months or years, during which time damage to the lungs may have begun. Cystic fibrosis affects about 1 in 2,000 children.

How is it caused?
Cystic fibrosis is caused by a defective gene. For a child to have the disorder, the faulty gene must be inherited from both parents (who are carriers, but have no symptoms of the disease). The defective gene causes the secretion of sticky mucus that cannot flow freely through the air passageways, leading to recurrent chest infections. The faulty gene also causes deficient secretion of pancreatic enzymes (which help in the digestion of food), leading to diarrhea.

What are the symptoms?
The main symptoms are:
• Failure to grow normally and to gain a normal amount of weight.
• Persistent coughing.
• Chronic diarrhea, typically with pale, oily, strong-smelling stool.
You should see a doctor if your child has any of these symptoms.

What might the doctor do?
If the doctor thinks that cystic fibrosis is a possibility, your child will be tested in a special laboratory, where a sample of his or her sweat will be analyzed; in cystic fibrosis, the salt content of sweat is higher than normal. Genetic tests may also be performed. If the tests confirm that your child has cystic fibrosis, the doctor will prescribe pancreatin (a replacement pancreatic enzyme preparation) for your child to take with meals so that food is digested properly. A diet high in calories and protein is recommended, and vitamin supplements will be prescribed. The doctor will prescribe antibiotics and recommend regular physical therapy for treatment of chest infections and to help prevent chronic lung disease.

What can I do to help?
You should start giving your child regular chest physical therapy as soon as a physical therapist has trained you to do it (see photograph at right).

It is vital that you contact your doctor at the first sign of any illness so that appropriate treatment can be given quickly. When your child is ill with a chest infection, you will need to do physical therapy more often than usual. To help your child to absorb enough nutrients for normal growth, encourage him or her to eat high-energy snacks.

How can cystic fibrosis be prevented?
Genetic counseling may be offered to any prospective parent who already has a child with cystic fibrosis or who is a carrier. Prenatal testing can be done, and termination may be considered if the fetus is affected.

What is the outlook?
There is no cure for the disorder, but the outlook has improved greatly due to earlier diagnosis and new methods of treatment, and most sufferers now survive well into adulthood. A few severely affected children have had a lung or heart-lung transplant, which has improved their quality of life and increased their life expectancy.

Chest physiotherapy
To help loosen the thick mucus in the lungs, clap your child's back with a cupped hand. Physiotherapy should be performed twice a day, and more often when your child is ill.

First Aid & Nursing a Sick Child

FIRST AID FOR BURNS

THIS SECTION provides a quick guide to treating some of the serious or life-threatening injuries. Don't wait for an emergency before studying these pages; familiarize yourself with these techniques now.

Another useful reference book is the Canadian edition of DK's *First Aid for Children Fast*. At the same time, be aware that first aid is a practical skill, and reading a book cannot replace practical training. Courses in cardiopulmonary resuscitation and first aid are taught by St. John Ambulance Canada and the Canadian Red Cross. Some CPR and first aid courses relate specifically to children. Please note

ARM SLING

the difference between CPR for babies and children in the following pages.

PRINCIPLES OF FIRST AID

The **A**irway–**B**reathing–**C**irculation check – called the **ABC**s of resuscitation – is the most important principle of first aid. If there is breathing and a pulse, treat other problems in the following order: BLEEDING and SHOCK (p.208), BURNS (p.209), FRACTURES (pp.210–211), other injuries. An unconscious child should be put in the RECOVERY POSITION (opposite).

ABCs OF RESUSCITATION: BABIES

Airway
To open the airway of an unconscious baby, tilt the head back slightly and lift the chin with one finger. Check for breathing; if breathing is evident, hold the baby in the recovery position (opposite).

Breathing
If your baby is not breathing, perform RESCUE BREATHING (p.205). If your breaths do not go in, your baby's airway may be obstructed (see CHOKING, p.204).

Circulation
Look, listen, and feel for movement, breathing, coughing, normal color, or any other signs of life. If there are no signs of a circulation, you should start CARDIOPULMONARY RESUSCITATION (p.206).

RECOVERY POSITION

ABCs OF RESUSCITATION: CHILDREN

Airway
To open the airway of an unconscious child, tilt the head back and lift the chin with two fingers. Check for breathing; if evident, place the child in the RECOVERY POSITION (right).

Breathing
If your child is not breathing, carry out RESCUE BREATHING (p.205). If your breaths do not go in, your child may have an obstructed airway (see CHOKING, p.204).

Circulation
Look, listen, and feel for movement, breathing, coughing, normal color, or any other signs of life. If there are no signs of a circulation, you should start CARDIOPULMONARY RESUSCITATION (p.207).

Any unconscious child who is breathing and who has signs of a circulation should be placed in the recovery position while you wait for the ambulance. This position allows fluids to drain out of the child's mouth so they are not inhaled. Check breathing and pulse frequently (see ABCs OF RESUSCITATION, opposite or left) and, if necessary, perform RESCUE BREATHING (p.205) or CARDIOPULMONARY RESUSCITATION (pp.206–207). If your child has a fracture, support the injury.

A child with a spinal injury should be turned only if the breathing is obstructed. Keep the child's head, neck, and back aligned at all times.

BABIES

Hold your baby
Hold an unconscious baby against your chest, head tilted downward to keep the airway open. Allow air to move around the nose and mouth.

CHILDREN

1 Roll child onto side
Grasp the farther thigh, pull the leg up to bend the knee, and roll the child over (pull the bent leg toward you). Keep the child's upper hand under the cheek.

2 Position child
Bend the top leg at a right angle and adjust the position of the bottom arm to prevent your child from rolling forward. Tilt the head back to maintain an open airway.

CHOKING

You may not realize that your child is choking. Initially, he or she may cough and gasp or make high-pitched squeaking noises, and then lose the ability to speak or breathe. A baby's face may turn red and then blue, and he or she may seem to have difficulty in breathing or appear to cry without making any noise. If the back blows and thrusts do not remove the obstruction at first, keep trying, since methods that are not initially successful may work eventually.

UNCONSCIOUS BABY OR CHILD

Call an ambulance. Open the airway. If you see an object, remove it carefully, but never poke blindly. Check for breathing. If there is no breathing, give 2 effective RESCUE BREATHS (opposite), making 5 attempts if necessary. If breaths do not go in, start chest compressions (see pp.206–207). Try to give a breath after 5 chest compressions. After every set of compressions and attempted breath, check the mouth again and remove any obstruction. Continue the sequence until help arrives.

BABIES

1 Give 5 back blows
Lay your baby face-down along one arm with the head lower than the rest of the body, and support the chin between your fingers. Give 5 sharp blows on the middle of your baby's back with the heel of your hand. Turn your baby over, look in the mouth, and remove any obvious obstruction.

2 Give 5 chest thrusts
If back blows are not effective, hold the baby with head low, put two fingers on the breastbone just below an imaginary line between the nipples, and give 5 downward thrusts. If an object is visible in the mouth, remove it carefully. Continue steps 1–2 until your baby can breathe.

CHILDREN

1 Position your arms
If your child is unable to speak, cough, or breathe, stand or kneel behind him or her, and wrap your arms around the abdomen at a position just above the hips.

2 Position your hands
Make a fist with one hand and place the thumb side of your fist against the middle of your child's abdomen, just above his or her navel.

3 Give abdominal thrusts
Grasp your fist with your other hand and press into your child's abdomen with a quick upward thrust. Continue to give forceful abdominal thrusts until the object is expelled. This is known as the Heimlich maneuver. If you cannot clear the obstruction, or your child loses consciousness, refer to box above right.

RESCUE BREATHING

If your child stops breathing, you must breathe for him or her, using a technique known as rescue breathing. This technique is effective because even the air that you exhale contains enough oxygen to sustain your child's vital organs until medical help is obtained. When giving breaths, take a deep breath yourself first and blow steadily into your child's mouth (or mouth and nose for a baby) and watch the chest rise. This is called an effective breath.

BABIES

1 Open airway, check breathing
Tilt your baby's head back slightly with one hand, and clear any obvious obstruction. Lift the chin and look, listen, and feel for breathing.

2 Give rescue breaths
If your baby is not breathing, seal your lips over the mouth and nose. Give 2 effective breaths, taking a fresh breath yourself after each one.

3 Check for signs of circulation
If your baby has normal skin color or movement, or other signs of circulation, continue giving rescue breaths for 1 minute, aiming for 1 breath every 3 seconds. Call an ambulance, then continue giving breaths until help arrives.

CHILDREN

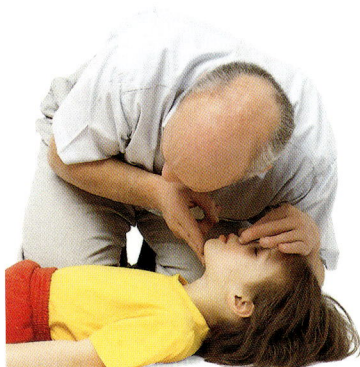

1 Open airway, check breathing
Tilt your child's head back slightly with one hand and lift the chin with two fingers of the other hand. Look, listen, and feel for breathing.

3 Give rescue breaths
Keeping your child's chin lifted, seal your lips over his or her mouth. Give your child 2 effective breaths, ensuring that you take a fresh breath yourself after each one.

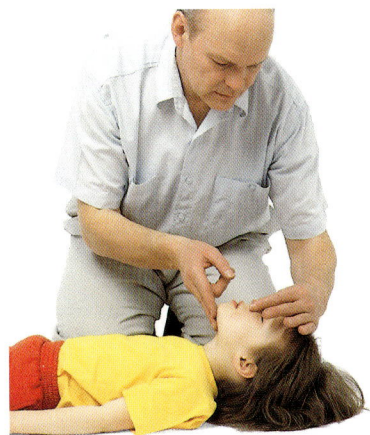

2 Pinch nose shut
If your child is not breathing, pinch the nose tightly shut. Keep the child's airway open by lifting his or her chin with two fingers.

4 Check for signs of circulation
If there are signs of circulation, such as normal skin color or movement, continue giving rescue breaths for 1 minute, aiming for 1 breath every 3 seconds. Call an ambulance. Continue giving breaths until help arrives.

CARDIOPULMONARY RESUSCITATION (CPR)

A child who is not able to breathe and has no signs of a circulation must immediately be given cardiopulmonary resuscitation (CPR) in order to keep the vital organs supplied with oxygen until medical treatment can be given in the hospital. Cardiopulmonary resuscitation is the combination of rescue breathing, to deliver air into your child's lungs, and chest compressions, to distribute the oxygenated blood throughout the body. If your child is a baby – under the age of 1 year – follow the instructions for babies (below); for older infants and children of all ages, follow the instructions for CPR shown opposite.

BABIES

1 Open airway, check breathing
Lay your baby down on a flat surface. Tilt the head back very slightly with one hand and remove any obvious obstruction. Lift the chin with one finger of the other hand. Look, listen, and feel for breathing.

2 Give rescue breaths
If your baby is not breathing, seal your lips over his or her mouth and nose. Give 2 effective breaths, making 5 attempts if necessary. Take a fresh breath yourself between each one.

3 Check for a circulation
Look, listen, and feel for movement, breathing, coughing, normal color, or other signs of life. If there are no signs of a circulation, begin CPR (steps 4 and 5).

4 Give compressions
Place your index and middle fingers on your baby's breastbone, just below an imaginary line connecting the nipples. Press down sharply with your fingertips, 5 times within about 3 seconds, to a depth of about 1.25–2.5 cm. Keep your other hand on the baby's head.

5 Give rescue breaths
Seal your lips over your baby's mouth and nose, and give one breath. Repeat the compressions and breaths for about 1 minute (20 cycles). Call an ambulance; if you have no helper, take your baby with you to the telephone. Continue CPR (steps 4 and 5) until the ambulance arrives.

CHILDREN

1 Open airway, check breathing
Tilt your child's head back slightly with one of your hands and clear any obvious obstruction. Lift the chin (with two fingers of your other hand). With your head positioned close to your child's face, look at his or her chest to check for movement, listen for sounds of breathing, and feel for breath on your cheek.

Tilt head back slightly and lift chin with two fingers to open airway

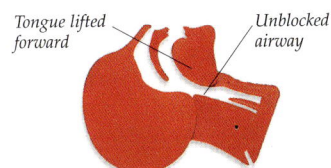

2 Give rescue breaths
If your child is not breathing, pinch the nose shut and seal your lips over your child's mouth. Give 2 effective breaths, making 5 attempts if necessary. Take a fresh breath after each one.

3 Check for a circulation
Look, listen, and feel for movement, breathing, coughing, normal color, or other signs of life. If there are no signs of a circulation, begin CPR (steps 4–6).

4 Find position on breastbone
Place your middle finger at the spot where your child's ribs meet, and put your index finger on the breastbone just above this.

5 Give compressions
Place the heel of your other hand on the breastbone next to your fingers. Press to a depth of 2.5–3.5 cm. Do this 5 times within 3 seconds.

6 Give rescue breaths
Seal your lips over your child's mouth, and give one breath. Repeat the compressions and breaths for about 1 minute (20 cycles). Call an ambulance, then continue CPR (steps 4–6) until the ambulance arrives.

TO OPEN AIRWAY
With the head lying flat, the tongue falls against the throat and blocks the airway. To open the airway, tilt your child's head and lift the chin.

Tongue fallen back *Blocked airway*

AIRWAY BLOCKED BY TONGUE

Tongue lifted forward *Unblocked airway*

AIRWAY UNBLOCKED

BLEEDING

In most cases bleeding stops quickly but if it does not, you may need to control it to prevent SHOCK (below). If an object is embedded in the wound, do not remove it – you might cause further bleeding and damage. Use disposable gloves to reduce the risk of infection, or avoid touching the wound. Wash your hands before treatment, if possible, and always afterward.

1 Apply direct pressure
Raise the affected limb and use your hand to press on the wound with a sterile dressing. Press until the bleeding stops. Treat your child for shock (below), if necessary.

2 Secure dressing
Fasten the dressing firmly in place. Support the injury in a raised position – for example, with a sling (see BROKEN COLLARBONE, p.210) – and take your child to the hospital.

EMBEDDED OBJECT

Cover the wound lightly with a dressing to prevent infection. Surround it with bandage rolls built up to the same height as the protruding object. Secure them in place by bandaging above and below the wound. Take your child to the hospital or call an ambulance.

This technique can also be used if your child has a broken bone that has pierced the surface of the skin (an open fracture). Be careful not to push the bone back into the wound.

SHOCK

Shock is the failure of the circulatory system to provide adequate oxygen-rich blood to all parts of the body. It can be caused by blood loss (from internal or external bleeding), infection, dehydration, or severe burns. The first signs of shock may be skin that is pale gray, cold, and sweaty; a rapid pulse that becomes weaker; and shallow, fast breathing. Later signs include unusual restlessness or agitation, thirst, and yawning or gasping for air. Shock may lead to a loss of consciousness. If your child has any of these signs, you should call an ambulance immediately, and then perform the necessary first aid for any specific injuries.

Lay your child down
Put your child on a blanket and raise the feet to a height of 20–30 cm on several pillows. Cover your child with another blanket if he or she is cold. Reassure your child, but do not give anything to eat or drink. If your child loses consciousness, place him or her in the RECOVERY POSITION (p.203) monitor breathing and pulse, and perform RESCUE BREATHING (p.205) or CARDIOPULMONARY RESUSCITATION (pp.206–207).

Legs raised to encourage blood flow to the head and vital organs in the body

BURNS

Whether the cause of a burn is heat or fire, electricity, or a chemical, the first aid is basically the same: the priority is to cool the burned area with cool water. If a child's clothes are on fire, wrap him or her tightly in a rug or blanket until the flames go out. (Remember: Stop, Drop, Wrap, and Roll.) After giving first aid, take your child to the hospital or call an ambulance.

PROTECTION IN TRANSIT:
BURNED HAND OR FOOT

To protect a burned hand or foot during a trip to the hospital, enclose it in a clean plastic bag after holding it under cool running water for at least 10 minutes. Secure the open end with first-aid tape, which should not touch your child's skin.

1 Cool burns under running water
Hold the burned area under cool running water for at least 10 minutes. For chemical burns, rinse the affected area for up to 20 minutes. If your child's clothes are not stuck to the burned skin, cut them off and flush the area again with cool running water.

2 Cover burned area
Place a clean dressing, pillowcase, or some other lint-free material over the burned area to prevent infection. Treat your child for SHOCK (opposite) if necessary. Take your child to the hospital or call an ambulance.

EYE WOUND

A child whose eye has been injured will be frightened and in intense pain. Movement of the wounded eye may increase the injury, so tell your child to look straight ahead. It will help if you keep your child calm and hold his or her head still with your hands. Cover the affected eye with a pad and then a bandage. Either call an ambulance or take your child to the hospital.

CHEMICAL IN EYE

Flush out the affected eye for 10 minutes under cold running water. Keep it from splashing onto your child's face or into the unaffected eye. Bandage the injured eye (left), then take your child to the hospital.

1 Cover injured eye
Use a pad to cover the injured eye. If an object is embedded, be careful not to push it further into the eye.

2 Bandage pad in place
Use a clean bandage to secure the pad firmly in place. Wrap the bandage around your child's head.

BROKEN LEG

If your child breaks a leg, you should support and stabilize it to avoid further injury while you await an ambulance (do not use your car). Do not straighten the leg. Place padding under and around a broken knee. Support it in the position in which you find it. Fractures may require surgery, so do not give your child anything to eat or drink.

1 Place padding
Call an ambulance. Put plenty of padding, such as rolled-up towels or blankets, or folded newspaper, on both sides of the injured leg.

2 Support leg
Hold the injured leg above and below the location of the fracture to prevent movement until the ambulance arrives. Excess movement may cause further injury and internal bleeding.

OPEN FRACTURES

If the broken bone has pierced the skin, the injury should be treated as an embedded object (see BLEEDING, p.208). Control the bleeding and bandage the wound before you continue with the first aid for a broken leg (at right).

BROKEN COLLARBONE

Before you take your child to the hospital, immobilize a broken collarbone by tying a sling around the arm on the affected side. A sling can also be used for a broken, bleeding, or bruised hand because it minimizes swelling by raising and supporting the injury.

1 Place triangular bandage
Put the fingertips of the hand on the injured side on the other shoulder. Hold one end of the bandage at your child's fingertips, and drape the long edge down the body. The point should be below the elbow on the injured side.

2 Gather bandage, tie sling
Take the bandage under the child's elbow so that it supports the arm on the injured side. Bring the bandage across the child's back. Tie it on the uninjured side with a square knot. Be sure you can see a few fingers.

Finished sling
The excess fabric at the elbow has been tucked in behind the sling; it could also be pinned to the front of the sling. Keep checking your child's fingers; if they become pale, cold, or numb, the sling should be loosened.

BROKEN ARM

A broken upper or lower arm bone or wrist and a dislocated shoulder should be immobilized with an arm sling before your child is taken to the hospital to prevent further injury and lessen pain. Avoid a sling if the fracture is in or near the elbow. Stabilize and support the elbow without changing its position.

1 Pad injury
Gently place your child's injured arm across his or her chest. Arrange a generous layer of padding, such as a folded towel or newspaper, around the injury, while supporting the injured arm with your other hand.

2 Place triangular bandage
Drape a bandage between your child's chest and the injured arm so that its long side extends down from the shoulder of the uninjured arm, and the other corner is positioned at the elbow of the injured arm.

Finished sling
The lower corner of the bandage has been brought up over the forearm and around the neck. The two ends have been tied on the injured side. Extra material at the elbow has been twisted and pinned to the front of the sling.

SWALLOWED POISONS

A child who swallows poisonous leaves or berries, a chemical, alcohol, or someone else's medicine needs immediate medical attention. Identify the substance and the amount that might have been consumed. If your child can't tell you, look around for telltale signs, such as an open medicine container or bottle of alcohol, and check the child's mouth for unswallowed material. Before treating your child, phone the poison information center in Toronto (1-800-268-9017), your regional poison information center, or an emergency medical service.

WARNING
IF YOUR CHILD SWALLOWS A POISON
• Do not try to make your child vomit. Some substances, such as bleach, can cause more harm if the child vomits.
• Have the poison information centre phone number handy and lock up medicines and household chemicals.

Determine what was swallowed
Ask your child or look for evidence. If the lips are burned, rinse gently with water. Place an unconscious child in the RECOVERY POSITION (p.203). Monitor breathing and pulse (pp.202–203), and perform RESCUE BREATHING (p.205) or CARDIOPULMONARY RESUSCITATION (pp.206–207) if needed.

NURSING A SICK CHILD

Most illnesses do not require any specialized nursing care. You should, however, make sure that your child does not become dehydrated, especially if he or she has a fever or diarrhea, or has been vomiting. A sick child may not have much of an appetite; small helpings of favorite foods may be tempting but you should not force your child to eat. If bedrest is not essential, your child may prefer to rest and read or play quietly in a room where other family members are present.

TAKING A TEMPERATURE

If your child seems sick and you suspect a fever, you should take his or her temperature. A temperature of 38°C or above is a fever. Measure your child's temperature every 2 or 3 hours until it returns to normal. Any of the thermometers shown in the box below can be used. Over the age of 7 years, a child can hold a digital thermometer under his or her tongue, but for younger children it is easier to use a digital thermometer in the armpit or a temperature strip on the forehead. Bear in mind that the temperature measured in the armpit or on the forehead is about 0.6°C less than true body temperature, so this amount should be added to the reading to obtain the accurate body temperature.

Using a digital thermometer
Hold the digital thermometer either in your child's armpit or in his or her mouth. Try to encourage your child to sit still. After 1–2 minutes, remove the thermometer and read the temperature from the digital display.

Using an aural thermometer
Place the aural thermometer in your child's ear. Hold the tip gently in position for the recommended time and then remove to read the temperature. The disposable tip should be replaced with a new one after every use.

GIVING MEDICINE

Always check the expiration date before giving any medication. Liquid medicine should be shaken before every use and measured carefully to ensure that the correct dose is given. Use a syringe (below) when you give medicines to young children to avoid spills and ensure that the right dose is given. A medicine spoon can be used to give medicine to older children.

Children find it hard to swallow pills. A chewable type, or one that dissolves or can be crushed and mixed with juice, yogurt, or apple sauce is best.

To prevent a recurrence of the illness, give all doses of a prescription medicine, even if your child seems better. Follow the storage directions carefully; some liquid medicines must be stored in a refrigerator.

Filling a syringe
The adapter is fitted into the bottle, and the syringe pushed into the adapter. With the bottle upside-down, the plunger is pulled out slowly until the syringe contains the dose.

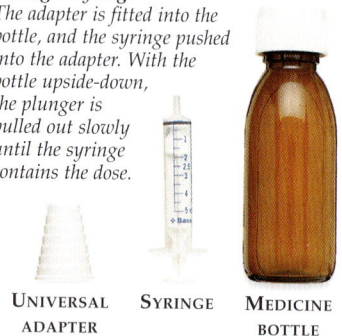

UNIVERSAL ADAPTER   **SYRINGE**   **MEDICINE BOTTLE**

TYPES OF THERMOMETERS

Three types are available – digital, temperature strip, and aural. Digital thermometers and temperature strips are easy to use and give a quick, accurate reading. Aural thermometers are more expensive. They are just as simple to use but are not considered accurate for children under 2 years of age. All the displays remain legible for a short time after removal and return to normal automatically after use. Mercury thermometers are no longer recommended as they are hard to read and are easily broken.

DIGITAL THERMOMETER

TEMPERATURE STRIP

| °F | 95 | 96.8 | 98.6 | 100.4 | 102.2 | 104 |
| °C | 35 | 36 | 37 | 38 | 39 | 40 |

AURAL THERMOMETER

Giving medicine with a syringe
Remove the syringe containing the medicine from the adapter. Place the tip of the syringe in the mouth so it points toward the cheek; slowly press the plunger. Aiming the syringe at the back of the throat may cause choking.

INDEX

Page numbers printed in **bold** type indicate the symptom charts. Page numbers printed in *italics* direct you to boxes or illustrations that explain self-help measures, first-aid techniques, or assessments.

ACKNOWLEDGMENTS

The author would like to thank his teachers, Dr. H.V.L. Finlay and Dr. R.J.K. Brown, whose experience and wisdom are reflected in these pages. He is indebted to Dr. Jackie Bucknall and Dr. Warren Hyer, his senior registrars, who checked the symptom charts and made several helpful comments. He thanks Dr. Robert Youngson for writing the articles on eye and vision problems, Dr. Bryan Lask and Dr. Sarah Benton for writing the articles on behavioral and emotional problems, and David P. Cocker, BDS for checking the information regarding teeth disorders. He also thanks Dr. Tony Smith, who has encouraged him in medical writing over many years.

DORLING KINDERSLEY WOULD LIKE TO THANK:
Additional medical advice: Ursula Arens, British Nutrition Foundation; Tam Fry, Child Growth Foundation; Prof. John A. Henry MB FRCP, St. Mary's Hospital; Joanna Tempowski, National Poisons Information Service; Dr. Frances Williams
Additional editorial assistance: Joanna Benwell, Dr. Amanda Jackson; Zak Knowles; Ruth Midgley; Cathy Shilling
Additional design assistance: Nicola Webb
Project photography: Andy Crawford
Photographer's assistant: Gary Ombler
Other photography: Mike Good; Steve Gorton; Dave King; Philip Powell; Susanna Price; Jules Selmes; Stephen Shott
Picture research: Christine Rista
Index: David Harding
Models: George Allen; Hugo Allen; Freda Belle; Charles Wilson Barnard; Emma Barnard; Rae Chen; Jane Cunningham; Max Cunningham; Anita Eade; Sally Evason; Lily Blawat Farr; Emma Foa; Lia Foa; Karen Good; Keiran Good; Olivia Grosvenor; Nicola Hampel; Jason Haniff; Ellen Harris; Joseph Lauder; Rebecca Lauder; Mary Lindsay; Michelle Papadopoulos; Nina Papadopoulos; Francesca Pritlove; Angela Rollinson; Joe Rollinson; Archie Walker; Aidan Walls; Mark J. Wilde; Amelia Wooding; Sally Wooding.

The growth charts, on pp.17–21, were derived from data collected by the National Center for Health Statistics in collaboration with the National Center for Chronic Disease Prevention and Health Promotion.

The first-aid information in this book has been validated by Dr. Vivian Armstrong. Thanks also to Jemima Dunne and Janet Mohun for their help on this section.

PICTURE CREDITS
Abbreviations: t=top; c=center; b=bottom; l=left; r=right.
Heather Angel 152; **AVS Imperial College School of Medicine at St. Mary's** 31br, 200bl; **Biophoto Associates** 31br, 79tc, 79cl, 120bl, 120cr, 134br, 139cr; **Bubbles** Loisjoy Thurston 79cr; **Sally Greenhill** 177br; **KeyMed** 184cr; **Medical Slide Library** 79cc, 122tl, 130cl, 135cl, 136cl, 163bl, 165cl, 166bc, 178cl; **National Medical Slide Bank** 79tr, 118, 132bc, 139cl, 141bl; **Dr. Price, Northwick Park Hospital** 183tl; **John Radcliffe Hospital, Oxford** 200tr; **Science Photo Library** 137bc, 180cl, 184cc, 187cl, 200tl/Alex Bartel 178br; Biophoto Associates 146bll; Biozentrum 148bl; Oscar Burriel/Latin Stock 173; Chris Bjornberg 155bc; Dr. Tony Brain, 123br; Scott Camazine 15ccl, 15cr/John Durham 146bl; CNRI 159bl, 184bc, 187br, 198; Eric Grave 199; John Heseltine 174; London School of Hygiene and Tropical Medicine 124tr; Dr. P. Marazzi 31cr; 119tl, 119bl, 137cl, 138bl, 140, 142bl, 151tr, 169cr, 175bl, 176tr; Will and Deni McIntyre 160br; Hank Morgan 172br; NIBSC 125, 151bc; David Parker 141tc; John Radcliffe Hospital, Oxford 143tc; Dept. of Clinical Radiology, Salisbury District Hospital 128cr; David Scharf 153cl; Garry Watson 88bl; Western Ophthalmic Hospital 166tr; **J. Sorrell** 184bl; **Dr. Bernard Valman** 79tl, 147tcr, 158bc; **C. James Webb** 143bl; **Timothy Woodcock Photolibrary** 176bc/Steve Horsted 172tc; **Mike Wyndham Picture Collection** 15bl, 15br.

All other images copyright © **Dorling Kindersley**